A HIMALAYAN TRINITY

BY

MARK KINGSLEY

Inquiries should be made to:
Seaview Press
PO Box 234
Henley Beach, South Australia 5022
Telephone 08 8235 1535; fax 08 8235 9144
E-mail: seaview@seaviewpress.com.au
Web site: http://www.seaviewpress.com.au

Printed by:
CM Digital
234 Currie Street
Adelaide, South Australia 5000

Front cover shows: My three porters — Ratna, Nadur and Chandra — spirit, mind and body on my trek
Back cover shows: A view of the East

National Library of Australia Cataloguing-in-Publication data
Kingsley, Mark.
A Himalayan trinity : a house in higher hills.

ISBN 1 74008 225 7.

1. Kingsley, Mark. 2. Cancer - Patients - Biography.
3. Himalaya Mountains - Description and travel. I. Title.

920.71

PART I – A HOUSE IN HIGHER HILLS

Dear Tom,

May this give you all the help it can, especially considering the father you have – who I know well.

Very best wishes,

[signature]

January 2004

In memory of
A beautiful Mother,
Who died too young;
But then the best often do.
Isobel Harriet Steyn
(17.11.1940 to 20.02.2002)

Foreword

By General Sir Sam Cowan, K.C.B. C.B.E.
*Colonel Commandant, The Brigade of Gurkhas and
Chairman of the Gurkha Welfare Trust*

Commanding Gurkha soldiers can have a profound effect on one's life and attitude. Many visitors to the Kingdom of Nepal will also attest to the fact that a trek underneath the high peaks of the Himalaya can have a similar impact. Those who have had to go through the dark valley of a struggle against cancer confess to similar life-changing transformation. Mark has been through all three of these experiences and in this remarkable book he tells his story of where it has left him in terms of outlook, values and attitude.

I have had the privilege of doing ten treks in Nepal, journeys which have taken me to most of the areas of the tribal people we call the Gurkhas when they are enlisted in the British Army. It is a land of amazing cultural, ethnic, geographical, linguistic and religious diversity. It is the place of the celestial snows – the great peaks that have captured so many people's imagination over the years. It is also a land of great poverty, and of course, it is the abode of impressively hardy, good natured and resilient people. Gurkha soldiers in the British Army often ask me why I keep going back and my initial response always leaves them a little dumbfounded when I tell them that they must understand that I do not go for trekking. When I tell them that my real purpose is a pilgrimage, the warmth of their smile indicates immediately that they have understood perfectly the importance of such journeys to me.

You will not read very many pages of this book before you realise that Mark takes the same approach, not just to his visits to Nepal but also to his battle against cancer. As Chaucer in his Canterbury Tales related so well, the point of a true pilgrimage is not to reach the shrine or to complete the journey: what is important is what happens on the trail in terms of the interaction with those one is travelling with, and, even more particularly, the challenging thoughts that can confront one when freed from the mundane reality of ordinary existence. Mark's extraordinarily wide ranging thoughts and ideas on a whole host of subjects reveal not only an amazingly versatile mind and very wide reading but also an ability to bring disparate thoughts together in a way which sheds new light on some extremely difficult issues. Nowhere is this more obvious than when he writes about his personal battle against cancer. This is really the central theme of the book, but it is one that is dealt with at many different levels and it is this achievement which makes the book such an interesting and challenging read.

In summary, Mark tells an intensely personal story but he does so in a way which will have wide and sympathetic appeal. He is very much a pilgrim who is still on the road, but his eyes remain alert, his mind remains open and he has already learnt much as a result of some searing experiences on the way. It is a pleasure to commend his insight to you.

13 July 2000

Acknowledgments

"Pray to God but row away from the rocks"

Indian Proverb

There are many more people to whom I would like to express my appreciation. Firstly to my wife, Ruth, and to my Father and my Mother's partner, John, who have all spent so much time, effort and concern on my behalf, through this difficult time for all of us. My two sons and Saki Kishimoto, our Japanese student, also bore this difficult time with courage and compassion. My thanks go too, to the leading international consultancy where I worked, and the people there, as well as the many friends, for their support.

Secondly I would like to express my gratitude for the professional medical advice and treatment provided by my doctor and my oncologist. I would also like to thank Cabrini Hospital and its staff for the excellent treatment and their refreshing sense of humour, on my rather too frequent visits.

I am indebted to my homoeopath and Chinese doctor, Professor Wang, for their wisdom and skill. I would like to thank Clif Sanderson for helping me to see the bigger picture through his healing, and Edna for her kind concern and advice to take high dose vitamin C in a particular form which I believe, amongst other things, helped me to cope with chemotherapy. My gratitude extends to Doctor Joe Reich for his quick diagnosis and effective treatment, which did much to save my left eye from the risk of permanent damage, and all the other medical practitioners of many disciplines who have helped me on this journey.

I would like to acknowledge the contribution of Colonel B. M. Niven whose beautifully illustrated book, *The Mountain Kingdom*, about his journeys through the high mountain villages, helped me to put a clearer perspective on so much of what I saw on my trek. *(A contribution will be made to the Gurkha Welfare Trust – registered charity No. 1034080 – from some of the profits arising out of sales of this book.)* As well as the contribution made by David Keirsey through his book, *Please Understand Me II,* which provided me with a very clear framework to describe the porter's personalities.

Lastly, my special thanks go to people who have given me advice about the book: my Father, John M., Peter H., Tony V., Azni T., Wendy B., Liat K., Nola B., Helen B-B., Magnolia G., Richard L., Bill P., Ruth, my Mother, and John Penn who died on 12 August 2002. They have all helped to make this a much better book.

About The Author

"Experience is not what happens to a man;
It is what a man does with what happens"

Aldous Huxley: author

Mark was educated in England, where he gained a Bachelor of Arts (Honours) and Master of Chemical Engineering from Cambridge University. He then served for eight years with the Royal Engineers working in Belize, Brunei, Cyprus, Germany, Hong Kong, Mexico, Nepal, South Korea and the Falkland Islands. It was an opportunity he was fortunate to have, for "Travel is fatal to prejudice, bigotry and narrow-mindedness. Broad, wholesome, charitable views cannot be acquired by vegetating in one little corner of the earth.[1]"

After that he moved to Australia, later setting up his own consultancy and working as a "human performance" consultant. While trying to work out what that means he goes hill walking.

The author's first two names are Mark Kingsley. He has not included his surname, to protect the privacy of those who have not explicitly stated that their names and details could be included. Mark can be contacted by letter addressed to: PO Box 193 Ashburton, Victoria, Australia 3147, or email: mark.kingsley@ozemail.com.au. (However, it may be worth remembering that email addresses, like people, have a habit of "falling over".) He will reply as the situation permits but cannot make any guarantees to this effect.

Disclaimer

"Dig a well before you are thirsty"

Chinese Proverb

The author may not be held liable or responsible to any person or entity with respect to loss or damage caused, or allegedly caused, directly or indirectly by the use of any information contained in this Trilogy.

I am not a doctor, a medical practitioner, an oncologist or a healthcare specialist. I am an ex-chemotherapy patient, who has had personal experience with cancer and who looked widely for the options around treatment. Book 1 – *A Sudden Trip Over Hodgkin's Disease* – does not attempt to interpret advice of qualified medical practitioners or their institutes. Cancer is a very serious condition and professional healthcare specialists should be consulted. To that end I believe my oncologist, my doctor, and Cabrini Hospital, all provided me with excellent conventional treatment. I also believe most alternative therapies I tried helped me very greatly.

The medical and nutritional information in this book is intended for educational purposes only and must in no way be construed as medical advice. I personally believe that many of the things I did helped me to recover from the effects of the disease and my treatment. I have included in the endnotes some scientific studies which support my views and a few which contradict them. However, it remains for you, the reader, to make up your own mind about suitable treatments for yourself or others. I hope this book helps you to make a much more informed decision about what type of cancer prevention techniques or cancer therapy you choose to adopt, however, I do not make any guarantees about the success of any particular therapy – be it conventional or alternative.

PART I: A HOUSE IN HIGHER HILLS

TABLE OF CONTENTS

A SUDDEN TRIP OVER HODGKIN'S DISEASE –
June to December 1999

A SHORTER WALK IN THE HINDU MOUNTAINS –
20 November to 22 December 1990

QUICKLY CROSSING THE HIGHER SELF –
1990-1999

PART ONE

A HOUSE IN HIGHER HILLS

A SUDDEN TRIP OVER
HODGKIN'S DISEASE
AND
A SHORTER WALK IN THE
HINDU MOUNTAINS
AND
QUICKLY CROSSING THE
HIGHER SELF

INTRODUCTION

"The real act of discovery consists not in finding new lands, but seeing with new eyes"

Marcel Proust; French writer

BOOK 1 – The Emotional Room

"Somebody should tell us, right at the start of our lives, that we are dying. Then we might live life to the limit, every minute of every single day… Whatever you want to do – do it now! Carpe diem… ! And expect miracles, because you are one."

Michael Landon; actor (from "Bonanza" and "Little House on the Prairie") who died from lung cancer

1999: 10 June, Melbourne

"**I**'m very sorry but it doesn't look good: it's cancer."

Not how you'd like to start any day, but that is how it started for me on Thursday 10 June 1999.

I feel the fear well up inside me after hearing a word I did not expect nor want. Doctor Iggy Soosay[2](Address) is our family GP and says that although he believes some alternative medicines are useful this cancer has a very good cure rate from conventional treatment. He concludes, "I will make an appointment for you to see an oncologist as soon as possible."

Shell-shocked, I feel more focussed than surprised, feeling the fear of not knowing whether my life is being measured in days or years. Now is the time for the advice I was given when growing up:

1. Never to lose sleep over small issues.
2. That all issues are small issues.

But it is a bit easier said than done at the moment.

How life changes in a moment! I recall the story of the gymnast who is approached by a zoo owner wanting to hire him out as a monkey because all of the zoo's monkeys have died. The gymnast feels a bit strange at first, sitting in the cage dressed up in his monkey suit. However, he soon gets the hang of things as he swings from tree to tree and plays up to the varied visitors. It is not long before he gets so carried away that he does an almighty swing which takes him out of his own cage and into the lions' next door. In absolute terror, as a lion bounds towards him, he runs up to the bars screaming "Help, help I'm a person not a monkey, get me out."

As the lion reaches him it suddenly stops, taps him on the shoulder and says, "Shut up mate; otherwise you'll get us all fired!"

I have experienced fear for fun – abseiling through waterfalls and out of a helicopter – but this is a different type of fear altogether.

I now understand a bit more how that gymnast would have felt. My lion is slowly walking towards me and I have four to six months to find out if it is real or not.

In a world of my own I turn into my drive as Ruth is walking out. She smiles at me despite my sombre expression. Her expression changes at my words: "The doctor says I have cancer."

I sit in the living room, thinking about perhaps not living and I look around my house.

There is an Indian saying: "Everyone is a house with four rooms – a physical, an emotional, a mental and a spiritual – and each one of us tends to live in one room most of the time, but unless we go into every room, every day, even if only to air it, then we are not a complete person."

So here I sit, my house within my house.

The real living room symbolizes the Physical for me. To my left is the study – a Mental Room of intellectual attentions where I write this diary. Behind me is my Emotional Room – the room of dreams and nightmares, where in times of stress, tiredness or ill health, I retire. I may even eat there as physical sustenance often provides emotional support. I am wandering into the garden, not escaping this bad dream I am living, just wondering where it will lead. If there is a Spiritual Room, this is it. A Room that is, in many ways, not a room and, in some ways, not part of the house.

I decide to act and change my diet to a vegetarian one, thinking if I do what I have always done, I am likely to get what I've always got. Earlier I had read Louise L. Hay's "probable causes" for diseases in her insightful book *You Can Heal Your Life*[3]. I read them again, and it is much more interesting the second time around. She lists causes for a whole range of illnesses.

I probably have Hodgkin's disease, and her possible reason is, "Blame and a tremendous fear of 'not being good enough'. A frantic race to prove one's self until the blood has no substance left to support itself."

Her suggestion for a new thought pattern is: "I am perfectly happy to be me. I am good enough just as I am. I love and approve of myself. I am joy expressing and receiving[4]."

My Mother has just had Non-Hodgkin's Lymphoma, diagnosed about a year before me, and her brother died two years ago from cancer. It gets me wondering whether there is a genetic link – all three of us being classic Ectomorphs[5]. Whether or not this is a factor, I am certain stress also has a part to play; but my Mother found this mind stuff all a bit fanciful, even when I explained to her that it is well established that more people die around 09.00 on Monday morning in modern society than at any other time of the week[6]. (Animals would seem to die at the same rate throughout the week.)

Remembering the old Army saying, "Time spent in reconnaissance is seldom wasted[7]," I decide to trawl my environment for information on a way out.

I take a little comfort from the first part of Churchill's observation that, "Most men occasionally stumble over the truth, but most of them pick themselves up and hurry off as if nothing happened …"

BOOK 2 – The Physical Room

"Like all great travellers, I have seen more than I
remember, and remember more than I have seen"
Benjamin Disraeli: British Prime Minister

The Kingdom of Nepal is about the size of England in
geographic area but has a third the population at 22.6 million
people[8].

As a Captain in the QGE (Queen's Gurkha Engineers) based in
Hong Kong, one of my less onerous duties was to design water
supply systems for remote hillside villages in East Nepal. This
relationship between the British and the Gurkha soldiers goes back
to the nineteenth century after the European and Sepoy Regiments
of the Honourable East India Company encountered the brave
Gurkha fighters in Nepal. The impressive fighting qualities of the
Gurkhas led to the first Gurkha Regiment (The Sirmoor Rifles)
being formed by the East India Company in 1815. Over almost 200
years of service with the British Army, thousands of Gurkhas have
died on foreign battlefields, time and time again showing their
immense courage and loyalty, under the cry of "Ayo Gurkhali!" –
"The Gurkhas are upon you!"

Trekking through Nepal, I was asked three questions:

What is my name and regiment?
What am I doing here exactly?
Where do I go after I am finished here?

The answers were pretty straightforward: "Captain Mark
Kingsley of the Queen's Gurkha Engineers – to design three water
supply systems – back to Hong Kong." Although I did not mention

in my reply to Question 2 that the fundamental purpose was "to support life", as I assumed it to be obvious.

BOOK 3 – The Spiritual Room

"You are your own master,
You make your own future"

Siddhartha Gotama; The Buddha

This Trilogy is not a light read as you will probably have already discovered. Its primary aim is to help those with a life-threatening illness, or those with friends and relatives suffering from one, and to help with life itself.

It is my belief borne out of personal experience, observing people and discussions with others, that most of us have issues in life; be they physical, emotional or mental. However, if you do not feel that you, or those around you, have any real challenges in life then this Trilogy is probably not for you. Reading this book is a possibly beneficial, but almost certainly challenging journey, and without the motivation to make this journey you are unlikely to see it through to the end. Never forgetting that those who don't read a book are no better off than those who can't read one.

This Trilogy is called *A Himalayan Trinity* because it is about mountains in my life (symbolized for me by the Himalayas). The word *Trinity* is used because it is composed of three different and separate volumes which are all part of the one tome. They are about three journeys of the one Journey we all make, called life.

If this book were a bungalow then on the next page would be its floor plan.

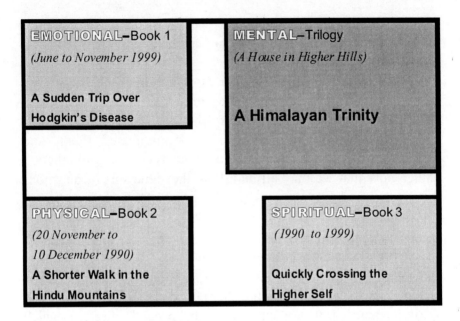

EMOTIONAL–Book 1	MENTAL–Trilogy
(June to November 1999)	*(A House in Higher Hills)*
A Sudden Trip Over Hodgkin's Disease	**A Himalayan Trinity**
PHYSICAL–Book 2	SPIRITUAL–Book 3
(20 November to 10 December 1990)	*(1990 to 1999)*
A Shorter Walk in the Hindu Mountains	**Quickly Crossing the Higher Self**

Book 1, about my journey through cancer and chemotherapy, was written from an electronic diary that I recorded at the time. The ideas expressed now are ideas I had then. A number of these seem to have been substantiated by studies reported in later medical or scientific journals, and where this is the case I have referenced my comments. Book 2 was written from a note book that I kept on my trek, although these notes have been interpreted from my current viewpoint which is not the same as the one I had at the time of making that walk.

Each journey has a time of *preparation* (although we do not always realize when we are preparing), the *journey* itself, and then a *home-coming* of some sort. These three books are about different mountainous journeys through sickness, foreignness, and awareness, but they are printed concurrently chapter by chapter because the chapters of each book are linked to the others. They are the same journey – just in different form. Book 3 takes the reader through a comprehensive model which can help to better understand the deepest human drives in all of us. It is a model to help with one's inner life in a similar way that the western scientific model can help with the outer one.

I have included a large number of quotes in this Trilogy even though I could have communicated the ideas in my own words. This is for two reasons; firstly, to recognize those who have come up with ideas and/or insightfully communicated them, and secondly, to sometimes show where my ideas concur with others. I realize now that we may all be asking the same sort of questions that I was asked on the trek – just in a more holistic form:

Who am I?
What is my purpose?
Where do I go to when my life is finished?

One answer to who we are, is "a four roomed house" which is another way to say we are "mind *[thoughts and feelings],* body and spirit." Again, it is the answer to the second question which supports life.

Why does death prompt us to think about and/or believe in the spiritual? Is it because we are desperate to keep living and so create an illusion of an afterlife? Or is it that we stop being distracted by the worldly things around us and are therefore able to see the Truth much more clearly? This is Part I of the Trilogy – the story of the *Preparation* and *Journey* in each Room. The *Home-coming* is in the second and final part.

Pierre Teilhard de Chaudin[9] asked, "Are we human beings having a spiritual experience or spiritual beings having a human experience?"

This is my experience, my story, in the last decade of the Second Millennium …

THE PREPARATION

"Proper   prior   preparation   prevents   piss   poor
performance"

The British soldiers' 7P's

*E**ach of these books is a complete book in itself, and can be followed without reading either of the other two. You may decide to read just one book, to explore only one Room, but might still find it worthwhile browsing the other two books and airing the other Rooms as you go!*

I have provided significant information on nutrition in parts of this book for those facing illness. For those readers not interested in the subject I suggest that you skim over or miss these parts.

CHAPTER 1

Pain is One Source of Courage

BOOK 1 – 1999: 11–13 June, Melbourne, Australia

The daylight wakes me as it streams into my bedroom. As I wake I totally forget that I am in the Emotional Room – ill and ill at ease. As I remember I get a very small glimpse of what it might be like to be waiting some day for execution. Here is the most dependent of my Rooms, about what I want and what I don't.

I go in to work. A friend there tackles me for getting a client to contact her directly, yesterday. I tell her I was in hospital at the time when the client phoned me on my mobile telephone.

She angrily retorts, "What were you doing phoning her from hospital?"

It's not what I need at the moment, and while I ignore her and her comments, my irritation grows. I begin to notice that both our breathing has changed. It is an example of connectivity; not between my friend and me, but between the mind and body. If you change your emotional state then your physicality in the form of breathing changes even if only subtly. It gives a clue as to the three primary negative emotions which manifest from the fundamental negative emotion – fear:

Breathing	Characteristic Emotion[10]
Lightly in and lightly out	Fear
Lightly in and harshly out	Anger
Harshly in and lightly out	Sadness
Harshly in and harshly out	Passion

Her anger is the fear of not getting something she wants, or of getting something she does not want. It seems to be a reaction blaming other people (or things) for an inability to control what is happening to her. Whereas the sadness I felt on my diagnosis was probably the same fear turned inwards – blaming myself while fearing the loss of my life. But now I feel another negative emotion at her reaction and it is certainly not passion, an emotion which might seem unfairly classed as a negative one. It is not to say it is inherently bad (or good); it is just that, like all negative emotions, it has a selfish focus. They all manifest from fear: when you focus on yourself and your own situation.

I hear someone say later, on another matter, that their sadness has turned to anger. They are not talking about a very great step.

That night I arrange to go and see a client and close friend at her home to tell her the situation. Joanna is a fellow Pom[11] who came out to Australia when she was twenty-one years old. She has worked for one of Australia's leading banks for many years in a range of roles, and is capable and considerate. She has demonstrated to me her ability to keep her eye on the bigger picture while remaining focussed on getting a fair and ethical outcome. We have been working together on a senior manager assessment project for a couple of years now. She had raised the issue before of who would take over from me should I be hit by a "London Bus". I go around to break the news. I have been hit by a red double-decker and still do not know what it's doing in Melbourne. She shows a great deal of sympathy for my predicament and I leave with more water in my eyes than when I arrived.

It is sobering talking to Peter that evening. Peter is a great friend from New Zealand and Godfather to my younger son. He is a big, rugby playing forward whose powerful physique belies his kindness. We first met when I came out to Australia to work for a mining company, and he has now moved back to New Zealand. Only last year I took my sons to visit his family and went out to a "batch" (what the Kiwis call a holiday home in the country). We took the time to talk about life. The discussion is more limited this time as I talk about possible death. Tact is not currently a strong point of mine and he is pretty upset, especially having just lost his elder sister to cancer a few months ago. I am no better with my Father, whom I phone in England later.

I start the conversation with, "Dad, I have cancer."

I finish the evening by phoning John, my Mother's partner, and tell him the news. He cannot believe it, having just gone through it all with my Mother. He has also recently been through a major health issue with his young son.

His immediate reaction is "Good God" and he agrees that we should not tell my Mother yet.

However, Ruth has her reservations. I feel life is going to change, and I tell Ruth this. I am into stating the obvious.

I turn on the television which happens to be on the Fox Sports Channel. There is an American cyclist being interviewed about the upcoming Tour de France – something I find uninteresting. Nevertheless I continue watching. Suddenly they flash up a picture of him three years ago when he was going through chemotherapy at 24 years of age. I become very interested. His name is Lance Armstrong and he is reckoned to have a good chance of winning this year. He says up until his cancer he was in the American squad but not one of the lead riders. His doctors told him he had a 50% chance of recovering from his testicular cancer and did not want to demoralize him by telling him he really had a 20% chance! After he had recovered from cancer he went back to the squad, mainly for the camaraderie of being with his team. He found his mind set had changed massively and he was now riding better than ever. He believes his mind was a very important part of his recovery.

I do not know exactly what caused this but not knowing the cause does not mean there isn't one. It seems to be a coincidence that I happen to see Lance on television, and where I am now is at some intersection of what I have done before – the decisions I have made. Perhaps coincidence is just God's way of performing miracles anonymously?

Saki Kishimoto, the twenty-year-old Japanese student staying with us, comes in and says the English equivalent of *"konnichiwa[12]"*, in her usual cheery manner. She is outgoing, lively and ready to try most things. Four weeks ago she joined the boys and me at an indoor rock-climbing wall, quickly getting the hang of belaying my younger son, Rob, while I belayed my elder, Olly. She has just come back after a day at her language school.

I tell her "I am afraid I have cancer."

She does not understand what I am saying so I ask her to get out her dictionary. She hands it to me and I find the word "cancer". Saki takes one look at it and bursts into tears.

I am having a basic question of life shoved in my face, "Where do I go to when my life is finished?"

There are only two mistakes, believing things which are not true, and not believing things which are; and with that thought I go to the Mind, Body & Spirit Festival. It is a three-day event in Melbourne, and is named after the three parts of all of us;

- The body which everyone agrees exists,
- The mind which most people believe we have, and
- The spirit whose existence is much more a matter of debate.

There, I hear of Morinda Noni juice for the first time[13]. The Noni plant is found in Tahiti, and has been used for hundreds of years because of its powerful therapeutic capabilities. Like most therapeutic nutritional "whole food" products part of the benefit is by helping the body to function in balance, allowing the body's own healing mechanisms to operate properly. I have little doubt that "Vis Medicatrix Naturae" – the healing power of nature – is worth tapping into. Noni juice, like other nutritional products, has been found to help, to some degree, a very long list of ailments. I see that one of the main "active" ingredients is also found in pineapple, but in much lower, and reducing, doses ever since commercially producing pineapples. The Noni juice turns out to be quite expensive. As I walk on, my mind mulls over the cost of life, vis-à-vis the cost of death. I return to buy a bottle, deciding to accept the research, which shows that it can inhibit the formation of tumours[14].

I feel the need for something optimistic and the views here are some of the most optimistic I have experienced to date. I go up to Jack Lim, a Grand Qigong Master. He explains that Qi[15] is Chinese for "Vital" or "Life Energy", and links the body of physical aspect of health to the "mind" aspect of health mirroring the connection between the individual and the universe. In Chinese medical philosophy, Qi underlies all living things and permeates nature. Qigong, the practice of Qi, is a systematic method involving personal moral (emotional) training, and mental and physical techniques. Mastery of Qi requires a respect of nature and goodwill to all living beings. It presumes an holistic Taoist philosophy but does not reject other religious perspectives. The idea of Qi is similar to that of Prana in Indian philosophy, or consciousness in western psychology. It sounds a pretty esoteric idea but he says that a physically measurable external Qi energy has been demonstrated in laboratory tests.

Jack looks nonchalantly at the tumour on my neck, which is about the size of a large lemon. He does not recoil from it, as I have got used to others doing. He sees the most effective cancer treatment is allowing the body to harness its huge healing powers. He shows me a tape of "walking Qigong". Much like Yoga, Qigong works by fostering the correct circulation of energy and blood to maintain, or restore, body rhythms. However, it is much easier to perform than many yoga or tai-chi practices I have seen. I buy it and leave with a range of "natural" medicines to start my home Pharmacy.

It has been good to have seen some different views of the world, and if I ever felt I had a handle on life, it has just broken.

From My Living Room to the Himalaya

"A ship is safe in a harbour –
But that's not what ships are for"

John A Shedd

BOOK 2 – 1991: 20 November, Hong Kong

The kettle screamed away but it was too late for my planned cup of coffee. Time was getting tight and my driver was downstairs. I took one look around the living room to check all was in order, and then leapt down the fourteen flights of stairs, four at a time.

I stood there at Hong Kong's main airport (Kai Tak) looking for Guy. He was a Lieutenant and a fellow Troop Commander of some thirty men in another part of my Regiment. It did not turn out to be such a hard task as he was somewhat incongruous in a rather natty blue Regimental blazer beneath his rather tatty green Army rucksack.

We went by Dragon Air, an exciting name for an exciting airline … especially at take-off and landing. Then we had a two-hour stopover at Bangkok airport. It was just long enough to be made to feel unwelcome as the Chinese and Thai customs officials seemed keen to maintain the reputation of Customs Officers the world over.

I have always wanted to see Sagarmatha in person, as the Nepalese call Mount Everest, and suddenly the pilot announced that Everest was on our right hand side. I was seated on the left side and so moved across to see the mountain range. I leant close to, and awkwardly, across some other passengers to take my photograph but had forgotten to turn it on. Just as I brought the camera back up to my eye again the plane banked away. So I took a rather grand photo of some relatively low ground and then I proceeded to fall into the laps of these passengers and made some new friends.

Once back in my seat I was served caviar for the first time. It looked like frogs spawn to me and did not taste quite as good as it looked.

Landing at Kathmandu is a fairly tricky procedure and a relatively large number of passengers visit the surrounding mountains earlier than planned. It is testament to the difficulty of doing it without modern navigation facilities and in bad weather. As it turned out the weather was okay this time and our descent was smooth. My sense of unease did not come from a fear of flying so much as the fear of crashing so I refrained from looking out of the window in case the view destroyed that illusion.

A slight ebb of people moved inside Kathmandu airport but it was awash with people outside as we exited with our baggage. Out of this torrent stood the Brigade of Gurkha's representative who ushered me through the Nepalese Customs in quick time and before they too could maintain the reputation of their brethren in Bangkok.

A flood of onlookers streamed forward as we came outside and out of them popped the ever smiling Corporal Narendra Rai, grinning from ear to ear. We were well acquainted from the British Forces Taekwondo Association, and with him was Lance Corporal Subasha, my trek guide. He shook my hand effusively giving me an inkling of what I was to find out – that he had an eagerness for life's experiences.

At this time, British Officers were usually provided with a guide from their Regiment who was in their Squadron or whom they knew. This was not always possible because any Gurkha soldiers acting as guides had to be on their triennial six-month leave. It was a carrot of a job (no plums up here) as the soldiers got additional pay, so most jumped at the chance. However, Subash fitted neither of the two categories.

We walked past two male, armed and uniformed policemen on our way out. They were strolling around the airport formally and full of an authority which was slightly dented for me as they were holding hands. I did a double take that my English eyes were not playing up, but in Nepalese culture it is quite acceptable for adult men to hold hands.

We drove into Kathmandu in the late afternoon to be greeted by a city of bright shapes against dull colours. The Valley of Kathmandu is a basin and former lake site in the centre of the country some 1300 metres above sea level. It is the only sizeable piece of flat land in Nepal apart from the Terai's[16] southern fringe-lands. Mountains ranging from 1500 to 2800 metres surround Kathmandu like picturesque prison walls etched with snow-white barbed wire. It symbolizes Nepal's occupation of one of the most mountainous parts of the world. Of the fourteen mountains over 8000 metres, and of the highest ten, eight are in Nepal – including Mount Everest which persists on getting taller (by 1/4 inch) each year.

Kathmandu is a city of 235 000 people, and once there we headed straight off to our four star Hotel – an international rating on price rather than quality. Six months earlier, a fellow officer went down with amoebic dysentery from eating eggs for breakfast while staying at the Hotel. So cooked breakfasts had moved down to the bottom of my menu for now. Guy and I found the bar tucked away to one side and ordered a drink, and increased the attendance by 200%. It was going to be one hell of a quiet night.

My hotel room was somewhat Spartan yet easily comfortable enough. I went through some of the details of the water supply systems and the three Eastern Nepali villages I would be visiting – Yakchuwa, Phakchuwa and Maimajhuwa. It is hard to overstate the importance of safe water in these parts of the world and things have continued to get worse. (Around the globe in 1999, 5.3 million people died from diseases caused by unsafe water[17], and many more were left maimed by water-borne diseases, such as parasitic worms, which often cause terrible pain.)

My job was to give recommendations for the construction of water supply systems. I was also to check the supplies and conditions of the AWCs (Area Welfare Centres), and record any hardship cases involving ex-Gurkha soldiers. I was not to forget the names of key persons met, distance and travel times for routes, local prices for land, building materials, livestock, the general state of the crops and land, and anything else which I deemed to be relevant. It might just be a big book.

Going Inside Our Garden

"Religion is the defence against the experience of God"
CG Jung: Swiss Psychologist

BOOK 3 – Awareness

"The experience of God" is another way to define spirituality but it is not necessarily the same as religion, as the latter is not always about "spirit as opposed to matter[18]". If God is in everything then He is in us, and spirituality would then be about experiencing god by "knowing thyself". At its essence, it is about self-awareness as we go to parts of life's rather large garden.

Coursing A Crevasse[19]

Chapter One: We journey along a mountain path and come to a crevasse. We fall in, but it is someone else's fault and it takes us forever to get out.

Chapter Two: We walk along the same mountain path and come to the crevasse. We pretend not to see it, but still fall in. We cannot believe it and get really mad.

Chapter Three: We walk along the mountain path and come to the same crevasse. Despite seeing it we still fall in, but we take full responsibility and get out immediately.

Chapter Four: We walk along the same mountain path and come to the same crevasse. We walk around it.

Chapter Five: We walk along another mountain path.

The world is good at convincing us that Chapter One is the whole material book, not just one chapter of the bigger spiritual story. Self-awareness helps us to realize that there are more chapters, but this is a "necessary", not a "sufficient" condition, as we still may not read them.

CHAPTER 2

Learning Lessons Too Late?

1999: 14 – 27 June, Melbourne & the Blue Mountains

I wake up on Monday; it is a public holiday, which would be nice under normal circumstances but it is meaningless now. At night I watch a fictional thriller on television. It manages to scare me in a few places. Funny how I can be scared by someone else's imaginary experiences of a pretend life. I am frightened by an illusion of an illusion. So how much more is this experience going to frighten me now?

I do little thinking yet think too much. I want to increase my wisdom around nutrition, but the more I know, the more I find I don't. It is true that we may not all be the same in what we know, but we are pretty similar in the extent of what we don't!

There is a well known, perhaps apocryphal story of a judge and a barrister clashing several times during a court case.

The barrister had given a lengthy summation at the end of the case, whereupon the judge said: "We are none the wiser for all that."

"Perhaps not, My Lord," the barrister replied, "but you are much better informed."

I hope to be both in trying a range of alternatives on this trek, and I am struck by a thought, "Why don't I go on a meditation course?"

In 1997, I had read a book about Vipassana meditation and decided then to do a ten-day course in May 1998. It was a shock to my system. Ten and a half hours of meditation per day. No talking, reading, listening to music, or any other form of communication was permitted. Up soon after 04.00 am each morning and to bed about 9.30 pm. Like most challenging things, there were some great benefits, although it is hard to describe them in words.

During the course I experienced some strange sensations. I got strong and continuous pains in one location in my back, in the very spot where the primary tumour has been diagnosed. Yet this was some 13 months before I was diagnosed with Hodgkin's. The pains were so strong and regular during the meditation that I mentioned them to Ruth when I returned from the course. What I did not mention to her, or anyone else, was that I got a strange feeling I would be returning to do another course in another year. This time with a serious illness. I don't think this meant that I created my illness, as I had some of the symptoms for Hodgkin's before I went to the Vipassana – although I did not know these were symptoms at the time.

The Vipassana course closest to me, just outside Melbourne at Woori Yallock, does not start for a couple of weeks. However, I find out that I can get on the one starting this Wednesday at the Blue Mountains, near Sydney.

Back at the Medical Centres for further diagnosis after a chest X-ray and an ultra-sound on the lump in my throat, the oncologist arranges a CT-scan and blood test. Yes, it is malignant. Although it is not clear whether it is Hodgkin's or Non-Hodgkin's lymphoma. Both are cancers of the lymph system but they involve different cells.

I tell my oncologist that I have now decided to go to a twelve-day meditation course.

He supportively says, "That's fine!"

But seems surprised by what is not so common a course of action on being diagnosed with cancer. He tells me that the primary tumour is grapefruit sized (some twelve centimetres in diameter) in my chest, behind the lungs.

My reaction is "That's the first I have heard of it," but Ruth assures me I was told initially.

I guess it was not news I wanted and "There are none so deaf as those who do not want to hear".

I was still thinking that the lemon sized lump on my neck was the sum of it. I am a temperamental optimist – sometimes I feel optimistic, sometimes not. The same day the ultra-sound image picked up an eight-centimetre tumour on my neck I thought it was just a swollen gland, even when told that they tend to be two centimetres, maximum.

The tests indicate Hodgkin's lymphoma. Potentially good news, as it is one of the most treatable cancers, and is very sensitive to radiation and chemotherapy. Although I remain unconvinced that this is so very different from the rest of my cells!

I see my oncologist again and he confirms that it is not clear when my cancer started. The Radiation Oncologist says 3 to 6 months ago. My oncologist thinks it is more like a year or so ago, but says it is hard to know. Books I am reading say it is about 1–2 years before the symptoms crop up. Some sources reckon a few cancerous cells are formed ten to twenty years before it becomes symptomatic. It seems no one knows for sure.

Professor Yong-Qiang Wang[20(address)], a slim, fit looking Chinese doctor greets me in his surgery. He seems to have an uncanny ability to diagnose medical ailments. However, it is his obvious state of good health which impresses me the most. He does not look anything like his 54 years of age and I did Kung-Fu training with him a few months back, and saw then how fit he was.

He listens as I ask for his comments about meditating for eleven hours a day for ten days.

He responds, "Good as long as you do not fear, fear is the friend of cancer."

He teaches Qigong[21] Chinese Medicine and shows me a few simple moves that he recommends I practise.

I spend some time reading his certificates on the wall after the treatment. Professor Wang is China's 24th Qigong Grand Master of the Traditional Branch of Emei School, with a doctor's licence awarded in 1987 by the Nanjing Health Department. The Emei School is actually named after a very famous mountain in Southwest China. This School has 24 Branches and a history of over 1700 years. Qigong absorbed the essence of the best techniques from many schools' traditions, concerning health preservation and "thought". The philosophical basis for this School is characterised by a combination of Buddhist and Taoist elements. Professor Wang's the guidance from his master was to "repay" the world by passing on his learnings.

Linda Cameron is the Managing Director of Nutricorp Industries[22]. This is the company which manufactures the shark liver oil I was told about at the Mind, Body & Spirit Festival. She shows great concern when I phone her. Doctor William Lane Ph.D., the author of *Sharks Don't Get Cancer – How Shark Cartilage Could Save Your Life*[23], believes shark cartilage can be very effective in treating cancer. Within all cartilage is a special protein, which inhibits the growth of a network of blood vessels, called angiogenesis, which cancer cells must do to grow[24]. Sharks have been on earth for 400 million years but remain relatively untouched by evolution, suggesting that they have achieved some form of highly evolved state in terms of survival. Sharks live for more than 100 years, and yet seem to have an uncanny resistance to growth of tumours and infections. In 25 years of research, the Smithsonian Institution has found only one malignant tumour in more than 25 000 sharks that they have studied. They seem to resist cancer even when put in water laden with carcinogens.

The "devil is in the details" and quality can be an excuse to charge more, but it can also be critical to do the job. I think of these products as tools for my body. I bought a cut-price screwdriver some time ago, thinking I would save money even if it did half the job. Unfortunately it bent first time. If I had never seen a screwdriver before then I might have been misled into thinking that no screwdriver works. Apparently there are large numbers of vitamin pills being found in sewage systems, which suggests that they have not done their consumers much good. The quality of the vitamin pills is critical.

Linda couriers over a large supply of shark liver oil capsules, some shark cartilage sachets and some information on studies carried out for both. She does not let me pay. Shark liver has been used for over 40 years as both a therapeutic and preventive agent. It appears that the liver may contain immunological substances called AKGs (alkoxyglycerols). The human body constantly produces AKGs in the bone marrow, spleen, liver and human breast milk but at very low quantities. Scientists have found that giving cancer patients small dosages of AKGs, before, during and after radiation treatment reduces the sharp and dangerous drop in white blood cells[25] – a common side effect of the treatment[26]. AKGs seem to elevate the non-specific immune response by increasing the level of white blood cells.

A study found that "Cancer patients treated with alkoxylglycerols [from shark liver oil] had a significantly higher five year survival than the control group[27]."

The uncertainty is beginning to sink in. We do not tell our boys much of my situation except to say that I have a temporary illness which will mean that I will not be very active for four months or so.

Ruth and I have not mentioned the word "Cancer".

We do not want either of them mentioning it to friends at school in case the friends say something like; "Oh, then your father is going to die!"

But children are intuitive and nine-year-old Olly asks at lunch: "What is cancer?"

Ruth and I are in a bit of turmoil. We do not sleep well that night but give each other a long hug. Ruth is becoming particularly upset, yet I am feeling too focussed to be conscious of what my emotions might be. It is true that the wisdom gained from experience provides good schooling but it is looking like a costly lesson. We go for a final, but I hope not too final, lunch at a local vegetarian restaurant, *Miracles Cafe*[28], before I leave for Vipassana. It is not so much that I am hoping for a big miracle, much as I would like one, but more because I see their organic food as offering some help in this fight. There are only a few people eating there and we chat with the owner, Martina.

The time comes for Vipassana and I pack my Nepali hat for this little journey (Vipassana) before the bigger journey (chemotherapy) – or is it the other way around? I tell a friend, Angus, that I am off to meditate for twelve days, staying in the Blue Mountains. He thinks the latter is a good idea but is less certain about the former!

The train to the Blue Mountains north of Sydney takes some four hours. It's uncomfortably hot in the carriage, so I open a window but it continues to do its impression of a mobile sauna. I am left uncomfortably deep in thought as I watch the scenery change through the window. It is a mountain range a world apart from the Himalaya, but beautiful in its own way. My mind churns over mountains bigger than those on which the train climbs.

It is late and cold when I arrive. As we wait to find out our room numbers, I start talking to a fellow "meditator to be". He is a quiet, quite inward focussed outward-bound instructor. After chatting for a while I come to a natural point to tell him why I am here while emphasising I know there is no point coming to such a course to be healed. Some people have reported becoming freed of terminal symptoms after attending these retreats, but it is not a reason to come! Telling him I have cancer reminds me of what is happening to me, and I feel a tremor of anxiety run down my body.

The meditation starts tonight and this is a serious meditation course. I wake up the next morning and it's like the film, *Groundhog Day,* all over again. The film is about an American salesman who stops on business in a small rural town for a couple of nights. His first day in town coincides with a US holiday, Groundhog Day. It is a bad day for him which he starts by falling into a puddle. Nothing goes right. The next morning when he wakes up he sees that the morning is starting exactly the same. He soon realises that time has gone back a day as everything is happening as it did yesterday. This happens day after day. I think I am experiencing my own "Groundhog Day". It seems like I have been here for three days but I am only on Day 1. By Day 3 I feel I have been here seven days. Shortly I realize that the course must have been extended, as I am sure that I have been here fourteen days. Unfortunately it is only Day 6. Time is not an objective reality.

I started consuming before the Vipassana course, Noni juice, shark cartilage (in much smaller doses than reported therapeutically for cancer cures) and shark liver oil. I drop the "shark oil" for now, because the Vipassana practice prefers students to stick to a vegetarian diet. In Einstein's words, "Nothing will benefit human health and increase the chances for survival of life on Earth as much as the evolution of a vegetarian diet."

I am hoping it will benefit one particular life while the silence gives me too much time to think about my illness.

As a second time Vipassana meditator there are small "cells" which I can meditate in. These are small rooms in the course set aside for solitary meditation. I prefer the idea of meditating in the hall with others, but reason the coffin-like nature of the cells will provide practice for confronting my own situation. It does it a bit too well. I am going to die sometime but it now may be a bit quicker than planned. Perhaps the lesson is to come to terms with it, so as to realize what is valuable just for its own sake.

The other thing about being on your second course is that you stay there on the condition you do not eat after 12.00 noon. This is to help with your meditation, although it probably has some health benefits too.

In the mountains of Georgia, where people often live well beyond 100 years of age, there is a saying, "Eat breakfast yourself, share lunch with a friend, and give dinner to your enemy!"

I have not had such extreme experiences as on the last course. I talked to a fellow meditator, called John, on the tenth day of the last course and he told me how he used to take drugs but was now completely off them. Interestingly, he has found that this meditation gives him as big a high as the recreational drugs he tried but this is *not* the reason for attending.

There seems to be no physical change at the end of the ten days. Everyone is allowed to talk towards the end of the tenth day, and most people are elated with the prospect of their own "freedom". Conversely, I feel trapped and upset, and keep to myself. I am not totally comfortable with the idea of dying.

Okay, the joke's over – I just want to be cured …

At the end of the course I try to find someone to pay. Just as on my last course you have to search someone out to pay them and paying is voluntary. Also as a taxpayer there is the advantage that Vipassana is a registered charity in Australia so payments are tax deductible[29].

Before I leave, I talk with Steve – one of the male helpers. As a helper he must not only be a volunteer but must also have completed at least one ten-day Vipassana course. He turns out to be an aerobics instructor who has become interested in counselling. He says we are all addicted to something.

The phrase of a fellow Gurkha Engineer officer, Lieutenant Andy, comes straight to mind: "What is the colour of the sky on your planet." But as I think more about it, I see some wisdom in

Steve's simple statement about human nature. The addiction is around one of three things:

1 Power – (*controlling ourselves, our surroundings or others, or gaining knowledge*) or powerlessness (*being a victim*).

2 Pleasure – (*having sex, gambling or taking drugs – though sometimes drug taking is more about "risking life"*) or being ascetic.

3 Survival or risking life itself.

I phone Ruth from Sydney. She has been very worried, as she did not hear from me, and my lack of empathy does little to enhance the communication. I buy two Vipassana books on the last day of the course; one for each of my sons. They are entitled:

- *The Power of Promise* for Olly, and
- *The Magic of Patience* for Rob.

Both are Jataka Tales, adapted for children, and first told by the Buddha two and a half thousand years ago. These tales celebrate the power of action motivated by compassion, love, wisdom and kindness[30]. I write in each of them:

"To a great, great son, and man. I hope the truth in this book guides and helps you to live your life to the fullest. And, when you are ready, I hope you too will take the chance to experience the wisdom in Vipassana. My very fondest love and best wishes – Dad$_{xxx}$"

For Ruth I choose a video tape called *Doing Time, Doing Vipassana,* an award winning video documentary about the use of Vipassana meditation in India's largest, and one of its most violent, prisons – Tihar Prison in New Delhi. It follows one thousand inmates going through a ten day Vipassana meditation together. The success of this course meant that it is used regularly in at least three other Indian jails. Taiwan and the US have followed suit. Lucia Miejer, the administrator of the NRF (North Rehabilitation Facility) in Seattle went on a ten-day course then successfully introduced it into the NRF. The San Francisco Jail also runs courses. It appears that the re-offending rate has been significantly reduced for prisoners who go through this experience.

Vipassana, like many of the best things, is simple yet difficult.

I turn up at Sydney airport on the Sunday when my flight to Melbourne is booked for 07.00 am on the Monday. I ask to be wait-listed but the lady at the check-in says everything is full for the next seven hours. I offer to show her my five-centimetre scar on my neck courtesy of the initial operation to check what type of cancer I had. She declines; either taking pity on me or not fancying the prospect of having it put indelicately in front of her, and she puts me on an early flight. Yet another advantage from being in my situation!

I know the world does not owe me a living but I am beginning to think an apology would be nice ...

In Nepal, Land of the Himalaya

"A Master is someone who started before you!"

Chinese Saying

1991: 21 November, Kathmandu, Nepal

As I came out of the hotel the next morning I was met by the fresh smell of mountain air heavily mixed with petrol fumes of badly tuned engines. Guy and I hopped into "put-put" which resembled a squashed three-wheeled robin-mobile – it was not big enough to be a bat-mobile. This cheap and efficient method of getting around took us to the British camp. We then paid Robin and went inside.

The camp was in the heart of Kathmandu and separated by a wall from the rest of Kathmandu. A diminutive physical obstacle compared with the emotional barrier between it and the outside. Inside there was physical security, enough to eat, adequate medical facilities and decent shelter. With few exceptions for those outside its walls, hardly any of these were possible and none were certain. I felt like I had been transported to a little England within Nepal, surrounded as we were by colonial buildings and British mindset.

We took the chance to catch up with a few soldiers from our Regiment before heading off to the bank. I checked the current exchange rate: US$1 to 30.3 Nepalese Rupees with each Rupee divided into 100 paisa. That was about half the value of the Indian Rupee. We then headed to Kathmandu airport where the Nepalese security official at Kathmandu airport was typically officious and smiled as he asked me if I had any matches.

"Yes" I said, proudly remembering that I had thought to pack my SAS specials – waterproof, windproof, bullet-proof, etc. He liked them too and they were swiftly removed from my person. Unfortunately they were not "airport-security" proof.

A rather old passenger plane of the RNAC (Royal Nepal Airlines Corporation) flew us to Pokhara in West Nepal where we were to get detailed trek instructions. (I am not sure what type of plane it was but if planes are reincarnated then it was a B15 Bomber in its last life!) I was sitting next to a British tourist who would have been sitting next to the rear gunner of the reincarnated plane. Perhaps that is why we started discussing religion or it might have been due to the sudden bouts of excessive vibration. He was quietly spoken and finally told me that he had personally met with God six months ago. Apparently God had sat down next to him and they had had a conversation. That beat anything I could say. Our conversation was killed dhungo[31] dead, although I remained mediumly unconvinced (as in "not convinced about this supernatural experience" rather than "moderately unpersuaded").

Pokhara is 700m lower than Kathmandu and set in a beautiful location which seems almost magical. The overlooking mountains of the Annapurna Range appeared to provide a grand view of life. These mountains seemed to offer a wisdom of the ages which was reflected in the large lake at their feet, called Phewa Tal, the second largest lake in Nepal. There, as I looked up at Machhapuchhare, I could see its name some 5000 metres further up, silhouetted against the sky. The crisp white snow of the peak was flanked by the more distant, and scenically awe inspiring, Annapurna Massif which dominated the Northern view. Machhapuchhare is lower than all the other five Annapurna peaks yet it is the only "holy" one. It is strange that its name came from the anatomy of a fish, when so many other "unholy" peaks are named after gods and goddesses. The late Colonel Jimmy Roberts attempted to climb it, way back in 1957, but had to turn back 50 metres from the summit when his Sherpas refused to conquer such a "holy" summit.

The contrasting contour of mountain and water joined by the simple shapes of Nepalese houses formed a pretty panorama. This beauty has its attractions and brings many tourists. Apparently the hippies in the 1970s were the first tourists to discover Pokhara in numbers. It was still a very popular destination and a melting pot of tourists, some beggars and lots of dubious wares for sale. Pokhara is one of the wetter places in the world but it greeted us dryly that day.

We got a staff truck to Pokhara Army camp which was like stepping back in time or onto some film set of colonial times, like the television program "The Raj Quartet". A Queen's Gurkha Officer Captain greeted us in a professional yet friendly manner. He was a Gurung, one of the main martial tribes in West Nepal. (Tribal names are used as we use surnames in the West.) He was of a typical broad and stocky build, with a swarthier complexion and more body hair than those we were to meet in East Nepal.

I was starving; probably a combination of my vegetarian diet and the diarrhoea that had already kicked in. We went to the Officers' Mess for lunch. Looking through the menu, there was a Nepalese fish dish which I had not tasted but which sounded delicious. After the waiter took my order I noticed other people eating the same dish. The way they are tucking in suggested I had made the right choice, and after a few more minutes I had the chance to confirm it.

We were primarily there to gain an understanding, some wisdom, about our trek and after a cup of coffee we went through the "Trekking Instructions". Unfortunately, I had not prepared well at this stage. When it came to asking questions, I asked questions from my list around how to design a water supply system – both of them. These gave rise to a couple of new questions which remained unasked, and unanswered. So I left about as ignorant as I was before, but at least I was ignorant on a higher level and about more important things!

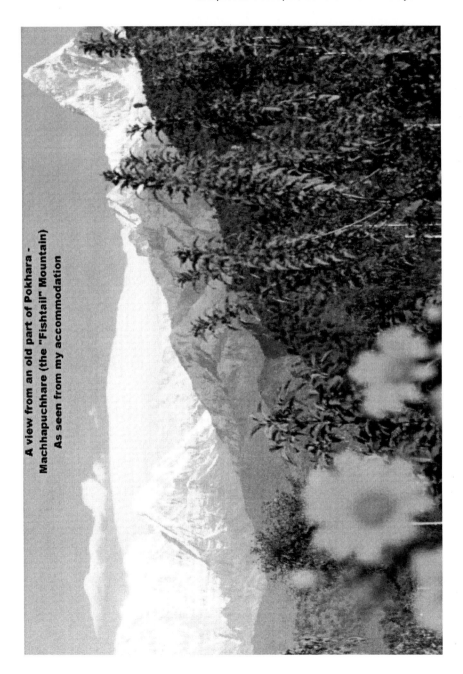

A view from an old part of Pokhara -
Machhapuchhare (the "Fishtail" Mountain)
As seen from my accommodation

A House in Higher Hills

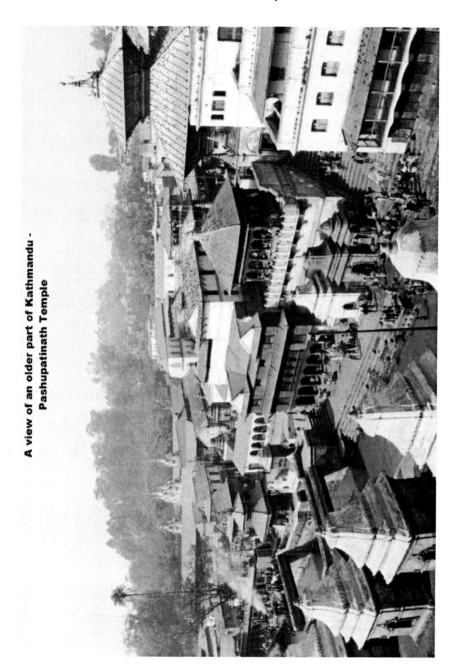

A view of an older part of Kathmandu -
Pashupatinath Temple

A House in Higher Hills

Back in my room I spent a bit of time preparing for my surveys. I marked out my route on a map. The water supply design "Bible" given to all Officers designing water supply systems was very good. It was called the *Handbook of Gravity Flow Water Systems*[32] – what I would have re-titled "The Idiot's Guide To Designing Water Supply Systems In Remote Areas When You Don't Know What The Hell You Are Doing and Don't have Much Time To Do it". Although I had meant to read it before arriving in Nepal, I was still going to be able to read it before the trek actually started and so should still be the "Master" by the time I got to the villages.

As the sun set and light faded over the surrounding mountains I watched the film, *Little Drummer Girl.* It all seemed slightly reminiscent of another time, and also reminded me that all films are illusions of reality; they only differ in how much they pretend not to be. Whether a film is factual or factional, they show partial reality to varying degrees. The film cannot convey 100% the reality of the situation it portrays, of what actually happened. The total reality includes what was not shown on the film and how each of us subjectively interprets it. The complete experience can only be gained by experiencing and living through exactly what happened, at the time it happened. Anything else is an approximation.

These thoughts remind me of Henry David Thoreau's comment, "If a man does not keep pace with his companions, perhaps it is because he hears a different drummer."

Observing in the Garden

"You can see a lot by observing"

Yogi Berris

Wisdom

We can turn to any of the World's seven major religions – Christianity, Islam, Judaism, Buddhism, Hinduism, Taoism and Confucianism – to gain insights as to who we are. Religion can be thought of as trying to identify some form of objective "Truth" with a capital "T", which is presumably universal, not sectarian. Therefore, it would seem reasonable to believe that where the world's seven major religions overlap is the essence of this "objective" Truth – such as compassion, tolerance, forgiveness and peace[33]. The rest of any religion may help by providing ways to understand truth, but they may hinder us if we take these symbols to be the Truth. This might be what Carl Jung meant about religion being the defence against the experience of God.

We can see the commonality when comparing the Christian prayer,

"Grant me the serenity to accept the things I cannot change, the courage to change the things I can, and the wisdom to know the difference",

with the Buddhist advice:

"Abstain from all unwholesome deeds [serenity/compassion], perform wholesome ones [courage], purify your mind [wisdom]."

The overlap in these superficially different religions extends to similarities in the lives and teachings of Jesus Christ and Buddha, although Buddha lived 500 years before Christ. Both went out into the wilderness and faced three temptations, and then both came back and brought together disciples to spread their gospel. This may not be a coincidence as there is a historical gap in Jesus' life and some believe that during this period he went farther east and encountered Buddha's teachings. John Paul II said at a general audience in St Peter's Square in 1999 that heaven and hell are states of being rather than actual places. The change is significant as previously the Church taught that heaven and hell were not similes of the truth, but physical realities in themselves. So much so that when the Russians sent up the first Sputnik, an English lady wrote in to one of the daily newspapers complaining that the satellite would be an obstruction between Heaven and Earth.

The Pope has recently said that God does not send people to hell, they send themselves. This is also what Buddhism describes. So heaven and hell are states of mind. They are relative and conscious experiences, not places.

The word Buddha means "One who wakes up."

Many philosophers would argue that there is no such thing as objective Truth as each individual's experience of life determines the nature of that truth. So another way to find truth is to look at the process of finding it. That is about wisdom and there are only three types:

1   Devotional Wisdom – the truth we gain from being told this or that, perhaps by reading books or listening to lectures. It is commonly stressed in religions, for instance by dictating that "you must believe ..." It was out of devotional wisdom that I selected a fish dish I had not tried before. It can lead to blind belief – my communication ability in Nepalese might have meant that I was not even eating the fish I thought I was eating in Pokhara. Perhaps it was not even fish!

2   Intellectual Wisdom – the truth we gain from understanding some basic axioms or truths, rationalising from these the validity or logic of the outcome. It is the wisdom of models and theories, such as the western scientific model. The better the

model the more accurately it describes reality. I talked to the waiter who had eaten the food before, and he explained why it was so good. I also watched the satisfied expressions of diners around me eating the same meal as I had ordered, and both these provided the intellectual wisdom of what my meal would be like. But it can lead to intellectual arrogance – thinking that I know fully what the meal really tastes like. The experience I had might be totally different from what I had expected, and, at the end of the day, no amount of intellectualisation could nourish my body.

3   Experiential Wisdom – this is truth that we have experienced in some way. It can only be experienced within our "body and mind" entity, as that is the limit of personal experience. By eating the meal I now really knew the food's taste and the satisfaction it offered. The experiential wisdom of eating the food was the only wisdom that could stop my hunger and fuel my body. This wisdom is gained from experience, and knowing what to do but not doing it is not a bad way to describe a lack of wisdom.

All three types of wisdom can be helpful, and all types can be misleading, but the most important and impactful wisdom is experiential.

Many years ago Aristotle noted that, "what we have to learn, we learn by doing."

We can use wisdom to increase our self-awareness, to discover who we are, rather than using a particular religion. There may be only one truth but we all see it from different angles and if we stand in some places we may not see it at all …

CHAPTER 3

"When it is dark enough you can see the stars"

Ralph Waldo Emerson

1999: 28 June – 11 July, Melbourne

I am feeling refreshed and a bit lighter having lost close to 6 kilograms in weight. Finally a weight loss program that really works… Ruth thinks I look pretty bad, but does not say anything as I come off the plane. She is probably right, as at 1.88 metres I weigh 70 kilograms. The meals at the Vipassana were sizable and very tasty, home cooked and mainly organic vegetarian food. However, with no meals after 12.00 noon you can get pretty hungry by nightfall.

At home I talk with Ruth about the course and say, "I don't know a better way to understand more about life – which really means 'know more about yourself' – than to do a Vipassana course." Ruth could be forgiven for suspecting that I just want others to go through the eleven days of boredom I have just been through! I explain;

> "It shows the 'chain' that can pull us into behaving irrationally or out of control. We are all conditioned in one way or another. Whenever we sense something with one of our six senses we have a sensation within our body. (*The mind is a 'sense' through which we can become aware of our environment, beyond what we immediately sense from our other five senses.*) The unconscious reacts by liking or disliking the sensation and this causes us to be pulled towards or away from the event. The more times the unconscious experiences this sensation then the stronger is its craving or aversion. It may be as simple as liking the sensations which arise when you look at the mirror, which may lead to becoming narcissistic. By

becoming both aware and accepting of these sensations as they arise we start breaking the sequence. It is a bit like the way NLP (Neuro-Linguistic Programming[34]) uses anchoring and collapsing anchors to 'break the chain'. However, the Vipassana process seems to me to operate at a much deeper level, and I have found it quite profound. The problem is how to be truly 'aware and accepting' and this is what you learn with Vipassana[35]."

I go straight to hospital to stay overnight for a bigger piece of my tumour to be cut out. I am directed to the floor but there is no one in reception, so I walk around to the ward and bump into a nurse.

I tell her, "I have come for an operation."

She directs me to a room which I realize as I arrive is the operating theatre!

Another nurse catches up with me and says "No; this way please." A couple of minutes later the other nurse comes up to me apologising saying she thought I was a "rep" selling surgical equipment.

I reply, "No, unfortunately I am at the other end of the knife!"

While I am waiting to be wheeled in the nurses comment on how relaxed I seem. Perhaps I should go into acting.

I am offered a variety of painkillers but before the nurse has reeled off her list, I interject, "Morphine will be fine."

Next is a lung function test. This is to check if my body can handle the chemotherapy chemicals, which are planned. I am going through a pretty thorough view of my disease from a "Western" perspective. The tests confirm that I have some structural limitation to my lungs. I know this as I suffered asthma as a child, although it was not enough to stop me serving later in the British Army for eleven years. I don't feel up to the heart blood pool scan, as it involves injecting a radioactive isotope, and I postpone it. Perhaps I will be better by then …?

Ruth and the boys pick me up from the hospital. Ruth has with her a beautiful bouquet of flowers organised by Kristen, my company's receptionist, on behalf of my office. Later, I go in to the office to thank Kristen and to see Kevin, my new manager. He and others ask how I feel. I tell them that Hodgkin's has a 70% cure rate. Good odds but not odds you would want to bet your life on.

Reading feeds my mind and I focus more on my diet to feed my body. I have experienced the major benefits this can bring. Today I start taking Sunrider foods. Sunrider products are packaged organic Chinese herb/foods, which I have used before and found very helpful[36]. I believe it is important to "listen to my body" to decide which help me. I am still taking Linda's high quality shark liver oil. The type is important as confirmed by John Croft, a marine researcher[37]. I am also eating organically produced Flaxseed and Canola Oils which are meant to provide an ideal ratio of Omega-3 *(alpha-linoleic acid)* and Omega-6 *(linoleic acid)* EFAs. These EFAs (Essential Fatty Acids) are critical because our bodies cannot produce them and need to gain them from food. Unfortunately, refining food tends to eliminate Omega-3 oils and this upsets the Omega 3/Omega 6 balance which is important for our health. Research indicates that the appropriate intake of these fatty acids may help to increase energy, while reducing blood pressure, blood cholesterol, and triglyceride levels. They may also reduce the pain and inflammation of arthritis and multiple sclerosis. The right fatty acids can have major benefits. I think back to the film *Lorenzo's Oil,* in which Augusto and Michaela Odone found that the disease Adrenoleukodystrophy (ALD) was killing their son, Lorenzo. There was neither treatment nor cure, and Lorenzo was given two years to live. Despite resistance from the medical experts at the time, these lay parents discovered a mixture of oils, basically 4 parts oleic acid (purified olive oil) to one part purified rapeseed oil, which stopped the effects of the illness. The message for me is not only that EFAs contain such powerful therapeutic properties, but also how resistant experts in any field are to ideas from outside their profession, no matter how good. Every society has its "paradigms" by which it models the world. These beliefs help it to describe and predict its reality but are always incomplete – they do not predict "reality" fully. New paradigms come into being according to three rules:

1   New paradigms will show up before the tough problems that they are able to deal with.
2   Someone outside the specialist field is most likely to identify and produce the new paradigm.
3   Those most involved with the old paradigms will find it hardest to see the new paradigms.

Of course, this is a paradigm itself.

I maintain my intake of olive oil supported by recent research in the Journal of Epidemiology and Community Health that has credited olive oil with significantly reducing the risk of bowel cancer. It was found that the protective effect of olive oil remained irrespective of the amount of fruit and vegetables in the diet.

I feel good and people say how well I look! Perhaps that is more a matter of relativity than reality, but I am further reassured when I read of a double blind placebo[38] trial in Patras University Medical School[39] in Greece, investigating the relationship between dietary fats and advanced cancer in humans. It was found that those taking Omega-3 had a significantly increased survival than the placebo group. This was enhanced further if the patients took both vitamin E and Omega-3.

I play "monster" with both my sons – a natural role. I give them ten seconds to scarper and then track them down in the house, catch them and hold them each for the count of ten. While I hold down one, the other hits me with whatever comes to hand, plastic sword, cushions, chair, table … I call it quits after four games.

I am going to be working from home and have had quite enough radiation as far as I am concerned. Therefore I replace my old VGA high radiation screen with a Daewoo SVGA "Low Radiation" model. I also use the extension lead and ear plug for my mobile phone.

Is it just that I am not so accepting of change? There was a huge outcry when the electric refrigerator was first introduced, with some claiming that it would cause an increase in cancer and infertility. The prediction has been proved right, even if the reason is not known. When it comes to mobile phones, a high profile study[40] concluded that,

> "It is not possible to say that exposure to RF (radio frequency) radiation, even at levels below national guidelines, is totally without potential adverse health effects, and that the gaps in knowledge are sufficient to justify a precautionary approach[41]."

A friend tells me to go and bet on Tattslotto, with its million dollar prizes.

He is Jewish and explains to me the tradition of "Mazel tov" or "Good luck."

For instance, in letting a plate fall and break you do not stop it, for it becomes good that you did not use up your good luck in keeping the plate from breaking.

"Mazel" he explains, "is more than fortune or coincidence; it is the lesser miracle which is part of the larger Miracle in which we are immersed."

Well getting this illness means that I must have a whole truckload of luck coming my way. Unfortunately it may just run me over! I prefer to stick to a surer way to double my money – I fold it in half and put it back in my pocket.

I have asked Olly to prepare everything for school tomorrow and to be ready at ten to nine. He has prepared everything but at 08.50 am is in the middle of "indoor volleyball", also known as "crash the ornaments". Ruth has to tell him three times to come. So that evening I tell him to donate A$2.00 to a children's charity.

I feel irritated and it is my attempt at punishment based on "This hurts me more than you!"

If true it is a sign of positive discipline – punishment for the sake of the child not the sake of the parent. Anyway, he is understandably upset as he sees his hard-earned savings dwindling away unfairly, and he heads upstairs. Fifteen minutes later he comes down, seemingly over it all, and asks if he can use the computer to write something. I set it up and he proceeds to write. He asks for some help as he has decided to write a book.

I say, "Great, what is it called?"

He replies, "Oh, What a Strict Life!"

I am finding things difficult at the moment and I guess I am being hard on them to make sure they do not love me too much – in case I am not here for too long. I am old enough to know the Johnny Cash song, *A Boy Named Sue*.

Back at the specialist I ask for another chest X-ray to see if the cancer has spread in four weeks. It is the same size – possibly slightly smaller? Reassuring in some ways, as this form of cancer can grow very rapidly; but I did hope to knock it on the head myself through my few weeks of meditation and nutrition. I am becoming resigned to the prospect of going through chemotherapy.

It is now off to see the Radiation Oncology Specialist. He is very professional but I find these visits to cancer departments unsettling. He says the twelve-centimetre tumour in my chest is large and that I will need at least one month of radiotherapy after the 4 months' chemotherapy. He informs me that the size of the tumours means that chemotherapy will not be enough on its own. That will take me to or through Christmas. What joy, something else to look forward to. He adds that my cancer is curable in 80% of cases.

I get a call from Jerry as I get back in my car. Jerry is a long-time friend who served in Military Intelligence – which I tell him regularly, is an oxymoron. He served in Hong Kong and coincidentally came to Australia at the same time as me. Through dint of hard work and clear thinking he has successfully set up his own international consultancy which aims to, "Build a legacy of leadership."

He now finds out I have cancer and reassures me, saying, "Mark, with your determination I am sure you will beat it."

I talk with my oncologist that night, who corrects what the radiation oncologist said. It is a 70% cure rate. I feel like a yo-yo, on the downward track.

I go to the office and it is clear that a number of my colleagues are, like me, not really sure what my situation is so I send a memo around my company.

> "... To update you all, I have been having several tests and I have cancer of the lymph (in the throat) but more tests are needed to ascertain what type exactly. My doctor says if you are going to get cancer it's a good one to get!! I'd probably prefer to pass but such is life's rich tapestry. The standard treatment is 6 months of chemotherapy and the cure/survival rates, for the type of cancer I seem to have at this stage, are somewhat over 50%. (Chemotherapy is almost, but not quite, as much fun as playing British Bulldogs[42] with Garry Hocking or Jonah Lomu!)
>
> ... My Father sent me a poem by Adam Lindsay Gordon – an English jockey of the 19th century who had to leave the country quickly because of betting irregularities and so of course he came to Australia where he became a politician (things don't change). It ends:
>> Life is mostly froth and bubble,
>> Two things stand like stone,
>> Kindness in another's trouble,
>> Courage in your own... [43]"

I see Doctor Wales, my surgeon, again today. He takes the large plaster off the scar on my neck and seems pretty pleased with his handiwork. It is a very professional job and I was in no pain after the operation. He says the tumour on the neck is right next to the artery and therefore he was not going to try to cut it out. It seems sensible to me. I have already worked out my after dinner story about the scar;

> "Oh this? Well I was walking home one night when I saw a young woman being attacked by seven thugs with knives and baseball bats. Unfortunately as I turned to run I fell over and badly cut my neck."

It is now time for more radiation and I have a CT scan first. It is pretty straightforward except that iodine is injected to give a clearer picture. I mention that I am allergic to shellfish. This might be a problem as shellfish have a lot of iodine in them which could be causing my allergy. The technician finds out that they have just injected iodine into someone else who has an allergy to shellfish without any problem.

So I tell them to "Go for their lives" (rather than mine).

As they inject it I feel a tremendous warm, fuzzy rush move along my arm then all the way down my body. Later it is a blood pool scan. They inject me with a radioactive isotope (half-life of 6 hours) and watch me on a camera. A starring role at last...

The last diagnostic that week is the "Gallium" scan. I happen to arrive wearing my bright yellow, fluorescent ski-jacket. A Gallium isotope is injected as part of the process. I find out that it is the most radioactive thing the practice of Nuclear Medicine injects diagnostically. I have found out already that seven chest X-rays equal a CT scan or, injection of blood pool scan isotope I had a few days earlier.

The nurse tells me that a CT-scan gives the same radiation as flying from Australia to England so I ask about the Gallium scan and she says she is not able to answer that question and will get a specialist to talk me through its implications. I find out later that it gives a radiation dose of over six times the radiation of a CT scan. As she injects it she asks me not to go near pregnant women or babies for a week. For a split second I think that she is joking. When I leave people think that I am still wearing my jacket...

Despite all the modern medicine I am not finding this situation easy to bear and it is safe to say that I am not the happiest teddy in the toy shop.

In Kathmandu, Capital of Nepal

"Give a man a fish and you feed him for a day;
Teach him how to fish and you feed him for a lifetime"
              Lao-Tzu, Chinese philosopher,
    or,
"Give a man a fish and you feed him for a day;
Teach him how to fish and you get rid of him at
weekends… "

                                        Anonymous

1991: 22 November, Pokhara, West Nepal

I woke up to a blue sky and crisp air, and Machhapuchhare rising before me in all her glory. Breakfast was on the veranda before a sea of bright pansies – not particularly military but very pretty. Afterwards I did some preparation for my trek. I had problems zeroing my Abney Level[44] and tried plan B… I read the instructions. I was there to teach the villagers *how to fish* – show them how to build their specific water supply system. Rather than just to bring them water – *give them a fish*. It would have been even better to train and fund them to make more water-supply systems – *educating and equipping them to make rods* – but the time and situation would not allow it.

The plan was for me to come back to Pokhara after my trek to give an immediate report, so having sorted out what I needed to, I went back to Pokhara airport with Guy to fly via Kathmandu eastwards on to Dharan.

While we waited we looked around at the offerings for sale. I noticed some Saligrams – black fossils of marine animals which are considered to be holy emblems. These ammonite fossils date back to the Jurassic Period over 100 million years ago when the Himalaya were under water. I resisted any temptation to buy them for three good reasons; it offends some Nepalese to barter these holy emblems, they are generally overpriced, and it is illegal.

At the airport an ex-Queen's Gurkha Engineer soldier, Tekbahadur, came up to say the Nepalese equivalent of "hi". He had recognised Guy and me from our Regimental ties. Tekbahadur was currently with Brunei's Gurkha Brigade. The Sultan of Brunei, the world's richest man, with an estimated wealth of US$38 billion[45], keeps a unit of ex-British Brigade of Gurkhas which he can call on if Brunei's sovereignty is threatened. The Gurkhas serve under similar conditions in this unit to those in the British Brigade in Hong Kong and are a critical force within the Brunei Defence Forces.

Tekbahadur was returning to Brunei and his wife and family were there to see him off. He had just finished his annual six-week holiday with his family and would not see his family for another twenty-four months; nevertheless he spent the remaining hour with us. He was a serious man and this was perhaps an indication of the Gurkhas' general sense of duty to the military.

I had already seen many signs of religion and spiritual belief around me in the form of Hindu and Buddhist temples, holy places and people. This was all very different from the way beliefs of Taoism and Confucianism manifested in Hong Kong. There it seemed much more under-stated in form, but more overstated in prosperity. Many shops in Hong Kong have a Taoist shrine somewhere at the back in the form of a bowl or piece of fruit and some joss sticks or candles. There the symbols stood on their own, jutting out prominently for God, and everyone else, to see.

Back in Kathmandu the city life seemed to lack the personal touch, and sense of meaning, that I experienced only a day before in Pokhara – the feeling I got as I sat on the edge of mountains. Kathmandu became the capital when the Shah kings from the little kingdom of Gorkha, halfway between Kathmandu and Pokhara, achieved their dream of conquering the rich and fertile Kathmandu Valley.

People all around me were getting on with their life. It was probably less complex than in western cities but seemed just as purposeful. My purpose here on the trek was pretty clear, and I could see my life was going to be about as complex as I wanted to make it.

We went into the main part of the city and I came across *The Mountain Kingdom*†, a beautiful pictorial guide of Nepal and the Gurkhas. It was written by one Colonel Bruce Niven. He knows the Gurkhas well, serving with the Gurkha Brigade throughout his Army career and commanding the 10 (Princess Mary's Own) Gurkha Rifles some ten years ago. Among many treks, he trekked 1800 miles across Nepal from 1961-62. It made my trek sound a doddle, but then all things are relative.

We headed to KC's restaurant for dinner in Doopalong … the name of a district and perhaps what you are meant to do there. I had done the nine-week Nepali language course but failed the final exam. Although I got the highest mark in the written part, I did badly at the somewhat more important aspect of the speaking part of the exam! Therefore I was due to re-sit after the trek. This did not stop me from making candid comments in Nepalese about some Swedes at the next table. My Nepali turned out to be good enough to be understood as after speaking Swedish initially they broke into fluent Nepali. I went back to English outgunned as I was

---

† Note: Colonel B Niven released the sequel, The Mountain Kingdom Volume 2 – The Gurkhas and their Homeland, in 2001. It is a "beautiful and penetrating pictorial essay of an enduring people". Profits go to the Gurkha Welfare Trust and it can be obtained by contacting the Gurkha Museum Trading Company Limited – tel: +44 1962 842832/fax: +44 1962 877597/ email:sales@thegurkhamuseum.co.uk/website: www.thegurkhamuseum.co.uk.

in language terms. We tipped 10% of the bill, which was customary in more expensive restaurants, (rather than giving some loose change as is generally accepted in smaller eating establishments), and left as it was closing.

It was 10.30 pm so there appeared to be time to visit a pakka[46] Kathmandu "night club" in the popular tourist area of Thamel. It was really a bar on several small floors and was great fun for three and a half minutes. We wandered back via Durbar (meaning "Palace") Square, which was the square in front of the old Royal Palace in Kathmandu. As the Palace was moved to Narayanhiti some hundred years ago, it is now a "Palace Square" without a Palace. In one corner of the Square is the Kathamandap, or "House of Wood" which gave Kathmandu its name.

There were some very unobtrusive signs of the prostitution which is found in any city. Kathmandu is no different in that respect or in that it has an HIV problem. A very unfortunate source of income for Nepal comes from about 100 000 Nepalese women working as prostitutes in Indian Brothels in conditions little different to slavery. Many are just children lured there under false pretences and some 30 000 are probably HIV positive[47].

We went back to the hotel bar but it had obviously not got any more popular and we did not hang around.

Inside the House

"You cannot keep your whole house clean
If you never go into some of the Rooms"

Mark Kingsley

The Rooms

Personal experience suggests that we have physical (aesthetic), emotional (moral) and mental (intellectual) aspects. In other words we act, feel and think. This trio is commonly accepted; what is not is whether we have a spiritual part.

We *act* through our "Physical Room or body" but if we lose a leg, a bit of skin, or any part of our body, our "essence" has not completely gone.

In the book, *The Human Brain,* Professor John Pfeiffer notes, "Your body does not contain a single one of the molecules that it contained seven years ago."

This makes marriage more exciting as we get a completely new partner every seven years! Perhaps that's the reason for the seven-year itch?

We *decide* through our "Emotional or Mental Room/body". Our mind is the summation of our feelings and thoughts yet we can observe our thoughts and emotions, so it is not the "*watcher*"? If we were our mind then we would have no basic identity but would be at the whim of the environment. If we take some alcohol our emotions are sent off in one direction, take other stimulants and our thoughts are sent in another. If we were our mind then we would change who we are every time we take drugs or even food.

So our physical body comes and goes, our emotions come and go, our thoughts come and go. Our body and mind are servants unless we become addicted whereupon they become our "masters". The body controls us if we become physically addicted and the mind if we cling to illusions.

One argument for some fourth entity is that we can directly observe our body, feelings and thoughts – which means that we cannot be any of them! Just like our eyes can only directly observe what they aren't! Sir Wilder Penfield, the renowned British neurosurgeon came up with the idea of a "watcher" as this fourth, or "Spiritual body".

The mind can make decisions but in *The Myth of Nine to Five,* Scott and Harker explain how it is only the watcher who makes really voluntary *"choices"*. They describe how,

> "Penfield… spent decades cutting and probing brains (while the patients were fully conscious!) after which he would ask them what they had experienced, when, for example, their arms would move or words were uttered as he probed. They told him that it seemed to them that they were voluntarily performing actions even though they knew it was the result of his probing[48]."

Others have discovered similar reactions. In 1929, a German surgeon, Doctor Forster, found that you could get a patient to involuntarily articulate a series of puns when manipulating a certain part of the brain[49].

Just because we think/feel we are voluntarily making decisions, does not mean that we are. Just as physical probing can cause us to believe physical actions are voluntary so too mental/emotional conditioning can mean apparently voluntary decisions, are in fact dictated by external experiences.

This argument is both comforting and challenging. For it seems to logically follow that if the Spiritual body exists then it cannot die and we do not need to worry, if it does not we do not either! For in the latter case we are, scientifically, just a collection of atoms and other elementary particles and we have died off completely by every seventh year of our lives.

Assuming that we have the four parts – physical, emotional, mental and spiritual – we can use them as the basis for a very complete personality model. Models help us to describe and predict; the better the model the better it does that. Now we can take a journey through this non-religious model built from these four "Rooms", to describe our inner reality. It is also a model that can be used in any religion including atheism …

CHAPTER 4

The Departure

1999: 12-18 July, Medical Centres in Melbourne

When I wake up I see that Ruth has written five affirmations from *You Can Heal Your Life* and stuck them next to my bed so I can see them clearly. Phrases like;

> "I lovingly forgive and release all of the past. I choose to fill my world with joy. I love and approve of myself (*to help get rid of cancer*) …"

and

> "I am the creative power in my world (*to help my glands*)[50]."

Ruth's first cousin, Keith, and his family have planned a trip to Australia for some time. When we told them the situation they said they would stay in a hotel but we insisted that they stay with us. They make very good guests, and Keith and Elaine's daughters, Nicola and Louise, are the same age as my sons'. This helps my sons as they have constant companions to play with, which distracts them from my situation. All in all it turns out to be a good chance to catch up and reflect on life, as well as spice it up with some northern English humour. Rob thinks they are putting their accents on, not believing that people could really talk like that.

I want some more Noni juice, and phone Bill Walsh who will not hear of my picking up the Noni in my situation. Instead he kindly drops it off the next day.

I ask John if he can get my Mother's specialist in England to have a look and comment on my situation. He says "no problem" as long as I fax a copy of my diagnosis to him. This I do before both families head off to some therapeutic hot baths at Hepburn Springs. Everyone except for me is hoping for a very relaxing time, I hope for a step change in my health – upwards. They end up getting the former.

My Mother had apparently said to John after the recent deaths of her father and brother and after her own illness, "Things could not get any worse."

John's instinctive reply had been, "Don't bet on it."

"What, next you will be telling me that one of my sons has cancer!"

John adeptly steered the conversation elsewhere.

Unfortunately now my Mother gets the fax before John. At first she wonders why I am sending a diagnosis of her illness, then realises it is mine. It is definitely not a good way to break the news and it was compounded by us being out when she phoned in a panic; nor could she contact John. She phones Ruth's parents, who seem to be the only people around, and they do a good job of calming her down until John arrives home. John then manages to persuade her that Hodgkin's should not really be called a cancer. This helps her to feel a lot better and leaves me confused.

I have started the laxatives as you need to take them for three days before the scan of the gallium. This empties the bowels in order to get a clear picture and an enema can help.

I ask, "Can I get an enema through the hospital?"

But I am told "No."

I have an incomplete television trace of the gallium in my body. Things are delayed 45 minutes and I get frustrated, or at least frustrate myself, while I wait. They take above body, then below body shots, each taking about 20 minutes. I find it very peaceful moving through the large camera and fall asleep. They decide not to take an around body view as there is too much gallium in my blood. I stress to them my feeling that they need to have a good picture so I can decide whether to go on to radiotherapy after the chemotherapy. They assure me they will get it in a couple of days and they ask me to up the dose of the laxatives but not so much that they caused strain on the bowels, as this might also confuse the picture.

After that it is off to see the oncologist and everything seems in order. His professionalism is reassuring and he asks whether I am happy to start next week. I confirm that I am keen to start chemotherapy on Monday and to start another of life's treks. I have long dreaded the thought of going through chemotherapy. It is strange how life throws up the things we fear most.

My oncologist tells me that my sperm sample was fourteen straws, I don't know what that means except that it is nothing to do with drinking. He says it is usual to get three sets of sperm samples, but I decide to stick with the one I've got.

People react differently to me once they know I have been diagnosed with cancer, and I have been acting differently to others since being diagnosed. Both at home and at work I have observed a typology in the way people react to me. I think it is to do with how a sense of "control" impacts our life. Cancer and other life-threatening diseases are situations which tell us quite clearly that, despite what we may think, we do not really control life. However, that does not mean it controls us, unless we let it. In a way it reminds me of the white water canoeing I have done. I could not control the river but by riding it I could determine where I ended up and how often I submerged.

There are various views of the way people think. D. Bannister summed it up,

> "Man is basically a battlefield ... a dark cellar in which a well-bred spinster lady and a sex-crazed monkey are for ever engaged in mortal combat, the struggle being refereed by a rather nervous bank clerk[51]."

There seem to me to be three types of personality, or curtains, behind which people view and interact with those who are ill. The first type is *"Curtains Open"* in this personality model I have just devised. These types can see the other Houses (other people). They know where they are, and they go and visit other Houses. Many people I meet fall into this type, and they have shown care and concern for my situation.

The second type is *"Curtains Partly Drawn"*. There are some other Houses and some other views, which they do not want to see. They are also concerned that other people may see into their House. So they half close their curtains. However, this type may suffer from "agoraphobia", and not be able to go outside. A few people found it difficult to have much contact with me. It seemed that in doing so they would have to face their own fears about life and death, which were understandably uncomfortable for them.

Finally there is the *"Curtains Closed"* type. They cannot see any of the other Houses because the curtains are closed which often means the light is on. They may know that other Houses exist because they know how to use the street directory but they do not know what the other Houses really look like since they never visit them. Bright may be "right" but only when it is natural light illuminating all the Rooms. A couple of people were so wrapped up in their own lives, their own situations, it seemed that they were unable to be concerned about my circumstances, or anyone else's for that matter.

In terms of reaching your full potential and "Being all you can be" – which Abraham Maslow described as self–actualization – you have to keep the curtains open.

I have felt the symptoms for at least 16 months (since February 1998). In March 1998 I felt unwell and started losing weight. I had heavy night sweats, lost my appetite, high fitness levels and felt continuously tired. In October 1998 I competed in the Victorian State Taekwondo Welterweight Open Black Belt Full Contact competition, down from my normal division of Middleweight because I lost so much weight. I felt something was wrong with me, and told Alfie that I might pull out. Alf is a very good trainer who runs an exceptional Taekwondo centre. He has coached me excellently in many fights and, in the end, I went through all four bouts of three rounds and won a gold medal. Not bad for an old man suffering Hodgkin's disease, who does not know it.

I end up going to Colon Irrigation Australia and see a lovely lady and colon hydrotherapist, Edna at the Colon Irrigation Australia[52(address)], for the enema. Edna recommends a full colonic irrigation rather than an enema as it clears further up the colon. When investigating enemas I read that fifty-seven leading physicians in Great Britain recently met at the Royal Society of Medicine and discussed alimentary toxaemia – the body's absorption of toxic substances through the mechanical and chemical process of digestion[53]. The speakers identified this as a factor in a whole range of diseases (including cancers) affecting many parts and organs of the body. The problem arises when the colon goes from being a "sewage system" to a "cesspool!"
I am reminded of the old saying, "Man digs his grave with a knife and fork", and despite one of the nurse's reservations about colonic irrigation I discover that it is not too bad.

It is late in the evening and we end up talking after the procedure. Edna is a mother of five and her oldest son was diagnosed in 1976, at the age of two, with a severe kidney problem and she was told that within eleven months they would stop functioning. In desperation Edna tried many things, including faith healers in the Philippines, before going to Linus Pauling, the American biologist and only person ever to gain two Nobel prizes independently. He said that he could not guarantee a cure with vitamin C, but he believed that vitamin C would improve her son's situation. Usually he advises that people take one gram of calcium ascorbate daily for each year of age up to a maximum of 10 grams. However, he recommended that Edna give her son as much as his body could tolerate and at least 10 grams per day because he had a medical condition. This was against the advice of the medical specialists who were treating her son, but she felt there was nothing to lose so she went ahead, and her son is alive and well today.

Her advice leaves me in two minds about things, which at least gives me a spare if I lose one! On the one hand, there seem to be great potential benefits in taking high dose vitamin C, on the other, there are apparently risks. In the end I ask Edna for some as she has access to very high quality vitamin C[54], made in Japan.

I have read that it is a fallacy to believe that ancient humans consumed large amounts of vitamin C from natural sources. Recent estimates put the consumption of vitamin C by Palaeolithic man at 400 mg per day. This is the basis for the article's argument that, therefore, modern man does not need larger amounts of vitamin C. However, you could look at it another way. Perhaps their low intake of vitamin C was a major reason for their very low average lifespan! Palaeolithic man did not have to wear a seatbelt either but the world has changed a bit since then...

When it comes to increasing your lifespan it seems a good idea to get ideas from people who have a long one. There are several communities around the world who routinely live to over 100 years. People like the Hunza's of East Pakistan, and the Tibetans. It is unlikely to be genetic as when these peoples move into the West, or adopt a western diet/lifestyle, the lifespan of their families quickly mirror those around them. The Hunza have a diet rich in vitamin C and vitamin B_{17}, the result of eating large amounts of apricots and apricot seeds.

> 'Sir Robert McCarrison, a surgeon in the Indian Health Service, observed "a total absence of all diseases during the time I spent in the Hunza valley [seven years]... During the period of my association with these peoples, I never saw a case of... cancer[55]".'

As a comparison, the average lifespan for American's in the mid

1990's was 75.5 years and the average lifespan for an MD, or Doctor, in the US was only 58 years!

I still feel it is worthwhile to supplement with this vitamin and I start taking about 45 grams a day orally, and on a few days as much as 80[56] grams (that is 1000 times the recommended daily intake!) Researchers at Cambridge University have concluded that "Vitamin C is a safe substance even with an intake about 100 times the RDA daily [6 grams][57]."

In addition, Sandra Goodman Ph.D. warns[58],

> "It is vital that vitamin C not be stopped suddenly, especially with individuals with cancer and AIDS … When large doses of vitamin C are taken, the entire enzymatic machinery, including metabolites, goes into operation … If vitamin C is suddenly withdrawn, the person's biochemistry will continue to produce these metabolites for a week or two."

This can lead to a state of severe depletion, which is dangerous as "Vitamin C is so vital for almost every body system, from the brain to heart to the immune system†."

This puts me straight into a select group of 22% of Australian cancer patients: those who try alternative, otherwise called complementary, medicine.

I have invited two friends, Corrie and Jen, around for dinner but they end up just coming for drinks, as they do not want to put us out at a time like this. Corrie and Jen are an independent couple with a maturity which seems to go beyond their years. They have both been to India to see Sathya Sai Baba several times. Some people believe that Sai Baba is an avatar – a Hindu term for a descendent, or even a manifestation, of a deity. Sai Baba manifested a ring for Corrie a few years ago and Corrie now wears

---

† Caution: Doctor Goodman advises to always reduce your dosage of vitamin C supplements over a period of time if you decide to reduce your supplementation and are taking 3 grams or more per day.

it permanently. A few years back, Ruth held this ring and it had such a powerful effect on her that she burst into tears! I want to see if it has any meaning for me now.

We are catching up after several years and we discuss many and higher things. They tell us about their last visit to Sai Baba, and how he told them again things which he could not have known. Corrie hands me his ring and I am disappointed that I get no obvious feelings or sensations from it. As they leave they give me Vibhoothi – a healing ash from Sai Baba's Ashram in India.

Ruth's been doing it tough, looking after three boys … , cleaning the house and doing her part time jobs. Chemotherapy's looming and to get into it I have been watching a documentary about cancer. To my mind it is classic black and white, or digital thinking. The documentary concludes that cancer is all genetic in origin.

It is a bit like saying, "Birth is the cause of death."

Even if we have a predisposition for certain cancers genetically it almost always requires environmental impacts to trigger it. In the same way certain ethnic groups appear to have a significant predisposition towards alcoholism. Despite this predisposition no one can become alcoholic if there is not any[59].

I phone Professor Wang's clinic and talk to his son, Bhin. I ask how TCM (Traditional Chinese Medicine) views chemotherapy. Bhin says in my case he would recommend I go through chemotherapy, but suggests that I might want to come to a TCM session once per fortnight as it can help my body to cope with the toxic effects of the treatment. He sends me a leaflet with more advice;

> "Take a Hot Foot Bath twice a day, before breakfast and before
> going to bed. Remember start with it as hot as you can bear.
> Put half a teaspoon of salt in the water and tap the feet up and
> down until you can stand to put them in. Finish the Hot Foot
> Bath while your feet and water are nice and warm. This will

help ground your energy and connect the kidney energy with your feet to achieve good circulation and assist your body in cleansing faster."

I have little doubt that it is good advice but I do not find the time to do it – or, more accurately, it is not a high enough priority for me. Bhin also tells me that Chinese medicines do not interfere with the effects of western medicine or vitamin and mineral supplements, but it is recommended that you take them at different times a day. I do not ask him the obvious follow up to that, "Why?"

I guess it is because western medicine and vitamin pills degrade the effectiveness of Chinese medicines and food. We talk about the different approach between western and Chinese medicine. He tells me how the Chinese system maximises the focus on preventive medicine. It is something I have already heard about – Chinese doctors are paid while their patients are well and not when the patients are ill: a good way to put the focus on prevention rather than cure.

Peter, phones to see how I am going. He offers to fly over from Christchurch to Melbourne any time I want his support. I thank him but say there is no need at the moment. He adds that he saw a news story about three men who survived cancer. They all said it was the best experience that ever happened to them. I am left wondering what those who did not survive would say.

Up in the Himalaya

"Don't expect mangoes when you plant lemons"
Nepalese Proverb

1991: 23 November, Dharan, East Nepal

I woke up feeling a bit rough, which was tough as I had only had three beers. I realized through my haze that I have paid too little attention to the 7P's. I did not ask about latrines and exactly how they were to be incorporated into the water supply system design. However, as I did not know the Gurkhali for latrine my communication might have stopped me from getting the answer, even if my memory had not.

After a vegan breakfast, Guy and I headed to Kathmandu airport for the flight to Dharan. It appeared that there was a run on knives and I replied: "No, I have not got a penknife" to the airport security official, and was pleased that he did not check my bag for the one that someone must have planted on me.

The sky was clear of cloud as we flew East. An RNAC pilot had said that they did not fly through the clouds in Nepal "because the clouds have rocks in them", and the Kingdom of Nepal showed itself as a series of voluptuous mountain ridges capped by the everlasting snows of the Himalayan peaks. I could almost feel the fluttering Buddhist prayer flags high up in the mountains as we passed over. These offer prayers to the God that each mountain has, and provide godly fortune to those who put them up there.

Dharan had recovered reasonably well from the major earthquake that hit it in 1988 and I saw no sign of the major upheaval. It lies on the Terai but at the base of hills which surround it to the North like some unfinished fortifications. Nepal can be divided into three parallel bands running north-west to south-east.

Closest to China is the Great Himalaya Range where average elevations exceed 4570 metres (or about 15000 feet). I was going to trek in the second band, which is dominated by the Mahabharat and Churia ranges. Elevations there average about 2500 metres above sea level. The third and southernmost region is the Terai on which Dharan rests. It is not much above sea level and its alluvial soils are generally more fertile than the soil of the higher areas. It is in these hills that a large mountain ape[60] roamed here half a million years ago. So I checked my camera in case I was to be the first person to get a clear photograph of a Yeti or "abominable snowman".

The air was hot and heavy in Dharan Camp. It was an old colonial military camp and formed a surreal window looking in on Nepal from the West. It still had much of its beauty then despite being closed a few years before and edging its way into a state of disrepair. Despite this, I could see why those in the Gurkha Brigade who had lived there, had had such fond memories of it.

We went to the AWC (Area Welfare Centre) by horse drawn rickshaw. The building stood out on the edge of Dharan Bazaar, some two miles from the Camp. The AWCs are set up and paid for by the British or Indian government. They are manned by ex-Gurkha officers, or sometimes soldiers, and provide welfare support to retired Gurkha servicemen. The AWO (Area Welfare Officer) greeted Guy and me, and then took us through some of the local history and culture over imported German beers.

The AWO was a mix of geniality and authority. We reminisced about life in the Gurkha Brigade. He had served for twenty-five years, but looked thirty-five and had the impish humour of one even younger. He symbolized for me the important work the Gurkha Brigade does in this area.

Later that evening the AWO treated me to a splendid Nepalese curry. Subash joined us. After a few pots of the local beer, and discussion about the different expectations people have in the East compared with the West, we crashed out.

Devotional Wisdom – Who Am I And What Is My Purpose (*In The West*)?

"I don't know. They always seem to me to overestimate the self-knowledge of the subject and to underestimate his sense of humour"

> *Sir Frederick Bartlett's* [61]
> *reply when asked about*
> *personality questionnaires*

Maslow's Hierarchy of Needs

We can look to a western model of personality to give us some idea of "Who we are".

Personality is generally defined as something like "A person's typical or preferred way of behaving, thinking and feeling[62]."

Our personality is clearly a combination of both "nature and nurture". Tom Bouchard, the founder and director of the Centre for Twin and Adoption Research at the University of Minnesota, is famous for his 20-year longitudinal study of identical twins who had been raised apart. He found that a minimum of 50% of what causes behavioural similarities in identical twins results from their having the same genes[63]. Although factors such as family and cultural influences appear to be less significant in the formation of personality than a person's genetic makeup, the result means that up to 50% of behaviour results from the environment. Bouchard's study also concluded that genetic factors continue to play a key part in defining our "qualities" throughout our lifetime, not just as a child.

Abraham Maslow's model the **Hierarchy of Needs**[64] helps us to understand "who we are" *(personality)* by considering "what is our purpose" *(motivation)*. His model has five floors.

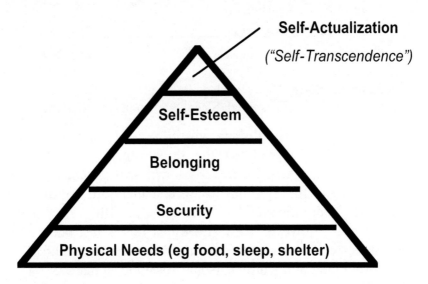

Maslow later changed the top level from "self-actualization" *(being all that you can be)* to "self-transcendence" *(being more than you are)*. He observed that one had to satisfy each level personally. To the extent that we have satisfied a level, we can then move up and satisfy higher levels. No level can be satisfied once and for all. Just as, physically, we cannot eat massively one day, and then go without food for the rest of the year, so each level must continually be satisfied. We can separate out the Needs into different parts of our life. For instance, if there is a fearful environment at work, we are unlikely to achieve a sense of belonging, pride, or meaning from it.

Later studies have indicated that the order of needs could be re-arranged with the order of the three lowest levels reversed. This corresponds to the differing importance individuals place on their four rooms. For some the Physical *(food and sleep)* is more important than the Emotional (*belonging or security*), for others it is the other way around.

Maslow's levels each fall largely in one of the four parts, or Rooms, we identified earlier.

Maslow' s Levels	Room
Self-Actualization/Self-Transcendence	**Spiritual**
Self Esteem	**Mental**
Security and Social Needs, such as Belonging	**Emotional**
Survival Needs, such as Food, Sleep, Shelter	**Physical**

Maslow seems to me to have missed other Rooms at the top Level and hence overlooked the three other ways we can commonly find meaning in life. Maslow's own personality type prefers to live in the Spiritual Room and therefore he saw that reality as pre-eminent – "self-actualization" or "self-transcendence". However, we can see that this is just one of the potential higher states – remembering the word "personality" is derived from the Latin word "persona" meaning "a mask".

Which says something about someone with a "big personality" and suggests that we may want to look elsewhere to answer the question, "Who am I?"

THE JOURNEY

"What is the use of running when we are not on the right way?"

German Proverb

You may want to go on one journey for now, and just read one book at a time. You can "air" the other Rooms by skimming through them briefly remembering that the other two books may become relevant at another time in your life.

CHAPTER 5

One Journey Starts – My First Chemotherapy

1999: 19-20 July, Cabrini Hospital[65](Address)**, Melbourne**

Almost nine years on from starting the 90s by trekking through the Himalaya, I am finishing the decade with an excursion up another mountain. I preferred the physical ones …

As Ruth drives me to the hospital I recite "Today's the day Mark begins his chemotherapy", but a teddy bear's picnic would be better.

I do not feel consciously anxious but I had a strong stomach ache last night which may indicate anxiety at some sub-conscious level.

Cabrini Hospital is named after Mother Cabrini who, from 1880 until her death in 1917, established foundations around the world to care for the disadvantaged and the sick. Mother Cabrini was declared Blessed in 1938, and in 1948 ten missionary sisters came to Australia to run a small private hospital called St Benedict's in Malvern. Cabrini Hospital with its healthy spiritual tradition grew out of this and I go in to see one of the administrators. She checks me in and apologises that I do not have the same room as I had last time I came in for the biopsy. I tell her not to worry, as I don't plan to be coming in with such regularity that it will become an issue.

I am led to the oncology (*study of cancer*) ward and sit on one of the beds. The nurses there are very bright and cheery.

The nurse, who is going to give me the treatment, arrives and looks at my lack of hair, "Oh! You've already started the chemo."

She is slightly embarrassed when I reply "Not yet."

She starts taking down all my particulars.

When she comes to, "How do you sleep?" – I tell her, "Usually on my back."

It's then into the two hours of administering the treatment – almost as much fun as climbing the Himalayas barefoot. I read an extremely helpful bit of advice from Ian Gawler, who was diagnosed with "osteogenic sarcoma" (bone cancer) but survived. He has written several books and recommends treating chemotherapy as your friend. To visualise the chemotherapy coming in and boosting all the healthy cells in your body and to see the cancerous cells as a mass of disorganised, lost cells, *not* a malignant aggressive force. It is also a good idea to visualise the chemotherapy going straight to the tumours and killing, dissolving or shrinking them into nothing.

I am put on two types of tablets, one for helping minimize the nausea from the chemotherapy (Zofran) and the other is a steroid (Dexamethasone). Both cause constipation, so I also get a Coloxyl and Senna laxative. Just in case the nausea is bad and the constipation not strong enough I also get Maxalon, which reduces the former and increases the latter. There are a myriad of other painkillers offered but all I feel the need for is Panadol and speed to get through this quickly.

I lie there focussing on "Getting rid of the tumour and being well".

Ali is a friend who happens to be a nurse on night shift at Cabrini, and she comes by about 9.00 pm. We know her and her husband, Bill, through Ruth's work at the Gym. She is articulate, with clear views, and we have a homely chat although the illusion is spoilt slightly by the drip and my distinct feeling of nausea.

A young female dietitian comes to see me the next morning to give advice. She is very considerate but I am feeling pretty assertive probably helped by the dose of steroids.

I tell her she has got to be joking to recommend chemotherapy patients put on weight by eating "Sweets, biscuits, jellies, etc."

I add that; "Cancer is a disease of a low immune system and making people fatter does not mean they have better immune systems, or are any healthier. In fact, just the opposite."

The recommendation appears to be on what gives people pleasure, what tastes nice, not on what they need. It is immersion in the superficial. One that puts taste before nutritional value, appearance before substance. Something is not right as research suggests that 30% of longevity is determined by your genetics and 70% is related to lifestyle and therefore controllable[66].

I lecture her, "People need to have their body in balance; they need to strengthen their immune system. Eating healthily must be appropriate for recovering from illness."

Ruth arrives in the middle of my soliloquy to pick me up. I continue saying that non-organic food content appears to have depreciated significantly over the last few decades due to modern farming methods. Doctor Walter Mertz from the US Department of Agriculture said in 1977,

> "In the future we will not be able to rely on our premise that the consumption of a varied, balanced diet will provide all the trace elements, because such a diet will be very difficult to obtain for millions of people."

This could explain some things happening around us. In the UK the number of cancer sufferers is rising by 10% a year. In the US between 1970 and 1990 the cancer rate doubled from 1 in 6, to 1 in 3 of the population. The Imperial Cancer Research Fund in the United Kingdom says most people think that they have a less than one in ten chance of getting the disease, whereas in fact four in ten will develop cancer in their lifetime. At least one million North Americans are diagnosed with cancer annually and 50% of those diagnosed will die within five years[67].

I tell her that I think GM (*Genetically Modified*) food is just going to make things worse. Natural whole food is what we have evolved to live healthily on, and large changes to it risk running counter to foods' real benefits. The dietitian listens very politely and Ruth takes me home after I have got all of this off my chest. Once there I continue to eat in a way that is very different to the dietitian's advice, staying away from products with added sugar, all dairy foods, potatoes and meat. However, there does not appear to be any simple philosophy on nutrition and the combating of serious disease. The Japanese eat very little fat and suffer fewer heart attacks than the Australians and Americans, but the Italians eat a lot of fat and suffer fewer too. The Japanese drink very little red wine and suffer fewer heart attacks than Australians and Americans, but the Italians drink excessive amounts of red wine and yet also suffer fewer heart attacks.

I read about a completely different philosophy in a very practical book about the Chakras by Peter Rendel[68]. Suddenly a whole set of patterns fall into place for me. It is known *(from Quantum physics)* that all living things are just energy in different states, or rates of vibration, and the Chakras describe how this manifests in the human body. Experiential wisdom indicates that this energy "concentrates" at seven specific locations in the body, and link to certain "human" drivers.

Chakra	Focus	Basic Human Motivations
7th		Meaning
6th	*Selfless*	Wisdom
5th		Courage
4th		Compassion
3rd		Power
2nd	*Selfish*	Pleasure
1st		Survival

On Sunday I hired the video of the *Wizard of Oz* starring Judy Garland for the boys. Its name suggests that it is for watching it in this country, and I thought my sons would like it, although I have never been interested in watching it in England. We watch it now and within twenty minutes they had both gone off to more interesting things, while I became enchanted by a story which I see is also the story of my cancer. It is about history or herstory.

Every experience has three parts; the *preparation*, the *journey* and the *home-coming*. For Dorothy, her *preparation* is being caught in a windstorm, mine is being told I had cancer and preparing by going on Vipassana meditation and changing my diet. Her *journey* was following the Yellow Brick Road; mine was chemotherapy and the alternative therapies I try. The *home-coming* was her waking up in her room, whereas for me it is yet to come. The experience of "*the journey inwards*" has to have certain essential ingredients; the key elements which are in all the great mythological and religious stories from around the world. The ingredients are each symbolised by a person in Dorothy's journey.

1   The Scarecrow who doesn't have a brain – only straw. He is trying to find Wisdom, while I can search the field of medicine for Wisdom in dealing with my disease.

2   The Tin Man who has no heart – only a hollow chest. He is trying to get to the Level of Compassion, while I can find Compassion by helping others in a similar situation or in the help others give me.

3   The Lion who is a coward – wants "the nerve". He is trying to get to the Level of Courage, while I can try different treatments so others may better save themselves if faced with a similar situation.

Dorothy said "Trouble stops over the rainbow."

She got lost and was now trying to find her way home.

In the words of the poet, T.S. Eliot, "We must not cease from exploration. And the end of all our exploring will be to arrive where we began and to know the place for the first time."

I feel confident that my eventual home-coming, whatever its form, is going to be around the question of meaning.

I have asked friends who are university lecturers or have Ph.D.s in psychology, what is the fundamental opposite emotion to love. They have replied words to effect, "Hate, I suppose."

This did not seem to be a very complete answer to me. I expect western psychology does not really consider the question and therefore, unsurprisingly, does not really have an answer.

Mythological stories try to take us to the higher levels of compassion, courage and wisdom. Whereas we live most of our lives at the lower levels of survival, power and pleasure – the "three F's" of motivation: feeding, fighting and fornication[69]. The "Basic Human Motivations" are linked to the primary emotions and our breathing, but it finally dawns on me, after much prompting from eastern psychologies, that they lead to a propensity for certain actions and arise from one of only two emotions – love and fear.

Put simply, love is selflessness, and fear is selfishness[70]. So the opposite of love is fear, as Eastern philosophies have said for thousands of years.

Basic Human Motivations	Characteristic Primary Emotion	Commonly Associated Action	Characteristic Fundamental Emotion
Meaning	-	Leading (in a specific way)	*Love*
Wisdom		Understanding	
Courage	Resolve	Saving	
Compassion		Helping	
Power	Anger	Fighting	*Fear*
Pleasure	Passion	Fornicating	
Survival	Sadness	Feeding	

Psychologists generally agree that there are the "Big 5" personality traits[71]. These are characteristic ways of behaving, thinking and feeling – which can be combined to define any of us (not to be confused with the "Big 5" African game animals[72]). Here are the "Bigger 7" individual motivations which apply to humans and all animals with a consciousness[73], and all motivation is some manifestation of these seven drives.

The Chakras are linked to physical points on our body. For example courage is at the throat level, you may gulp when nervous, and your sense of power is at the solar plexus – that is where you get butterflies when things seem out of our control. It describes many things, for instance bullies are about "Power". They operate from the 3rd Chakra. They like to appear brave but their energy comes from power not courage, which is a very different focus and outcome. As I have found in life, when bullies are confronted with a higher energy like courage – standing up to them to stop them mis-treating others – they retreat very quickly. Bullying is not only detrimental for those bullied but also for the bullies. (I heard a psychologist presenting on the topic say that by the time bullies are 24 years of age one in three has been in prison at least once, and the other two have become politicians …)

In this model, the higher Chakras are not better nor worse than lower ones, but they are more powerful. We must be selfish at times, for instance if we did not eat then we would not live to do unselfish things. Life is all a matter of balance. We can also use the simile of notes. Each Chakra is like a note, the higher the Chakra the higher the frequency and greater the energy. No note is bad or good in itself, and it takes a combination of notes to make music. However, any note in the wrong place can have an adverse effect on the melody.

Caroline Myss Ph.D. describes how the Chakras relate to lessons to be learned in life:

- 1st Chakra – "lessons about the material world"
- 2nd Chakra – "lessons about sexuality and desires"
- 3rd Chakra – "lessons about ego and personality"
- 4th Chakra – "lessons about love and forgiveness"
- 5th Chakra – "lessons about will and self-expression"
- 6th Chakra – "lessons about mind and insight"
- 7th Chakra – "lessons about spirituality[74]"

I have often sympathised or empathised with people in very difficult or life threatening situations, believing that I fully understood their plight. I see now this was only an intellectual understanding of their experience, and therefore has to be incomplete. Anything that happens to us, any experience, involves things that cannot be described by words alone. How can we convey by words the full extent of our feelings? Part of any experience is beyond thought. That is why experiential wisdom is greater than intellectual wisdom can ever be. Doctor Ainslie Meares[75] once came across a venerated yogi in Nepal. Yogis are "spiritually disciplined individuals" in the Hindu faith and Doctor Meares asked him what it was like to meditate. The yogi replied by asking him to describe the taste of a banana.

For if you know what a banana tastes like then you do not need to ask, if you do not then words can never be enough to describe it.

Symbols are a powerful way to convey meaning, and a friend, Helen, expands on this, "Surely this is the significance of the arts in any society. Art seeks to transform and communicate human experience through the imagination."

I read to Rob that evening about the lives of animals. We get to one of the African "Big 5" and I say you must be very careful around lions, "They are very dangerous because they have very good eyesight."

I turn the page to "Saltwater" crocodiles and he says, "You must also be very careful around saltwater crocodiles because they have a very good sense of humour."

I realize he has confused his words and does not mean that there is a high risk of dying from laughter!

Trek – Day 1

Nepali Trekking Truism: A Nepalese bus is never full.

1991: 24 November, The Himalaya, East Nepal

The next morning I met up with Subash, who introduced me to my porters; Nadur, Chandra, and my head porter, Ratna. Ratna was a wiry man with the weathered facial features of someone in their fifties. I never found out his age but I believed him to be at least 10 years younger than he looked. He had a combination of humane enthusiasm and fleeting imagination, and broke into a smile as we met. Chandra was in his late teens, lean and fit. He quickly conveyed a sense of industry and dependability, someone who was happy with the routine and detail. I also noticed he was an onychophagist[76]. Nadur was the same age as Chandra and turned out to be just as fit although he was a bit more thick set. He was an introspective man but gave me a friendly greeting.

It was usual for an "officer sahib" to have four porters. Subash told me that he could get another porter here in Dharan Bazaar but they would not have been vetted by the Gurkha Brigade. The Gurkha Brigade paid more than the usual going rate for porters and selected them using a pretty rigorous assessment process. Ratna made it clear that they would carry whatever was necessary to avoid having an additional porter. They wanted to get a share of the 66 Rupees a day that the extra Porter would be paid, and I was happy to help by carrying my 60 pound Bergen; not that this compared to their loads of almost 100 pounds.

I bumped into Lieutenant "Iron Stomach" Guy just before boarding my bus. He was merrily chomping away on a meat pasty, or "kal"[77] burger (as I felt like calling it) which he had bought from a street stall. He not only wanted to live the Nepali experience but eat it as well. I thought that if that burger was as good as it looked then he might die the Nepali experience instead. We said our farewells and then I boarded the bus for my next stop; Dhankuta.

Nadur had made sure that we had booked seats but "booking" did not have quite the same meaning in Nepali or in Nepal.

I guess we say "Get on a bus or train" because it used to be open topped, and you get on a horse (and cart).

My porters used the term appropriately for this bus as I could see several people hanging on the back of what was little more than a large minibus.

I asked Subash how many there were and he commented cryptically, "As many people as there are Chakras."

After almost five hours the bus arrived at Dhankuta, the halfway station. The town was rather precariously strung from south to north along a ridge. We were one hour late and were just in time to see our connecting bus preparing to leave an hour early. So much for the two-hour stopover and missing this would make our tight schedule too tight. Subash suggested we stay the night and sample the delights of the town. I gazed around and thought "delight" was probably more accurate and wondered what we would do with the other ten hours. I told the porters to try to get onto the departing bus which they did to the letter. They had little problem transferring roof to roof, this time keeping all the rucksacks with them. The bus was packed out inside and it was obvious that insisting on taking a booked seat would be an unpopular and unsuccessful move. Instead, Subash and I joined the porters on top of this single Decker. It was more a cosy than a safe ride.

As we travelled along I asked Subash what the Chakras were. He replied that the body is thought of primarily in terms of energy in this part of the world, and that the form of the human body meant that there were seven concentrations of energy, each located along the spine. The 1st Chakra is at the base of the spine, 2nd at about the level of the abdomen, 3rd at the level of the solar plexus, 4th at approximately the level of the breastbone, 5th at the throat, 6th at the point of the forehead between the eyebrows and 7th at the top of the head. I knew that Einstein's discoveries confirmed that the body was just energy in what might be thought of as 'frozen form'. I had also done enough biology to know that the Chakra points are at the levels of key components of the hormonal system[78]. The second through to the seventh Chakras relating to the gonads, adrenals, thymus, thyroid, pituitary and pineal gland, respectively. It seemed one way to explain why these points might be so significant, but it also sounded a bit too superstitious for me as we drove ever upwards in mountains which cradled the rivers far below.

I could occasionally see the rivers mass of moods. Sometimes they would run smooth and deep, at other points there would be a fiery surging of melt water boiling and foaming around rocks. But as darkness fell the scenery disappeared and my primary sensation became one of iciness. I spent three hours on the roof before the combination of the warmth and available seats pulled me down below. Subash and the porters soon joined me. About four hours after leaving Dhankuta we arrived in Basantpur.

This was the first of my hill towns and I was impressed by the surprisingly stylish architecture of some three storey Nepalese houses. We stayed in hotel Yak which could have been used for a scene from *Raiders of the Lost Ark*. The hotel charged like a "wounded cow"... not very much at all. Ten pence a bed for a porter in a shared travellers' dormitory. A whole twenty pence for my single room complete with some secret trap door in the wall.

Looking at the dining area, I wondered whether the hotel had put the wrong vowel in its name. We cooked our own food in the back courtyard. I was getting a bit tired of the Nepalese food but the added variety of the tinned tuna I had brought from Hong Kong gave it a whole new life.

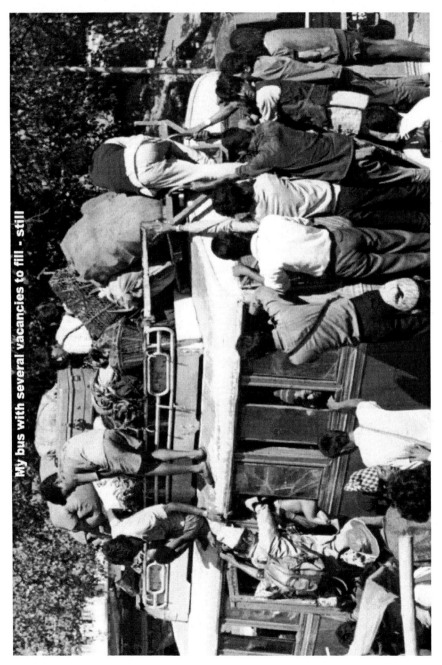

My bus with several vacancies to fill - still

A House in Higher Hills

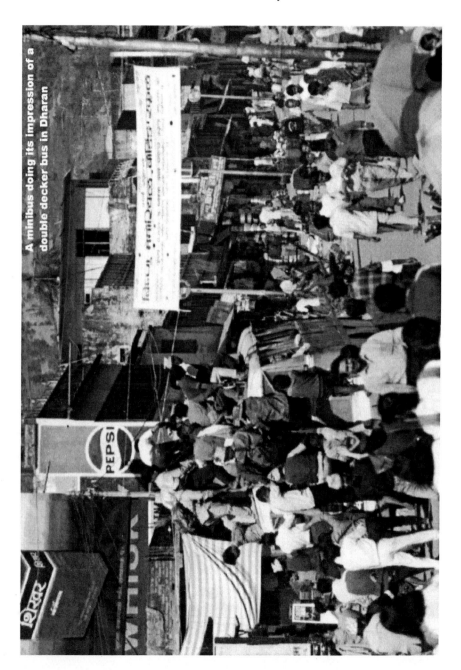

A House in Higher Hills

After dinner I joined my team in drinking tongba. I had decided to give the commercial beers a miss. It was worth acquiring the habit of having bottles opened at the table as diluting drinks was not unheard of, but using clean water was. Tongba is the name of the traditional Limbu drinking vessel. It is made of special wood and banded with metal. The vessel is filled with fermented millet, on which boiling water is poured and it is drunk via a wooden "straw". I found it to be a very pleasant drink, bearing in mind that the straw is reused and usually washed out in a semi-ritualistic but functionally ineffective manner.

At this stage I handed out some thermal tops which I had bought in Hong Kong for the porters. Size-wise I had definitely played on the safe side. Ratna's fitted okay but Nadur and Chandra could have been fairly accused of cross-dressing. Despite this, they all thanked me profusely and put them on immediately, keeping them on for much of the trek. A few hours later we departed to our separate rooms. I was firmly in the land of Hinduism, a good religion to bet on as with so many gods one has got to be right, and I was soon in the land of nod too.

Intellectual Wisdom – Who Am I And What Is My Purpose (*In The East*)?

"People travel to wonder
At the height of the mountains,
At the huge waves of the sea,
At the long courses of rivers, at the vast compass of the
ocean,
At the circular motion of the stars,
And they pass themselves by without wondering"

St Augustine

The Chakras

We can look towards the East for a model on self-awareness. Their thinking about spirituality may have been overlooked because the West's advances in technology helped its religious practices to be extended in the last few hundred years. Missionaries were able to preach in countries dominated by western force and their ideas were often well received because, to some, western power was dominant and appeared "god-like". The fact that we have focussed so much on science in the West – a focus on the Mental and Physical Rooms – is perhaps the reason that our spiritual insights may be less extensive than the East's?

The eastern idea of the Chakras provides a framework that we can combine with the four Rooms, to make a house of seven floors. In each level, one room is most significant and predominates, and this is the "Main Room". The Levels between the basement and top floor also have one Room which is smaller than the Main Room but larger than the others. This is because at each Level the Main Room represents the dominant energy – be it physical, emotional, mental or spiritual. This "radiates" to the next Level up and increases the significance of the same Room at the next higher Level, which I have called the "Auxiliary Room".

Why upwards not downwards, or why not both ways? This direction makes sense to those of us whose experience suggests that the "life force" in each of us tries to take us up to the next Level – try to resist as we may.

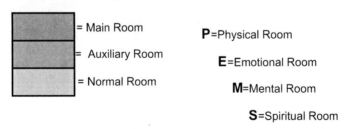

Meaning of Shading and Letters:

= Main Room

= Auxiliary Room

= Normal Room

P=Physical Room

E=Emotional Room

M=Mental Room

S=Spiritual Room

"Chakra" means "wheel" in Sanskrit – the ancient language of the Hindu civilisation and religion – and Chakras are thought to be centres of vital energy in the body, which manifest as vortices or wheels of force. Each circles in either a clockwise or anti-clockwise direction.

We can see that the Ground and 1st Floors have only three rooms, whereas the others also have a "Spiritual" Room. This is because at the Levels of Pleasure and Power there is only a focus on ourselves. There is no "connection" to anyone, or anything, else; this connection is partly what the spiritual is about.

The Main Room varies depending on the Level we are at, as shown in the figure below, and the higher the Level then the higher the potential energy.

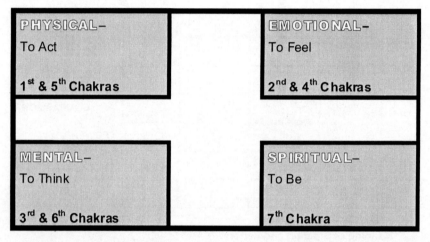

Below is an example of the symbolic representation of the "House" which will be used throughout Book 3.

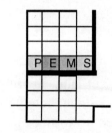

In this example it indicates that the chapter is discussing the fourth Chakra – the Level of Compassion. The shading indicates the Room size at this Level. The darker the shading the bigger the Room. The letters stand for Physical, Emotional, Mental and Spiritual.

A House in Higher Hills

This model, like western science or any other model, can only provide an intellectual understanding and approximation on life. It is like describing what a banana tastes like. The description of the banana is not the actual taste. However, by describing it we will know better what the banana looks like, and where it may be found, and so improve our chances of finding it so that we can "taste" it fully. The Levels in this model are similar to those in Maslow's but the structure is more accurate and better describes and predicts human motivations/needs.

Having built this model we can now see how predictive it is.

CHAPTER 6

What Cannot Be Measured May Still Exist!

1999: 21–24 July, Melbourne

John continues to be very supportive. He has a very good knowledge of conventional therapies for cancer and is a veritable fount of helpful advice. He sent me a long letter in June, after my diagnosis. I read it properly for the first time. It starts,

> "I cannot begin to tell you how sorry I am to hear your dreadful news today. There never seems to be any peace for the good. After the trauma you had with your mother last year, now this. It's all so unfair."

He then goes on to give me a wealth of useful advice. I only skim read it as I find it difficult to read this clinical information which reminds me so much of my situation.

However, some of his advice, as he knows, contradicts my beliefs, "… Eat everything that you can think of that is fattening like fry-ups, steaks, pork chops etc.†"

I do not see how being overweight can help. Excess weight is associated with a significantly increased incidence of cardiovascular disease, type 2 diabetes mellitus, hypertension, osteoarthritis and some cancers[79]. Yet getting fat seems to be part of the conventional nutritional advice for my situation. Conversely, I believe strongly that with little effort and cost you can adopt a diet

---

† Note: As I write this at the end of 2002 it seems to me that the conventional advice now seems to be changing and becoming more in agreement with what I was advocating in 1999.

which helps you significantly, and is much better than the "Food Pyramid". John does not have much time for the alternative therapies I am trying, but he clearly understands the importance of optimism making sure that he is always positive at some level. He sends me lots of the latest information on the conventional treatment of Hodgkin's. He also suggests I look at the mass of information on the World Wide Web, but I do not follow that up, as I do not feel the need to do so – yet.

John finishes,

> "One last thought from me today. Logic tells me since your mother made such a satisfactory recovery you will do much better for all the obvious reasons. The next 4-6 months are going to be tough on you, on Ruth, on your mother and all of us who care. You must remain strong in the knowledge that any sign of weakening from your side will be exaggerated or misconstrued. On the other hand you must also be selfish. Decide what is best for you and act unswervingly towards it … Do not settle for second best because of over-riding circumstances or responsibilities. For once, be selfish. I want you to know that I'll do anything to help. All you have to do is ask."

John is talking about going into survival mode and putting myself first[80]. My Mother is not so impressed with how things stand in England at present. "It is good in some ways that you are in Australia. The health care system like the overall quality of life generally seems better in Australia than it is in England." Although she remains happy in the UK she says she is sure there are more opportunities and chances for an enjoyable life in Australia.

I replace the Sunrider[81] with Usana[82] vitamins reasoning that now my body is being assaulted by harsh chemicals I will probably want significantly more than the recommended daily dose of vitamins and minerals, especially as my appetite may reduce. There is a great deal of evidence indicating that antioxidants reduce the risk of cancer[83] or protect normal cells during chemotherapy/ radiotherapy[84].†

Ray D Strand MD, said in 1999;

> "I believe all my patients with cancer should be on the most potent antioxidants available. The results that I have seen in using nutritional supplements in my patients have all been positive. I personally believe that within 5 to 10 years all physicians will be recommending their patients with cancer should be taking nutritional supplements."

However, I find the advice in this area contradictory.

In the Australasian Nutrition Advisory Council's (ANAC's) booklet, entitled *Food for Cancer Prevention*, it says, "Dietary supplements are of no value in reducing cancer."

It seems to me to be poor advice considering all the research I have come across, although I am not an expert in this area. I write to ANAC's chairman saying:

> "It does not appear that the Australian Nutrition Advisory Council is aware of a wealth of research which shows strong evidence to the contrary, or it is just ignoring it? The evidence covers a range of vitamins and minerals, and the research includes articles indicating that antioxidant vitamins protect against cancer (Cancer Research 56:1291, 1996). We can take one, selenium, as an example … Cancer is a disease of a 'low immune system' so Doctor Margaret Rayman's comment in Lancet (the United Kingdom's leading medical journal) in July 2000 is indirect support for using it as a supplement, 'selenium is of fundamental importance to human health. We need it for proper functioning of our immune system' …
>
> However, all this could be ignored if it were not for research reported in an article published in JAMA (the Journal of the American Medical Association) in December 1996. A 10-year study showed that selenium can reduce the risk of

---

† Caution: you should take professional medical advice before taking high doses of vitamins especially if you are ill or undergoing medical treatment.

cancer by 50%. A double blind, placebo-controlled study showed that men might significantly reduce their risk of developing prostate cancer by taking 200 micrograms of selenium each day. Even better, this study also showed that both men and women may lower their risk of developing lung and colon cancers. Compared with the placebo group, there was a 37% reduction in the incidence of cancers, and a very significant 50% reduction in the number of total cancer deaths among those who were given the selenium ..."

It is mid-morning when Bernie, a close friend and fellow Taekwondo competitor, comes around to visit me. Bernie is one of those gifted athletes who, when you give him a new sport to try, picks it up as if he has been doing it for years. He has been Australian Taekwondo champion several times which can surprise as it is his friendliness which strikes you most when you meet him. Ruth lets him in and he waits expecting to see some ashen, pale and hairless figure stumbling around the corner. He is happily surprised how well I look and remarks as such.

"Isn't it just typical that we have in our mind how bad things are going to be, and it is often not the reality?"

I agree that often our fears are worse than the reality.

I am taking Zyloprim[85] so that, should the cancer reduce quickly in size, my body can cope with the large production of uric acid. Otherwise, this can cause gout and kidney problems. The former manifests as the formation of uric acid crystals. I gather it is like having ground glass in your joints which sounds worth giving a miss. But nothing is all bad; apparently uric acid is a very good antioxidant.

Mark, a friend at work and fellow Pom, left me a voice mail and email message yesterday wishing me well for the chemotherapy.

"First lot today? Didn't want to bother you with a phone call. Thinking of you. Mail or call whenever you fancy having the piss taken! Well we nearly managed a serious conversation last time so you never know!"

Quite a few people wished me well a day or two before the chemotherapy, or a couple of days after the chemotherapy. However, Mark was the only one who did it on the day of the chemotherapy. Logically this is a minimal difference, but it made a marked difference emotionally. If you want to build up a reservoir of goodwill then phone someone up the day they go into chemotherapy.

I email back: "It was as much fun as chewing tacks."

My oncologist confirms what the nurse said, saying that chemotherapy works mainly in the first pass around the body. It is broken down on reaching the liver and subsequent passes of the chemotherapy around the body kill less cancer. This means that after 24 hours maximum you want to get it all out of your body. Hence their advice to drink at least 3 litres of fluid a day.

Ever one for a challenge I say, "Watch me drink," and drink like I was made to drink.

I have four litres in the first 3 hours of chemotherapy!

I wonder whether a Turkish sauna and lymphatic massage will help me two days after my first chemotherapy. I am now feeling relatively great and looking like Nepalese frost! Although we see things differently when it comes to alternative therapies, I have confidence in much of my oncologist's advice. I ask him what he thinks of saunas and lymphatic massage for my situation. He says it should be alright although the sauna may dehydrate me a bit and the massage should avoid pressing the lump on my neck. I also ask about whether he has anecdotal evidence of high dose vitamin C helping people undergoing chemotherapy. He says that he cannot really comment until proper double blind statistical experiments have been carried out.

Later I go to see Doctor Soosay. I have just found out that he is the President of the Australian College of Herbal Medicine[86], something which I take to confirm my belief that he is a very good GP, and so I expect him to accept alternative remedies more than my oncologist. However, he advises me not to go for either a sauna or massage, and I err on the side of caution. He recommends vitamin C and selenium, in the form of sodium selenite. He also suggests a North American Indian herb – Essiac – which seems to have anti-cancer properties, but is yet unproven. He also advises I take very light exercise, like gentle walks. I am confident that Doctor Soosay's advice is sound, especially about gentle exercise. A few months ago I heard that Helen Rawlinson, a BBC sports commentator who had been diagnosed with cancer, was doing hard physical exercise with a personal trainer as part of her therapy. This sounded very unwise to me as the body uses very large amounts of energy to fight any serious illness.

I wrote to her on 25th January of this year saying, "Another consideration is please do not exercise too hard, your body needs the energy, and consider meditation – I know this may sound a bit wacky, more so coming from an ex Army Officer… "

Little did I know I was in the same boat. (Helen was unfortunately to die of liver cancer a number of months later.)

I am frustrated by the two opposite bits of medical advice about the sauna and massage.

I talk with Peter about it and he agrees, saying, "Western medicine is absolutely bloody brilliant and bloody arrogant."

I was talking to a friend who spoke about a terminally ill lady.

She had been told by her doctor (*not mine*) that she should listen to what treatment he was recommending, saying, "I am responsible for your health."

My immediate retort was, "I hope the doctor added 'therefore I will commit suicide if you die'."

We know healthy people can be markedly different. I have an allergy to shellfish; if I eat any then I am pretty ill. But most healthy people would be fine. A trace of peanuts can kill some people whereas I and others can gorge on them to our heart's content. Medicine knows that the mind (e.g. stress) has a major impact on the health of the human body – how often does it say that major illnesses, such as heart disease, cancer etc, are caused by stress? Knowing these things conventional medicine sets up statistical tests which involve undifferentiated groups of people with treatments for a disease without taking into account mental and environmental differences affecting the people in the sample, nor does it account for different body and blood types which can respond subtly but crucially to different stimuli. Perhaps that is why there are concerns that doctors and patients are being misled by the results of drug trials published in major international medical journals. Analysis at the University of California suggests that a significant number of drugs and procedures are reported as more effective than they actually are[87]. If weird treatments work, their success is often labelled as psychosomatic. This may be true, yet stress lowers the immune system, so all disease starts in the mind. Doesn't that make most diseases and cures psychosomatic at some level?

I say to John that most modern medicine is palliative; he is not so sure, "While some modern medicine is clearly palliative, for example aspirins for headaches, others, such as chemotherapy, are curative."

I disagree;

"Well if western medicine is curing cancer then it is by accident because they don't know what causes it! If you doubt this just talk to your local blood bank. I cannot give blood now that I have had lymphoma presumably because they are not sure of the 'mechanism' that causes lymphoma and fear I may pass on some form of 'agent'.

Chemotherapy treats the symptom – in this case the anaerobic cells growing unchecked in the body. That is a symptom, not the cause of cancer. If there is one cause then it triggers the formation of cancer cells and keeps them growing unchecked. Normally the immune system eliminates cancer cells. Who can tell us what that is, or if it is only one thing?

Even if we take smoking and lung cancer, the cause is not clear. Clearly smoking is a major factor but it is not the 'sole' cause. If smoking was the only cause of lung cancer then only people who smoked would get it. But this is not the case and was one reason the link between smoking and lung cancer took some time to be established. The cause is not the smoking. It is just a factor, albeit a major one.

If chemotherapy gets rid of the cause then it is by chance because western medicine does not know what is the "trigger". I believe chemotherapy is an extreme palliative. It kills the cancer cells giving the body/mind entity time to get rid of the cause. If it does not then the cancer comes back again after the treatment!"

A manager of a global IT company and friend, Paddy, comes round to see how I am going. He is a fellow Pom of my age but still plays a very solid game of soccer. He offers to take my boys to their soccer training, and he, Ruth and I chat about life rather than its opposite.

The boys are beginning to show signs of being unsettled by the situation.

Olly is not sleeping either and comes down the next night saying; "I can't sleep as every time I am almost asleep something crawls up my nose and buggers me. I keep getting buggered!"

I think he's talking about being bugged.

Trek – Day 2

Trekking Truism: Just because the path is a good one does not mean that it goes anywhere – even if it says it does.

1991: 25 November, Jirikhimti, The Himalaya

B reakfast was tea at two New Pence a cup. I splashed out and bought two cups for everyone.

The vehicular road finished about half a mile past Basantpur. It stopped dead – not quite what the signs had suggested. It was a true road to nowhere and perhaps a portent of things to come. The funding had run out for the road and there were plans to continue the road when more cash became available. Nepal only has about 2800 kilometres of paved roads in total.

While we were stopping for a rest a high caste traveller, a Baun, passed us with his porters. He bore the countenance of someone who had an assured place in his society. I knew a bit about Nepal's Hindu caste system, but Subash told me more:

"There are four classes of society or castes. The supporting philosophy of svadharma – one's spiritual duty in accord with the cosmic law and order – believes that each caste is born to do a particular job, marry a specific person, eat certain food, and have children who will have their svadharma. It is better to live in line with, and enjoy the pleasures of, one's own dharma – the cosmic law and order – than be led astray by others onto a different path. The fourth caste is the Harijan caste – the Untouchables. 'Outside the system' are parents and children of forbidden marriages, killers of cows, lone hermits, scavengers and you!"

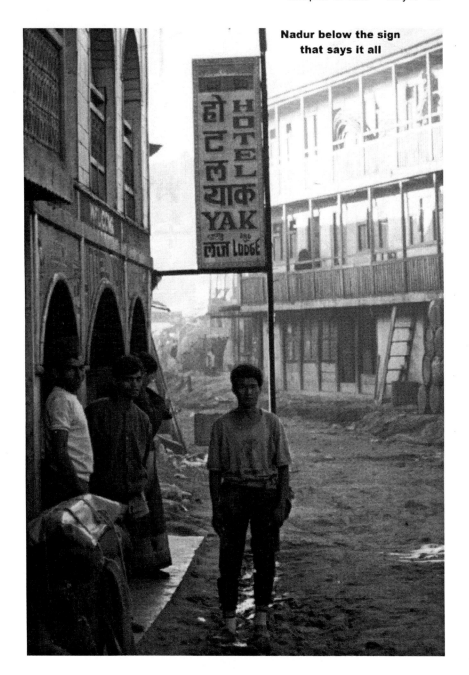

Nadur below the sign
that says it all

A House in Higher Hills

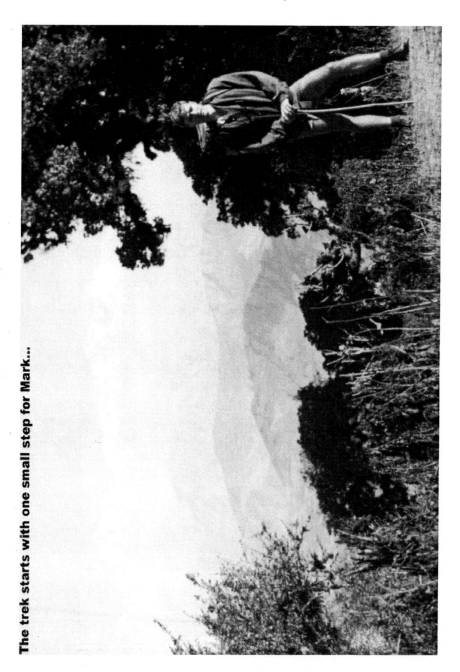

The trek starts with one small step for Mark...

A House in Higher Hills

I felt rather pleased to be differentiated from "scavengers!"

Shortly after we had set off, we in turn passed the Baun as he stripped and washed before preparing his lunch with his own hands. The Gurkhas largely ignore the caste system in the Army, but in the hills a high caste will not eat with a low one, or even allow the shadow of a lower caste to fall onto his food.

As was to become the custom for lunch, we stopped on a mountainside overlooking some of the grand old "hills" of the Himalaya. My porters' meal time preparation was in stark contrast to that of the Baun's. They removed their hats, spat on their hands and wiped them over their face. Their ceremony ended there and they then tucked into their food. As we sat there I could see distant Lasune clearly.

The military treks took place between August and December, between the unrelenting heat and rain of summer and the cold of winter. Nepal has a monsoon climate. The "Wet Monsoon" starts in early June and continues until late September, owing to air overheating in the plains of India and absorbing lots of water moisture. The water laden monsoon winds are drawn up the Ganges Valley from the Bay of Bengal and drop their load as heavy rain. These rains enable the rice culture to exist but on a landscape devoid of trees to break the force of the rain or stabilize the soils, the rains turn quickly into surging rivers. By October the water is draining off these terraced paddy fields and the rice ripening. Now starts the "Dry Monsoon" when the hill farmers are busy with the cutting and threshing of the rice crop. They then have to carry heavy loads of rice seed and straw up hundreds of feet to their homes. The mother of the house then meticulously rations out and stores the seed over the next twelve months.

I was at first strictly teetotal, I just drunk tea. My porters look suitably jaded as they drink Jard, a wine made from millet. I use the term "wine" loosely as it looked like muddy water and it was aptly named as when I sipped it jarred my taste buds. I call it "Wonse" as in "only once".

We arrived at Jirikhimti AWC after some seven hours of walking. The only crops around appeared to be tobacco. The villages in the area were pretty poor and for them this was a cash rich crop. The AWO greeted me. He was a Rai, one of the main warrior tribes of the East, the other being the Limbus. He had a typical physique for this part of Nepal, small stature with black hair, dark eyes and a ruddy brown complexion. He had little facial hair, again typical of the Mongolian stock. With a flash of his pearly white teeth he told me he was new and unfortunately did not know the exact requirements of the local villages. In true Gurkha style he was very hospitable. Subash and I settled down to a traditional meal of bhat – cooked rice – the staple diet up there in the hills. Pronounced "bhaat" it was also a term used to describe the local curry. However, the social customs were pretty clear, and the porters ate outside. I supped tongba, a drink that I had taken to. I also tried raksi – a Nepalese spirit made from millet. I decided tongba had the most attractions which included its price: 8 New Pence per pint.

After dinner we sat with the porters. I asked what prompted them to come on this trek and they talked about enjoyment but in different ways. Subash saw this as the chance for play, his was an emotional approach. In contrast Chandra enjoyed the work so he could feel justified in relaxing afterwards. For Nadur, the work seemed to be the play. He enjoyed the learning. Ratna seemed to be uninterested in the question, or the answer, and remained quiet.

I had been reading the trekking "Bible" but was not clear about all the implications. I brainstormed a few possible options and it is a minor tempest.

I was still feeling a bit like a fish out of water but remained wary of going too much with the flow; as Malcolm Muggeridge once said, "Never forget that only dead fish swim with the stream."

The Journey Inside – Step 2 – Who Am I?

"It's not that having money is so good; it's that not having it is so bad"

Yiddish Saying

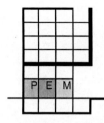

Level of Pleasure – Physiognomy

The Level of Pleasure is the second Level in this model, and each Level can be described by a typology. We know that in some ways we are the same as everyone else, in other ways different, but there are patterns in the human population where some are the same and others different. It is the understanding that there are important qualitative differences among individuals which is the key to typologies. Typologies can provide a framework which helps to see how some people's apparent random behaviour is quite consistent. The British Army's experience supports the idea of typologies. The Army teaches that officers and soldiers must lead in their own style – not as people outside the Army might suspect. If we were all the same type then, for a given situation, there would be just one way to lead.

The most significant room at this Level is the Emotional Room although when it comes to pleasure it is not surprising that there is a significant Physical element. We can use a typology based on "Physiognomy" – the art of observing bodily features to determine inner characteristics, to help us look around this "floor" more closely and to identify the different types. Although the typologies covered in this book apply across several levels to a certain extent, they are used at the Level where they give the clearest picture of the House.

Physiognomy shows the range of "Styles" when we are operating at the Level of Pleasure and helps us to answer Question 1: "Who Am I?"

Floor Plan for Pleasure

(Where we enjoy ourselves)

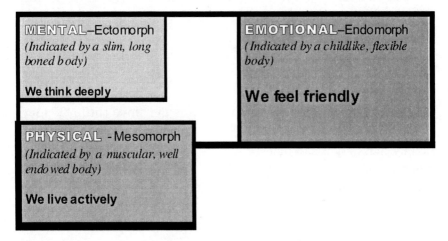

The information in the floor plan above is derived from *The Varieties of Temperament*[88]. The style descriptors have been deduced by the author from information about this book.

Turn to Annex A at the back of this Book and there is a blank diagram of a working diagram of your House, a model which I have called *Mark's Mansion* – a 2M model, one "M" short of an innovative company!

Although it is the same design for all of us, we each live in it differently. Now put a circle in the Room or Rooms that you tend to spend the most time in.

1 Look at the Styles in the floor plan above.

2 Decide which one, or ones, you adopt significantly in your life.

3 Identify which of the three Rooms it is in.

4 Go to Annex A and look at the second Level.

5 Mark a circle in the corresponding Room(s) at that Level.

6 *As a guide – it is probably most accurate to circle only one or two of the three Rooms, at this Level.*

To decide which Rooms to circle at this Level, look at the floor plan above and the adjectives associated with each Room.

Ask yourself: "Which of these adjectives best describe me? Which of these adjectives would other close friends or relatives use to describe me, if any?"

Money is linked to the Level of Pleasure but it is not "The root of all evil."

Money is just an entity, neither good nor bad in itself, which may be used positively or negatively. It is the "love (little "l" love) of money that is the root of all evil" – the attitude we take towards money that may mean that we "*l-i-v-e*" backwards. In other words, when as an adult, we remain totally selfish rather than selfless. The former being the characteristic state of children. If we have "*l-i-v-e-d*" backwards as an adult for long enough then we may be described as a devil!

CHAPTER 7

Deciding is not the Same as Doing

1999: 25 July–1 August

I am feeling a lot lower than I did nine years ago when trekking through the Churia ranges of the Himalaya and it is not just physically. John remains supportive, but finds it hard to believe that I would try alternative therapies (for such a relatively treatable cancer) when they may adversely affect the treatment. We differ as I see no point waiting to see if the conventional method works and then saying I should have listened to my intuition. Especially as I am concerned about the long term affects of the treatment should I survive. I need to listen to it now – rightly or wrongly – and then take action.

I have received a letter from my Father saying he has just been to a Royal Military Academy Sandhurst 50th anniversary reunion for his intake. When he joined the Royal Air Force Regiment, officers were trained at Sandhurst.

He notes that fully one third of his intake went either into the Gunners or the Sappers (my Corps) and follows this up with, "Apparently the Army was rather short of intelligent officers in 1949!"

I wonder why he uses a non sequitur about Intelligence Corps officers before realizing it is a compliment to the officers of these two Corps. The Army was trying to increase the number of officers in these two key "Teeth Arms".

At last I get diarrhoea! Some specialists say that the "bowel tolerance technique" is the best way to judge your own vitamin C requirements. Diarrhoea may occur when excess vitamin C reaches your intestines because in the presence of a concentrated solution of a substance – in this case vitamin C – the intestinal cells pull water in from the surrounding cells, loosening the stool and producing diarrhoea. However, excess vitamin C only reaches the intestines when it is not absorbed through the stomach first, which happens if the body needs it because it is depleted. So using some simple calculations it would have taken me over 6 years of only eating the RDA for vitamin C to reach saturation assuming that I did not use any of it up during that time!

John tells me about newspaper articles reporting that high dose vitamin C can cause cancer.

However, 10 years ago a Cambridge University research paper[89] stated that concerns about vitamin C causing kidney stones, excessive iron absorption or causing cancer, and interfering with B_{12} metabolism or triggering rebound scurvy, have been disproved by "An extensive and very thorough analysis of the data during the past years."

I tell him the newspapers are at least 10 years out of date and the apparent cancerous effect was found to be caused by impurities that had been left in the equipment. I add that we have been going through a gradual change in the quality of our food. Apparently if you boil a frog in water hot enough to kill, it will immediately climb out and save itself. But if you put it in cold water then boil the water slowly it will lie there until it is boiled to death. This seems to be a good simile for the approach of some conventional health organisations.

Some experts consider a vitamin C intake of 1300 mg as a sensible prophylactic action. That would require 16 medium sized oranges a day. In the mornings, I mix half a teaspoon of vitamin C with a teaspoon of organic Spirulina, a microalgae and another part of "God's kitchen" (I use *Hawaiian Pacifica*[90] in powdered form). It feels like a supercharged food combination to me[91]. Spirulina offers more nutrition per acre than any other food; 20 times more protein per acre than soybeans and 200 times more than beef. It is a 95% digestible and complete food – a Japanese philosopher, Toru Matsui, is reported to have lived for 15 years exclusively on Spirulina in a retreat near Mount Hakone, close to Tokyo. My reasoning for mixing the two is that Spirulina provides GLA (gamma-linoleic acid), cislinoleic acid and zinc which are essential raw materials for prostaglandin production. This stimulates the T-lymphocytes – a critical component of the immune system – and the vitamin C also helps in the metabolism of collagen, which is the essential constituent of fibrous tissue and cartilage which the body uses to encapsulate the cancer. Phycocyanin is found only in blue-green algae and has been proved to stimulate the immune system function. It also contains two polysaccharides which have been shown to "supercharge" the immune system[92].

Peter has sent me three books about "beating" cancer. One, *Interrupted Innings* by Helen Mitchell, looks a bit too good. It is an account by Helen of her 18-year-old son's struggle with lymphoma, and final victory. It is a bit too detailed on what may be my future for my liking, and I put it to one side.

At work I am left wondering whether a smart friend realises how easy he is to see-through; but this transparency is best seen in the Emotional not the Mental Room. Trevor[93] comes up to greet me and asks me how I am. Formalities out of the way, he asks me for some technical information I have. I tell him I will email it to him later that day. A few days after he receives it he has not said anything to me.

So I send him a gentle reminder email with just the heading "What Trevor, no thanks?"

He comes up to me rather quickly afterwards, apologising and I advise him that it's best to treat people on chemotherapy tenderly. It is not enough to know how to construct a bridge; you have to go and build it before you can cross it. I sum up his style as "Curtains Closed" in my model although I do not think my email helped the communication. It only provided the words, missing out on the more significant channels of body language and tone[94].

Lance Armstrong won. John H., a close friend from England phones me up. I first met John at Cambridge University through the Officer Training Corps. He stuck me as an engineer with a big-picture perspective thinker who quickly spotted the flaws in arguments and was not backward in coming forward, as the saying goes. However, he did it in an inclusive way, helped by a very good sense of humour.

He tells me how he was watching when Lance was in the lead pack with only a few kilometres to go and then "He seemed to say 'okay I have had enough, bye', and he just left them for dead."
I write to congratulate Lance, "Brilliant news to hear you won today. Many congratulations on being the first US winner[95]."

I feel calm in a way about my situation. Many people say to me how well I seem to cope. Is it a show fooling them or me? Yet what I am living is too important to waste on a show. It is life and I have no real choice but to face it. I do not believe in submissive acceptance of what happens to me but believe that if we do not accept where we really are, then we cannot know what direction to go in to get where we want to be.

Typologies are about awareness and I think up another typology for people who do not accept typologies. Either they:

1 Do not believe typologies have any scientific basis, or
2 Do not want to be boxed in (but if you don't know you are in a box you may never try to get out), or
3 Do not want others knowing what they might be like, or
4 Do not want to know what they might be like!

The first reason is largely refuted by empirical data and theory. You have a consciousness which means you can choose what you focus on in life. But although we have 60000-70000 thoughts each day, ninety-five per cent are the same as the previous day. Therefore you have a "preference" for the same thoughts – you tend to keep the same mental focus. This is the basis for typologies. Of course some typologies are better than others. For instance a commonly used typology in the West is the horoscope.

My company has an annual conference in Sydney. It will be nice to have the simple pleasures of living a "normal" life for a bit. My Mother has impressed upon me the problems she had at the start of her chemotherapy. I spent a week with her in England soon after she was diagnosed. She commented then that most people there seem to be surviving rather than living. (Which means that they are sticking to the basement of the house!) My Mother's blood count was reduced to nil after her first chemotherapy and she very nearly died from complications. The day I left her to fly back to Australia, she became seriously ill.

John had phoned a doctor who said "Don't worry, just get her to come in on Monday" – it was Friday afternoon.

Fortunately John rarely takes an "indefinite no" for an answer and insisted that she be taken to hospital immediately. It was only when he got her there that they saw how close she was to dying. It took two days before they were sure she would live. That is a lesson for me so I check my blood count and it is all right.

I feel a bit guilty, as my Mother would be very unhappy if she knew I was flying off to Sydney at this stage of my treatment. I have told Ruth to tell my Mother that I am asleep if she phones – irrespective of the time of day.

Over in Sydney I give a short talk on my current view of life. I try to make it motivational. I tell everyone that I have agreed that my presentation will last ten minutes and I was going to get everyone to hug for the first eight minutes, but was beaten to it by the external facilitator of the day. My talk ends up being very well received; some come up to me and say that I should do more motivational speaking. I think the outcome just resulted from when the truth in you connects with the truth in others. There is a party after the day-long conference but I leave others to go through that pleasure.

On the flight home I read more about GM food. It seems that the jury is out on its risks and rewards and that both positions are yet to be confirmed.

On one hand, "GM crops haven't ... put more food into the bowls of hungry people[96]."

In fact, 24 African scientists at a United Nations' conference in 1998 produced the statement,

> "We do not believe that ... [companies producing GM food] or gene technologies will help our farmers to produce the food that is needed in the 21st century. On the contrary, we think it will destroy the diversity, the local knowledge and the sustainable agricultural systems that our farmers have developed for millennia and that it will thus undermine our capacity to feed ourselves."

However, the critics concerns been not been verified either. Professor Arpad Pusztai's study showed that rats fed GM potatoes had shrivelled brains, livers and hearts, and their immune systems had been damaged. Many eminent scientists supported his findings, yet Pusztai's findings are now generally considered to be "irrevocably flawed[97]". Scientists at Cornell University found that GM corn killed monarch butterfly caterpillars in laboratory experiments although, in field studies, it appears that caterpillars do not eat enough GM pollen coated leaves to be affected. A variety of GM corn was found to have a structure that might cause people to develop an allergy and was therefore it was approved only as animal feed, but there is no definitive evidence that it would cause actual problems for humans. The fear that genes from GM crops might jump to weeds, making for "superweeds" has not happened yet, although a milder version of the same danger has turned up in Canada[98].

A major argument in support of GM food is that it will help to address world starvation. However, world starvation comes more from blockages at the 3rd Chakra – the *3Po's* (*Po*verty, *Po*wer and *Po*litics) – not the single *OPo* – *O*ver-*Po*pulation, which is more about a blockage at the 1st Chakra. Also it is widely accepted that the world currently produces enough food to feed everyone, (albeit the Earth's population is likely to increase[99]).

The ability of gene technology to improve the survivability of plants is highly questionable. The making of bug-resistant crops will very likely go the way of antibiotics and be beaten by evolution in an even shorter time[100].

In the end I think Erwin Chargraff asks a good question, "Have we the right to counteract, irreversibly, the evolutionary wisdom of millions of years?"

We may answer "No" at the Level of Survival or "Yes" from the Level of Power.

"Typologies" can be applied to both energy and food. *Nuclear Fuel* is similar to that of *GM Food* in this way. Energy, for movement, heating and cooling, can be put into the same three categories as food: *Natural*, *Evolved by Humans*, and *Artificial*.

Category	Energy/Food	Example	Benefits	Problems
Natural	Energy	Wind, wave and solar energy	Natural resource – cheap to run and has very limited adverse effects on the environment	Inflexible and difficult to harness in certain circumstances
	Food	*Wild and edible, flora and fauna*	*Natural resource – high in minerals and vitamins (including B_{17}) with very limited adverse effects on the environment*	*Inflexible and difficult to maintain consistent supply*
Evolved By Man	Energy	Fossil fuels (Petrol/diesel engines and oil/gas heating)	Engineered resource which has facilitated the Industrial Revolution and benefits of a modern lifestyle	Produces poisonous chemicals. Mass use has led to environmental problems such as the "Greenhouse Effect"
	Food	*Domesticated crops and animals*	*Biologically refined resource which has facilitated an agricultural evolution with the benefits of modern nutrition*	*Dispersal of toxic pesticides. Mass use has led to environmental problems such as reduced biodiversity and allergy problems from over-consumption of certain foods, such as wheat*

Category	Energy/ Food	Example	Benefits	Problems
	Energy	Nuclear fuel for electrical generators and nuclear submarines	Scientifically engineered and can provide cheap energy. Is without some of the polluting effects of fossil fuels	Can cause very severe damage to human health; this was not recognised initially. Concerns about long term adverse effects to the global environment of this new form of serious environmental contamination – **Radioactive pollution**[101]
Artificial	Food	*Genetically Modified food*	*Biologically engineered and can provide cheap food. GM crops are being produced which are aimed at reducing losses from pests and diseases, especially viruses*	*May have the potential to cause very severe damage to human health; although not universally recognised. Concerns about long term adverse effects to animal life of this new form of serious environmental contamination – "**Live pollution** (GM Genes have already "jumped" across species)*

There is no contingency action for nuclear energy or GM food – neither of them once released can be taken back out of the environment. In a few decades I think we shall see that GM food has done for nutrition, what nuclear fuel has done for energy, and with similarly severe side effects for our planet Gaia[102]. It seems to me that we do not know nearly enough about the interaction between normal nutrition and the human body to begin using genetically modified food.

Companies have been genetically modifying plants to contain vaccines, drugs and industrial chemicals ("pharmed" crops). It is universally agreed for obvious reasons that such crops must not contaminate food crops yet, despite safeguards, it has been discovered so far that "pharmed" crops in the USA have twice contaminated fields of soybeans used for food[103]. Another unexpected consequence that opponents of genetic engineering warn about has occurred with a fungus which was genetically modified to be more deadly to the weed it blights, ending up killing the crop it was meant to protect[104].

I had contacted Bob Phelps, the Director of the GeneEthics Network[105] to find out about the "tryptophan affair" and he suggested that I look on the internet using the Google search engine. There I found an article[106] by John B Fagan Ph.D. It recounted how one amino acid, tryptophan, produced in genetically engineered bacteria resulted in at least 37 deaths and 1500 more people being permanently disabled. There was a delay in realizing what was causing this major problem because this tryptophan was not labelled to distinguish it from tryptophan produced without genetically modified bacteria. Over 200 studies have failed to establish with certainty whether the problem arose from the genetically engineered bacteria or from an inappropriate purification procedure. However, if it was the filtration process, then why has the company never tried using this method of producing tryptophan again?

This episode seems to support the need to identify on food labels if GM food is included in the ingredients and a descriptive way to label GM food would be something like, "No natural flavouring, colouring or preservatives!"

We live well on simple, natural food yet the preoccupation with GM food fits with Thor Heyerdahl's[107] belief, "Progress is man's ability to complicate simplicity."

In contrast there is a route generally accepted by all sides and which uses the genetic data from scientific research to dramatically improve how conventional plant breeding is carried out. For instance in 2002 researchers made headlines when they genetically engineered a tomato that could grow in water almost half as salty as sea water, yet equally salt-tolerant tomatoes have been produced by scientific conventional breeding[108] but without the fanfare.

A *New Scientist* report comments, "[conventional breeding using plant genomics] promises progress that's dramatic and fast enough to make GM irrelevant for many problems.[109]"

It seems much better to nudge nature rather than to knacker it.

As I enter my home I hear the none-too-dulcet tunes of a musical instrument waft downstairs. Olly has just started to learn the saxophone, and he is doing his bit on it.

A few minutes later he follows his music down, says, "Hi Dad, are you feeling okay?"

He then tells me that when he grows up he might want to be a rock musician.

I do not want to disappoint him by telling him he cannot do both!

Trek – Day 3

Trekking Truism: A mile on the map will feel
like two on the ground,

or,

A day's walk takes 48 hours.

1991: 26 November, Churia Ranges of the Himalaya

I had fallen to sleep quickly, but got up a few times with
diarrhoea. I think it was thanks to the raksi but remained
confident that the bottom had not fallen out of my world: I was just
not sure if it was the other way around.

I checked the AWO's medical supplies in the morning. They
were in a pretty good state but unfortunately had nothing to offer
me for my trouble during the night – the nearest thing was a cork!

The AWC book indicated a regular attendance at sick parade and
this Centre seemed to be providing a much-needed service to the
community. I decided that it was not necessary to check the
accounts as the AWO had recently taken over and carried out a full
handover.

Shortly after leaving we came upon two small children playing
in the dirt in the middle of nowhere. There was nothing but the
vaguely scenic backdrop of tombstones on the summit of the hill
one hundred metres away. They had grubby cheeks and smiling
eyes which lit up as I handed them a couple of biros from the box
I had specifically brought for this purpose. They grabbed them
elatedly. A woman, I presumed to be their mother, called out for
them. She used terms like "third-born" rather than their names. In
the hills a boy seldom hears his name used or shouted over the hills
as a witch or some "evil-spirits" may get to hear the name and

thereby have power over him. A captured name can lead to a captured soul. The two children did a "Harry Houdini" and disappeared in front of my eyes. The trick was made even more impressive, as in a few minutes a much larger group of children appeared. The hill telegraph worked much better than the phone! Forty biros, brought as trek gifts for the whole trek, lasted less than one day.

The children followed us for a while, all the time laughing and giggling. I asked Subash whether children from different castes played together but I did not fully understand his answer. I guessed they do unless taught otherwise, because children are generally born "colour blind". It takes conditioning by others to make them racist or any other "-ist".

We stopped for bhat near the shimmering green of new coniferous trees. I could see mountain ridge after mountain ridge, each a day's march for a heavily laden man. Around me were a few of the 6500 known species of shrubs and wild flowers in Nepal.

A large proportion of the people (about 42%) lived in poverty and nearly 75% were illiterate. It all makes Nepal a land of both great beauty and great challenges. Subash told me that he believed we all have the choice to be optimistic – a quality epitomising the Gurkhas. I agreed with him that the view of any situation was more a reflection of us than the world. I told him a tale on optimism.

"Two men are sent to a remote part of the Himalaya to sell boots. After a week one sends back a message which says, 'big problem out here, the Sherpas don't wear boots'. A week later, the other one sends back the message, 'fantastic opportunity out here, the Sherpas don't wear boots.'"

As all routes appeared to go more uphill than down I was sure we would get to Everest eventually. There was the constant backdrop of the mountains with their brutish beauty which no photograph or two-dimensional panorama could hope to capture. Despite this, I could not resist trying and started snapping away about twenty-five photographs a day. Much of the time there was little sign of agriculture and the vegetation was sparse. It was all too evident how man and goats have ruined the natural tree cover of the hills, and set up the environment for the yearly landslides which take a terrible toll of life as they sweep communities into raging rivers during the wet monsoon. The dichotomy up in the mountains is that to have hot water, see at night, cook food or keep warm; then, wood is the only fuel available. Therefore to live in the mountains, trees must be cut down, and yet this leads to death in the Himalayas.

We came to a rise at 9900 feet but the evening was closing in and the view disappointing. We had made far less distance than I had planned, or had been indicated by the locals when asked. If my map reading was poor enough then there might be another 19128 feet up before we started going back down.

The porters used large wicker woven baskets called "dokos", which have narrow bases opening out towards the top. They are a flat conical shape and carry a great deal but require expert packing. The porters used the shoulder straps which keep the baskets on their backs when the namlo, or jute headband, was removed. Usually the headband takes the full weight, so their forehead and neck must take most of the force. Each time we stopped, the porters rested on their third leg or "tekuwa" – a "T" shaped walking stick which slotted beneath their baskets so it took the weight off their shoulders. Chandra had garlanded his basket as an offering to the gods for safe journey. I was feeling the load of my more mundane green army rucksack and was tempted to hand over a rather large book to my already heavily laden porters, all 526 pages of the hardback biography on Field Marshal Sir Gerald Templer;

"As things get tough;
Perhaps rough and I'm out of puff,
Or I've just plain had enough,
Preferring even the awkwardness of being in the buff;

I'll pass over the Templer book and other stuff,
Quite off the cuff,
Even if it puts the porters in a bit of a huff."

This ditty belied the fact that the porters would have accepted whatever I gave to them, with good grace.

We stopped after about nine hours in a field oddly reminiscent of *The Grand Junction at Southall Mill* by Turner[110], less the windmill and canal. Another group of foreigners also liked the spot. A team of about ten trekkers and forty porters turned up led by an American with two surnames: Anderson Smith. I wondered why everything's always more in America. He had gone on an Overland bus tour from London to Calcutta twenty years ago, had stopped in Nepal on the way, and stayed. He was a convivial fellow, a bit larger than life and he invited me over for a drink. We talked about how the essential things in life are as much emotional, mental and spiritual, as physical. Tired as I was, I remained deeply awake back in my tent to the sounds of raucous talk from the others at the camp fire.

The Journey Inside – Step 3 – Who Am I?

"… Man in the distant future will be a far more perfect creature than he now is, it is an intolerable thought that he and all other sentient beings are doomed to complete annihilation after such long continued slow progress. [Yet] to those who fully admit the immortality of the human soul the destruction of our world will not appear so dreadful"

Charles Darwin

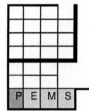

Level of Survival – Social Darwinism

The Level of Survival is the first Level in the model. Again it can be described by a typology. As well as a sound empirical base, typologies also have a strong theoretical one. Humans have a consciousness which by definition means that we can decide what we focus on. However, we tend to focus in the same way each time and it is a well validated psychological construct that past behaviour is the best single predictor of future behaviour. This tendency to have the same focus means that we have a "preference" and this is the basis for typologies.

The Level of Survival is about physical survival which, if necessary, is at the expense of those around us. It is a selfish not selfless focus of higher "Levels". An example of selfless behaviour was shown by a young British padre captured by the Japanese and working with his unit on the Burma railway in World War II.

> At the end of another gruelling day building the railway line, the prisoners were formed up and the shovels, etc, counted. One shovel was found to be missing, and the Japanese officer in charge became incensed, threatening to kill several prisoners at random if the culprit who stole the shovel did not own up. The young padre stepped forward and said: 'I stole it.' He was immediately beheaded. On re-counting the shovels it was found out that there had been a counting error – none were missing.

The young padre's example was one of great "Courage" – a higher energy.

At the Level of Survival we all tend to stay in the biggest, the Main Room, which is the physical one. Wherever we are at, we can quickly be brought back into this Room by the environment and once at this Level we do not concern ourselves with higher things. For instance, if all the air is taken from our surroundings so that we cannot breathe, it does not matter what pleasures are around us, we will only concentrate on one thing – getting more oxygen. But if we have enough air, then air does not motivate us any longer – only unmet needs motivate.

Turn again to Annex A at the back of this Book. Circle the Physical Room at the Basement (Level of Survival) as we *all* have to spend a significant amount of "doing" something or other, in order to survive.

Social Darwinism theorised that people, like animals and plants, compete for survival and, by extension, success in life. Social Darwinists classed individuals who became rich and powerful as the "fittest". Therefore it followed that the lower socio-economic classes were the least fit. They believed that human progress depended on competition. It was used by some as the philosophical basis for racism, imperialism, capitalism and the like. However, new scientific discoveries have reduced the role of natural selection in evolutionary theory, and its application in the social sciences has largely been discredited.

CHAPTER 8
Chemotherapy Number Two

1999: 2–6 August, Cabrini Hospital

Twice the fun today – it's my second chemotherapy. I have found something else makes time go more quickly apart from velocity. A fortnight goes faster when chemotherapy is at the end of it.

I am feeling a bit tired because I took my two sons and Saki to an Australian Rules football match yesterday at Waverley Football ground. It was something they were both keen to do. It is not a sport I follow although there are some very impressive displays of athleticism.

I re-watch the six part series called *Joseph Campbell and the Power of Myth.* Joseph Campbell was a leading authority on world mythologies and religions. He describes lucidly how symbols can have a power over us, especially when we are not consciously aware of them. George Lucas asked his advice when producing *Star Wars* and it is believed that one factor in its phenomenal success was the inclusion of symbols which have been used through the ages in mythologies and religions, and which have a fundamental effect on the human psyche. These include the Dark Side and The Force which of course represent the powers of bad and good, the manifestations of Fear and Love. Campbell describes the essential need we all have to be heroes or heroines, and how this need manifests through conscious or unconscious choice. To actualise this drive we all have to have "the Adventure of the Hero", which involves three steps – a *preparation, journey* and *home-coming.* Mythologies are simply descriptions of external journeys and battles which represent the internal feelings and struggles common to all of us. I would be quite happy to swap chemotherapy for a different battle.

I have readily agreed that a research nurse can interview me about the alternative nutrition and medicines that I am taking, and she arrives around two o'clock. I have gathered a number of books for her and suggest it may be a long interview as I am almost dying to talk. I reassure her that she is investigating a very important area, adding that more people could recover from serious illnesses if they did the appropriate alternative therapy in conjunction with the conventional treatment. I talk about the weaknesses and strengths of alternative therapies' anecdotal rather than statistical approach. I am being pretty forward and she returns the serve asking me why I think I got cancer – a question related to my very survival.

I think it is linked to my mind and body. I think stress depends a lot on how you see reality and becomes harder to deal with when you have them both at work and at home. I tell her about the Holmes-Rahe Scale of stress ratings which gives point scores to forty-three common life events, ranging from 100 points for "death of spouse", 47 points for "being fired at work", down to 11 points for "minor violations of the law". Holmes and Rahe found that 80% of the people who exceeded 300 points in a single year became seriously ill, or suffered severe depression, within the next two years[111]. "Good" stresses like marriage (*50 points*) still aggregate towards this total. Doctor Bernard Siegel, author of *Love, Medicine and Miracles,* found similar results. Ninety-five per cent of his patients with serious illnesses experienced some significant life change just prior to their affliction.

Emerson once said, "The measure of mental health is the disposition to find good everywhere[112]."

I tell the nurse that I believe that happiness comes to us more by choice than chance, whether conscious or unconscious. You cannot avoid many of life's changes but the way you react to change is much more important than the change itself. I have tallied up my score on this scale and it was over 400 points for the period February 1997 to February 1998, and this might have indicated that there was a fair chance I would become significantly ill before the year 2000?

This was compounded by some physical interventions which I believe are significant factors. In 1996, I drank some tomato juice which I had left in an opened can for about three days. Not a good idea. In the Army we would regularly half eat cans of rations and save the rest for later. Unfortunately I did not realize that these cans were made out of a particular metal alloy which made this relatively safe to do. Normal tins are made from a very different alloy therefore it is always a good idea to empty tin cans of all their contents straight after opening them. (It is also not a bad idea to avoid buying dented ones.)

After two tapes worth the nurse asks what I see are the benefits of alternative therapies and I reply, "First, and most importantly, they give hope, second they treat the individual not the group. So they treat the specific not the general, and therefore may provide gentler remedies."

She leaves after thanking me for my time and wishing me well.

It is 6.30 pm before I start getting the treatment for chemotherapy number two. The chemotherapy nurse asks me how I am going.

"I have not had this much fun west of the Himalaya," I reply.

She advises me again on "do's and don'ts" for chemotherapy. She says I should double flush the toilet at home so no family members get splashed with any of the chemotherapy chemicals I pass from my body when they go to the toilet. It may cause others some skin irritations.

I say, "Great, what is it doing inside of me?"

She does not talk about that. But I expect one way to kill the cancer is to kill the body it is in!

She also says it is particularly important that I wear a condom if I have sex within two days of chemotherapy as it comes out in all bodily fluids. She also recommends that I use a condom at all times. It is amazing what you learn on chemotherapy and I do not think it will be a big issue for now.

I am in a ward with three other men, all sixty years plus – Neville, Paul and Ian. It turns out to be Neville's third series of cancer treatments. I think it is with a different cancer each time. He is on morphine pain release and has gone through twenty-two sessions of chemotherapy. He accepts it with a smile – a brave man confronting his own survival.

It reminds me of what someone once said, "Growing old is like being punished for a crime you did not commit!"

I finish the last chemotherapy drip at about 10.10 pm and am not happy. Chemotherapy treatment time varies very significantly depending on the chemicals – Neville's took a grand total of 5 minutes. But there are always pros and cons, and he has to have a colostomy bag. I am having this treatment as an in-patient to get an early night's rest and have an overnight drip to saturate my body with water, a more friendly fluid, while the chemotherapy is injected.

"This is not working", I tell the nurse, "I know it is not your fault as at 8.00 pm they replaced the nurse who started my treatment".

She reacts defensively to what I thought were well considered words. "I know it does not make it any better for you but we are one sister down" and mentions some other reasons which, in my state of frustration, I only see as excuses.

I say abruptly, "Good, I can then expect it not to happen again". She does not react to this comment but carries on describing the exceptional circumstances which made it late.

As she continues, I focus on my own sensations wondering why I am feeling so offended by her not apparently seeing my point of view. My company teaches customer service using a four letter acronym. Lying there I imagine this nurse must have been trained using another about being "MEAN" (*M*ake excuses/*E*mpathise as little as you can/*A*ccept that the patient may not be interested in your excuses/*N*o action is to be taken under any circumstances). I look away, and she picks up on my body language. She apologises and starts to empathise with me.

I do not sleep particularly well. Steroids, apparently if given late, tend to keep you awake. It is probably exacerbated by my frustration, although I am clear that neither the nurse nor anyone else can make me feel that way.

My oncologist visits me at 07.00 am in the ward to check on how I am and I am reassured by his efficiency. I get the irritation off my chest about last night and tell him I do not want a repeat of last night to happen. He listens graciously.

We are soon talking about Lance Armstrong, who I think is the first US winner of the Tour de France. My oncologist says that the usual diagnosis for straight testicular cancer has about an 80% chance of survival. He also says that he thought Greg Lamont, twice winner of the Tour de France in previous years, was the first American winner. I say I think he must be Canadian as he leaves. A couple of minutes later he is back to tell me Lance was not the first US winner (it was Lamont) but that this is the first US team to win. I like having an oncologist with good attention to detail even if his facts spoil my story.

I do not know how I am feeling. It may sound strange but I am not feeling that tired or sick, but not great either. I went to get a blood test eight days after my first chemotherapy. The oncologist happened to be behind reception and looked at the result.

He said, "This is well within normal range" then paused and said "This is fantastic," and asked me how I felt.

"I say I'm okay and don't really know how I feel."

Funny thing is I went away feeling worse emotionally with no idea why.

I am still pretty tired a few days later. I take a sedative, but not the ones the hospital gave to me. Instead I use Valerian *(Valeriana officinalis)*. This is a herbal sedative which has been used for thousands of years. There have been well over 200 scientific studies on it over the last 20-30 years. It is not as powerful as the modern sedatives but is gentler. Unlike barbiturates, it does not interact with alcohol, which is yet to be an advantage in my case. I also use a trick with a lavender essential body oil (in diluted form). Before going to sleep I put a small drop on my fore-finger and then rub it for a few seconds into my forehead and back of my neck. I find this is a surprisingly soporific but also think that high quality lavender oil is necessary so I order very reasonably priced oil from Zurma[113(address)].

My illness is a chance to sleep more. I have built up a debt in the sleep department partly having been working very long hours and effectively not taking any leave in the two years leading up to being diagnosed. I thought I would save my leave for later in my life! This deprivation is not uncommon as our sleep time has reduced by about 20 per cent over the last one hundred years in our modern society[114]. In 1959 the American Cancer Society started a massive study, surveying more than 1 million people about their exercise, nutrition, smoking, sleep and other habits. After tracking the group for six years, researchers found that short sleep time had a high correlation with mortality. If people had originally reported sleeping less than seven hours a night, then they were far more likely to be dead within six years than those who slept an average of seven hours a night. After years of further research, the results still stand. Although sleep needs vary, people who sleep about eight hours a night, on average, tend to live longer. But more is not necessarily better. Adults who said that they slept for ten hours or more per night also had shorter lives[115]!

At 6.00 am, four days after my second chemotherapy, I am still awake, having not slept well. I awoke at 3.15 am thinking about things to note in my diary. Two days ago I got up at 5.15 am to write it as well. I am on a slightly downward roller coaster at the moment, a bit fearful of my progress. I sweated last night – is that a bad sign? It is one of the possible symptoms of lymphoma. I have spent 2 hours on and off visualising my immune system melting away the cancer cells.

I have not felt particularly well since my second chemotherapy. I become anxious. Is this a sign of the Hodgkin's returning or is it a good sign that my body is getting rid of the toxins and cancer cells?

That evening, Saki gives me a simple Buddhist/Christian charm which she made at a Japanese temple in Melbourne. It is very touching, and very characteristic of her caring nature. I feel that we could not hope for a better student to live with us at a time like this. She has a great sense of fun and is incredibly patient with Rob, who is constantly vying for, and getting, her attention.

She asks me what the difference is between the English words "concern" and "worry". A good question to which I reply both are a focus on something or a situation, but worry includes more emotion or anxiety. I think that they can nicely be described by the different Rooms, even if it is not totally in synch with the Oxford Dictionary definition! "Concern" is a trouble in the Mental Room, whereas "worry" indicates an issue in the Emotional Room.

I am also getting strong pains in the reflexology point on the foot related to the lungs, just below the middle three toes on the sole of each foot. This is something that has been very noticeable for the last 18 months. In fact they were so strong that I mentioned them to a doctor, some six months before being diagnosed. I first got a very strong pain in the sole of my foot at the reflexology points for my right lung *(on the sole of the foot)* and, to a lesser extent, my glands *(on the heel)* in 1992. This was three years after having large blisters in these two places injected with tinc benzene for four days. It was so painful that I was unable to walk on it properly although a doctor and physiotherapist could find no sign of any bone or tissue damage. It lasted on and off for six months and I believe it was a sign of this illness starting way back then. Is it a coincidence that I now have cancer in the glands (the lymph) behind the lungs? What I am sure about is that benzene is the most important physical factor in getting my disease.

Are my current pains a sign that the lungs are moving back into their normal position as the tumour shrinks or is it that it is growing again? I am worried and focus on the negative, thinking about a possible early demise. Yet, worry is too often what happens when you take your eyes off your goal, which in my case is to get 100% better.

I phone the stand-in doctor at the weekend and he says to check if I have a temperature as it could be the early signs of an infection. I use the new fan-dangled computer thermometer that Ruth has bought.

It shows my temperature is normal, but I am still concerned, "I feel the fear but am not sure whether I'll do it anyway[116]."

My oncologist comes back to me saying the sweating is nothing to worry about. His words help me to settle my mind. Consciously or unconsciously he knows the importance of maintaining my optimism.

At work some friends there say I look well, but not Mark, my pommy friend at work, who asks me how I feel.

When I say, "I feel tired."

He replies, "Well you look like shit."

It is typical British humour. I rather enjoy the interaction and ask him whether he has ever kicked someone who was standing up[117].

I hired the film *Patch Adams* on video some time ago not realizing how relevant it would be although my Army experience showed me how important humour is to general healing, or even a cure. When Norman Cousins found out that he suffered from a disease that was virtually incurable, and that would kill him, he got his family to bring to his hospital room as many comedy films as his family could find, then spent all day watching them. In his best selling autobiography, *Anatomy of an Illness,* he describes how he was cured of his terminal illness by the "medicine of laughter". When we laugh we actually change our body chemistry. Our body produces peptides and endorphins in our blood stream that can heal our body. The endorphins released are the body's own opiates and are many times more powerful than morphine and hundreds of times more powerful than heroin[118]. Tears of laughter actually have a different chemical makeup to tears of sadness.

Humour can also heal psychologically. It is now ten years since 270 people lost their lives when Pan Am 103 exploded over the town of Lockerbie. I read one report which described how the police were overwhelmed when trying to collect all the body parts so they called in the local Scottish infantry regiment.

Whereas the Police solemnly did this difficult work the soldiers did it with typical humour, saying things like, "I've got the hand who has the matching arm!"

In the end a significant number of Police officers needed counselling for PTSD[119], whereas the soldiers suffered a much lower rate.

What the heck, I have decided to adopt Charles Schulz's[120] viewpoint, "I've developed a new philosophy – I only dread one day at a time."

I am still not sure what feeling right is like. People ask me how I feel and I say "I don't know."

It seems a non-answer, but is an honest one.

A more difficult question is asked by some, "Am I clear that I will get better?"

For me what really counts is how I am sub-consciously.

It is not enough to go around superficially mouthing words to the effect that "I am going to get better" since if I don't believe it deep down it is unlikely to help.

I don't want to crawl across the finishing line at the end of chemotherapy. I want to sprint across the line fast and free.

Trek – Day 4

Trekking Truism: If you cannot read a book a day your porters are going too fast.

1991: 27 November, Churia Ranges of The Himalaya

I woke early to the brisk air and stepped out of the tent and into "shit" – frost in Nepalese. Fortunately, I had also managed to narrowly avoid some mammalian animal waste by my tent. I wanted to go back to the peak, so Subash quickly offered to come with me back up the 300 vertical feet. This time the view was superb, although I was a bit disappointed that I could not see Sagarmatha. The mountains before it were clearly visible but the air is not clear enough to see the apex of the "roof of our world".

It was déjà vu for breakfast. Not wanting to suffer Montezuma's revenge I was rapidly consuming my twenty cans of tuna and managing to reduce the weight of my Bergen as well as my body. At least I would die from monotony before dysentery. It seemed like it was feeding time at the zoo and I was the key exhibit. The track we were near was on the main route between two relatively large market towns; Basantpur and Taplejung. I was a bit of an oddity for locals and indigenous travellers as tourists did not come this way as a rule.

We got on the track at 07.00 am as usual. It took nine hours to get to Sirijung Ward/8, our destination for the day. I had again underestimated the time it would take by some margin. I was finding the map reading difficult and had got Subash to ask the locals for some directions. They demonstrated an uncanny ability to contradict each other's directions. I knew it was not planned … it was done too well for that. My GPS – Gurkha Positioning System – was simply not working. Neither my porters nor Subash spoke the local dialect and I had learnt to take care when translating such directions. I was comforted a little to read that Gerald Templer also encountered language difficulties;

> "Sometimes Gerald ... was less fortunate in his interpreters ... The story is well known of his descent on the New Village of Kulai, ... where a terrorist band had succeeded in overawing some Home Guards and had got away with twenty shotguns and ammunition without a fight. Gerald blasted the villagers. 'I trusted you – and you've let me down. You're a lot of bastards.' (Pause for interpretation, which came out as 'His Excellency says that your fathers and mothers were not married when you were born.') Gerald continued: 'You may be bastards, but you'll soon find out that I can be an even bigger one!' ('His Excellency admits, however, that his father and mother were also not married')[121]."

Along the route we passed a Buddhist shrine perched high on a pass. Some have brightly coloured prayer stones surrounding them. This one had the prayers etched in Tibetan lettering and was probably set up here by Tibetan refugees. My porters always kept them to the right as they passed as one should always walk clockwise around such shrines. I followed suit out of a sense of cultural propriety.

The terraced mountain slopes signalled that we were close to our destination. A "burho manchhe[122]" hobbled stiffly up towards us, fully using his walking stick. His name was 65573 Gopilal Limbu. He must have been over 65 years old and looked every day of it. He saluted me and then talked to the porters. He had walked some distance to meet us; whether by coincidence, telepathy or a more planned means.

He did not hold an official position in the village, and talked about his nine years in the British Army before leaving in 1947.

"What a time to pick military service," I thought to myself.

He had fought the Japanese in Burma for three years. I knew it to have been a severe campaign but he did not mention that. Then he started to cry as he told me he only got five rupees a month, about 15 Pence. It only bought five hen's eggs up here in the Hills. I felt sad as I looked at the old man, while the porters seemed somewhat embarrassed. Despite this all, he bore himself proudly. For him the pension was about survival – about his very existence. It is ex-soldiers like this that organisations like the Gurkha Welfare Trust[123] try to help†.

He described his situation without any bitterness but rather an acceptance of what life hands out. He knew well the human truth that even the moral right to bitterness does not avoid the inevitable outcome – damage to ourselves.

I commented over dinner how tough it was at times for the locals to survive here in the hills. In reply Ratna told me the Indian story of two princes whose father had died. Subash translated.

> "As is common in India the two brothers continued to live together in a single household. However, they soon quarrelled and decided to split the possessions in half. After they had allocated everything they came across a small packet hidden in the house, which had two rings. One was a silver ring studded with precious gems. The other was a similar silver ring but with only an inscription on it. The elder brother, out of greed, declared that the valuable ring was obviously a

---

† Note: Currently the Gurkha Welfare Trust is trying to remedy the situation. The plight of these old soldiers is really no government's fault. Many Gurkhas served only during the critical period of the Second World War, returning to a normal life in their Himalayan homeland. Unfortunately, they did not serve the 15 years necessary to qualify for a British Army Service pension. The British "Tommy" did not get a pension either after the War, but at least he had a social security system to fall back on. Nepal has no state welfare system. So "Johnny Gurkha" had to go back home and take his chances. Something which they did, and continue to do, proudly. Fortunately, thanks to the generosity of people all over the world, the Trust is now paying a welfare pension of some 20 pounds a month to many of these old Second World War veterans and their widows.

family heirloom and should not be sold. Therefore keeping with tradition, he, as the older brother, should take it and the younger son could have the other silver ring.

The younger brother smiled and said, 'All right I am happy with the silver one'.

After they parted the younger brother thought, 'I can understand why my father kept the valuable ring, but why did my father keep this ordinary silver ring so securely too'?

He read the inscription on it, 'This will also change'.

He thought, 'Ah, this must be the mantra of my father', and he replaced the ring on his finger.

As their lives continued both brothers faced life's ups and downs. When spring came the elder brother became very happy, when autumn and winter came he fell into deep depression; every time losing the balance of his mind. In time he became stressed, suffered panic attacks and eventually needed to take drugs to manage his emotional state, and the physical ailments that arose from them. Meanwhile the younger brother enjoyed spring when it came, but remembered his father's mantra, smilingly.

When autumn and winter came he remembered, 'This will also change'.

With all the ups and downs, all the changes in his fortune, he knew nothing is eternal, that everything that comes has to pass away. With this attitude he lived a happy and fulfilled life[124]!"

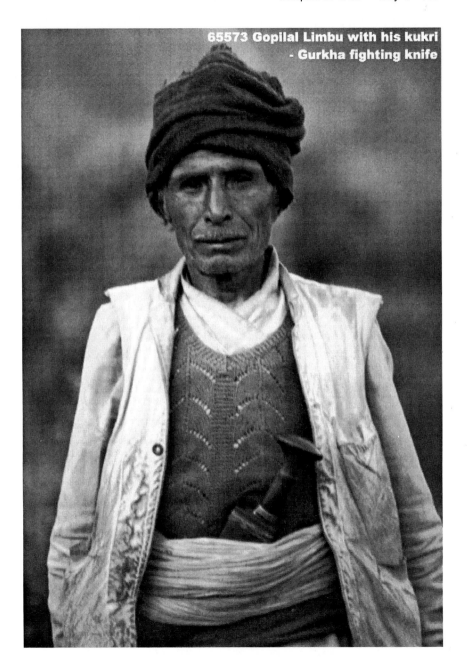

65573 Gopilal Limbu with his kukri
- Gurkha fighting knife

A House in Higher Hills

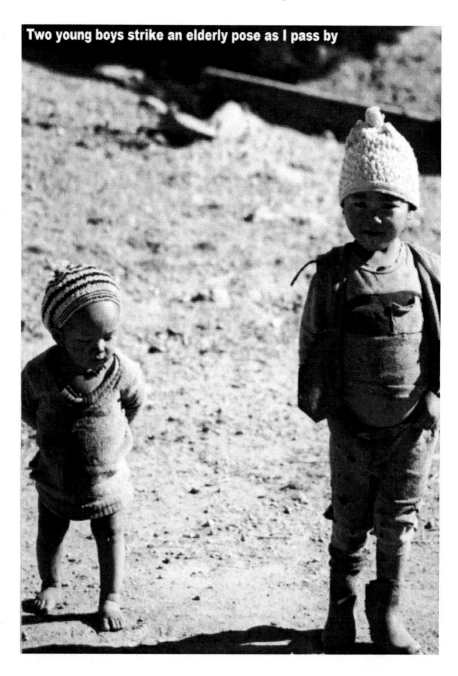

A House in Higher Hills

The Journey Inside – Step 4 – What Is My Purpose?

"He who has the 'why' to live for can bear almost any 'how'"

Friedrich Nietzsche; German philosopher

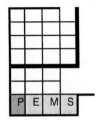

Level of Survival – Twelve Archetypes

B aptism could be considered as the Christian Sacrament which symbolizes this Level. This act may be thought of as the expression of grace which gives us life in this physical world. Our aim at this most basic level is to exist.

At Annex A we see that there is a Fire Escape Ladder connecting the Basement to the Top Floor. However, it is not accessible at any other Level and all Levels are connected by a set of stairs.

The Basement is the lowest Chakra yet it is linked to the 7th, the highest in this framework. In fact the 1st and 7th Chakras are two ends of the same Chakra. So there is an element of the highest in the lowest (and vice versa), and an element of the Spiritual at the Basement too. The Physical Room is the Main Room at this Level.

Carol Pearson Ph.D. describes the archetypes or "inner guides" which guide us through our journey of life and each of these twelve archetypes offers a route to exploring the Emotional, Spiritual or Mental Rooms.

The Purposes shown below can help us to answer Question 2: "What is my Purpose?" at this Level.

Floor Plan for Survival

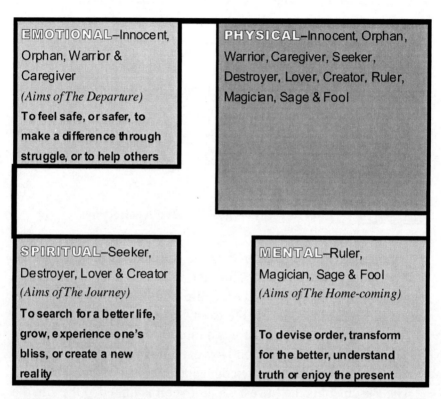

EMOTIONAL–Innocent, Orphan, Warrior & Caregiver
(Aims of The Departure)
To feel safe, or safer, to make a difference through struggle, or to help others

PHYSICAL–Innocent, Orphan, Warrior, Caregiver, Seeker, Destroyer, Lover, Creator, Ruler, Magician, Sage & Fool

SPIRITUAL–Seeker, Destroyer, Lover & Creator
(Aims of The Journey)
To search for a better life, grow, experience one's bliss, or create a new reality

MENTAL–Ruler, Magician, Sage & Fool
(Aims of The Home-coming)

To devise order, transform for the better, understand truth or enjoy the present

This is taken from one of Carol Pearson's books[125]. In it Carol describes how archetypes can help us to prepare for the journey, embark upon the quest, and return to transform our lives. (And this typology can be applied to other Levels too.)

Turn to the "House" shown in Annex A at the back of this Book again. Although it is the same design for all of us, we each live in it differently. We are now looking at how Purpose is defined at each Level.

1 Look at the Purposes in the floor plan above.
2 Decide which one means the most to you.
3 Identify which of the four Rooms it is in.
4 Go to Annex A and look at the first/Basement Level.
5 Mark an "→" in the corresponding Room at that Level.
6 *Mark only one room with an arrow at this Level.*

To decide which Room to arrow at this Level, look at the floor plan above and the verbs associated with each Room.
Ask yourself: "Which of these do you most want to achieve in your life, if any? Which of these is most important to you?"

You may find that none interest you; then just leave this Level "unarrowed". If you want to explore the Rooms at this Level in more detail then Carol Pearson's book is helpful.

Remember we do not need to try to go into the Physical Room because, at this Level, while we are alive we are already there.

CHAPTER 9

Where I Am Decides What I *Can* See, Where I Look Determines What I *Shall* See

1999: 7–16 August

My Father arrives from England early in the morning. Ruth offers to pick him up but I insist on doing it. I get up at 06.00 am to leave for Melbourne Airport – feeling knackered and on the not so great side of good. It is his first time out, but of course he knows the convict heritage of the Australian population.

Therefore if asked, when passing through Australian Customs, "Do you have a criminal record?" The answer is, "I didn't realize it was still compulsory."

My Father stays at home for much of the time he is out here. He and I discuss a wide range of issues including how the preservatives we consume in our lifetime; also affect our "death time".

According to Doctor Nancy Corbett, "The average Australian consumes from 2 to 7 kilos of chemical additives in food each year."

This is probably why human livers are unsafe for human consumption. It puts us in a similar category to polar bears whose livers are toxic because of extremely high levels of Retinol (*vitamin B*) and polar explorers have died from eating them. My Father tells me that a friend of his, who is an undertaker, has told him that they don't need now to fret so much about refrigerating dead bodies. Nowadays they last a week rather than the 2-3 days they did a few decades ago. His friend believes that this is because of the amount of preservatives in them. So our modern food may not help us live longer, but at least it helps us to die longer.

On Monday I go to a Traditional Chinese Medicine doctor and I persuade my Father to join me. He does, and finds it an interesting experience. It leaves me with large, painless red marks on my chest which, in TCM terms, are a sign of blocked energy. Professor Wang emphasises to me the importance of the mind state; that fear supports cancer.

He says, "Everyone has cancer, you have cancer, I have cancer but do not worry, be confident for the body and mind, when it is strong, eliminates cancer."

It strikes the chord of truth with me. Having "no fear" is a very powerful tool in your fight with cancer, or any serious disease. Difficult though it might be.

In Australia there is the Aboriginal practice of "pointing the bone", where members of the aboriginal community who have seriously transgressed the rules have a "bone" pointed at them. Perfectly healthy offenders have been known to go off and die in a short space of time. It is easy to dismiss this as only possible with people from primitive cultures. Yet cultures, such as the Aboriginal one, are in many ways more enlightened than our western urban cultures[126]. Western society also points the "bone", for instance saying we have cancer which is enough to kill us[127]. Of course cancer can kill us, but one that would not normally kill us, might because of our beliefs about this illness. The mind state is pervasive and even knowing this intellectually (in the Mental Room) may not be enough to stop it manifesting in the Physical Room.

Western sciences strength is that it asks for reproducible results, and this is also its weakness. Conventional medicine knows that stress is a major factor in many serious diseases. But stress is purely a "mind phenomenon" – one person's terror is another's delight (take for example public speaking). You cannot measure it exactly so in that way you cannot know for sure if you are reproducing the same situation. How then can you know if you are measuring like with like in any situation?

My reasoning goes like this,

> "To be an objective truth it must be quantifiable, predictable and provable. But things such as spiritual healing are about subjective/personal truth as are many things that impact our lives. Things such as love cannot be quantified, predicted and proved objectively. Does that mean that love does not exist, or it is an illusion? If so, then some illusory things are more important than real things. There are many examples of people becoming better after visiting a spiritual healer, and others where they have not. Does that mean it was a coincidence with those who are healed? Or is coincidence just a subjective truth? But if it is a coincidence that some people were healed and others not, then it is no different to conventional medicine… for treatments such as chemotherapy must work by coincidence too, unpredictably working for some and not for others!"

When I see my oncologist later so he can check me over, he is rather taken aback by the bright red spots left by the acupressure.

I say, "Don't worry; it is not another form of cancer."

I suggest he try TCM but he misunderstands me thinking I mean try treating his patients with it and replies that it would be a good way for him to be struck off. He says that it is important to consider any treatment which has led to a cure within reason. If a man claimed to be cured from cancer by rubbing his back against a tree, then he would not be inclined to follow it up.

Although I can understand this view, the alternative can be low risk and cost, with little to lose and lots to gain.

I thought, "I would look closely at the tree first, and may give it a go myself."

Aspects of Chinese medicine that were dismissed by western medicine are now accepted, like acupuncture which the FDA[128] recently announced was "As good as, or better than" western medicine in treating a variety of ailments.

Allopathic medicine has significant downsides too. A recent study by JAMA (the Journal of the American Medical Association) found that in one year, hospitalised patients experienced approximately 2,216,000 serious drug reactions.

An estimated 106,000 patients died annually from what was thought to be *appropriate* use of pharmaceuticals[129] – described as "Non error, negative effects of drugs!"

It is much the same in other first world countries. "Over one million Britons end up in hospital each year due to bad reaction to prescribed drugs or medical error[130]."

It is not to say that nutritional supplements are not to be used with care as seen from American Journal of Emergency Medicine compiled statistics from Poison Control Centres in the US between 1987-1994. There were five deaths from Nutritional supplements. However, this compares with the 4065 deaths from prescription and non-prescription drugs over the same period.

In fact an article in the JAMA said, "Drug reactions are now the fourth major cause of death after heart disease, cancer and stroke[131]." This may run counter to current thinking but "A great many people think that they are thinking when they are merely rearranging their prejudices[132]."

I am continuing to find TCM beneficial. Early Chinese philosophers described the world in terms of flow, judging the most important aspects and impacts on life as those signified by movement or rhythm. Therefore, they emphasised energy flows in medicine, believing health had to be a balance of energy. For movement to "happen" there must be two opposing forces, the passive – Yin *(coldness, the female principle)* and the active – Yang *(heat, the male principle).* In this medicine the Law of Nature is Yin and Yang – becoming and unbecoming. Yin and Yang run through everything and move all the time. They cannot be independent of each other. Just as "high" has no meaning without "low" or "rich" without "poor". If you have a Yang foundation you will develop Yin symptoms. A strong fit athlete is Yang, they have a strong foundation, and they will develop a Yin condition, a weak immune system. If you have a Yin foundation, say you are sickly, you will develop a fever when stressed – a Yang symptom.

Western medicine focuses on the physical composition of the human body. This physical/chemical makeup of the body can indicate disease. Since Einstein's revelations we know that the human body is just energy in a specific form. Although we may be described in terms of matter, at the moment of our most major change of health, at death, there is a much larger change in energy flow than physical composition. TCM also provides a philosophy for eating based on this understanding of energy.

Lin Yutang commented, "The Chinese do not draw any distinction between food and medicine."
Professor Wang tells me that an ancient Chinese emperor[133] who compiled much of the basis for Chinese medicine, taught, "It is diet which maintains health and is the best drug."

The oncologist says I seem to be progressing as planned and asks if I mind delaying going to the hospital from Monday to Tuesday next week, to have my third chemotherapy. That night I sleep badly again and wake up at 03.15 am sweating. The lump seems to have grown a bit and got harder so I relax as much as possible and visualise it melting away for some time. However, later I have an X-ray and the result appears to show that the tumour has reduced by some 60%. The oncologist is pretty pleased with that but it is safe to say I am probably more so!

Ruth has lent a friend a book about relationships called *Men are from Mars, Women are from Venus*[134] (apparently it is not unknown for it to be filed in the astronomy section!) The friend phones up Ruth and starts talking about Doctor John Gray's book. It has sold millions of copies, and she feels it is a great book. It makes some very perceptive, and humorous, points about typical ways the different genders behave in relationships. Conversely when it comes to processing information, MBTI (*Myers-Briggs Type Indicator*) studies[135] indicate that there are some cross gender similarities with most women, and some men, preferring to make decisions based on feelings, while most men and some women tend to base them on facts. While basing decisions on feeling is not necessarily logical it can be very rational, and neither evaluation method is universally better or correct.

The MBTI also highlights some key relationship issues such as criticism. If we prefer logic then criticism (and praise) is like emptying and filling a bucket up with sand. A bit of praise – put a couple of spoonfuls in the bucket, a bit of criticism – take a couple of spoonfuls back out. Hence our emotional levels move up or down more gradually with feedback. Of course, the bigger the bit of praise or criticism, then the bigger the spoonful. However, for those of us who make decisions based on feeling, giving praise is like blowing up a balloon, giving criticism is like popping it. Another friend says it is best to be just who she is, inferring that it is up to other people to accommodate her however she is. That's fine but it has consequences. It may just mean that they leave her as her boyfriend did a few months back. He tended to base decisions on feelings and he may have left her after she had popped his balloon once too often.

I get a feeling of morbidity when starting to read *Stalingrad,* which my Father has given to me. It is a compelling account of this World War II campaign which tells of the experience of battle and I can identify with some of them. I get to page 223 in no time, and then I decide one battle is enough for the moment.

Ruth comes home and tells me she bumped into a friend and very experienced dentist.

When she told him that I had Hodgkin's, he replied, "There is a body of dentists who think mercury-amalgam is a factor in many serious diseases such as cancer!"

I recently had all my mercury amalgam fillings taken out but look for information anyway. As in many areas, experts seem to have opposing views. This is not so surprising as, to a certain extent, experts know more and more about less and less – whatever their area of study.

"Mastery is acquired through resolved limitation[136]" which can end up meaning that there are more experts but less expertise!

On one hand, silver amalgam has been in use for over 150 years, and is proven by experience? In the UK over 800 million amalgams have been placed in people's mouths since the start of the NHS (National Health Service) in 1947. On the other hand there is not one research article which proves the safety of dental amalgam as a non-toxic substance. In 1991 the WHO[137] published its report in Environmental Mercury – Criteria 118. They concluded that the single greatest source of mercury exposure for the general population is dental amalgam. Up to ten times more than all other dietary and environmental sources combined[138]. The WHO also states there is no safe level of mercury vapour. There seems to be a general move away from amalgams. Since 1997, the Swedish government has stopped recommending mercury amalgam for fillings in children's or teenagers' teeth, and it helps to pay for the cost of removal of amalgam fillings where the person is over-sensitive to it[†].

---

† Caution: Be careful about rushing off and changing your mercury amalgams, especially if you are in good health. It might help just to take an appropriate dose of selenium and vitamin C – but as always see a health professional for advice. The process of removal may lead to releasing more mercury into your body so if you do decide to remove your mercury amalgams then I would recommend seeing a qualified dentist who specialises in doing this.

I am beginning to understand what is happening to health in our modern society. The general build up of toxins in the environment, and in people nowadays, means that toxic interventions, such as amalgam, which people could cope with in days gone by without obvious ill effects, are now pushing people below a "Threshold of Health", and causing serious illnesses in them. Experts have frequently told us that substances are much safer than is accepted later. For instance DDT was developed in 1932[139] and widely used by farmers until the 1970s. In 1969 an Australian Doctor, Warwick Raymont, warned that DDT would promote cancer and reported the results of a WHO study concluding that DDT has been found in human breast milk from all corners of the globe[140]. An expert commented that in many cases women's breast milk has such high concentrations of DDT that, if it was not in such a "lovely container" it would be banned as being unfit for human consumption[141]. Yet it took 60 years before it was acknowledged as a carcinogen[142]. Why couldn't DDT (and other pesticide) contamination be a major factor in the dramatic rise in the rate of breast cancer?

Doctor Raymont's also predicted that DDT would promote osteoporosis and increase global warming. It interferes with calcium metabolism in animals and hence plays a part in osteoporosis. Some medical experts recommend increasing the intake of calcium to help reduce the symptoms of PMT as well. I wonder whether an increased severity of pre-menstrual tension may be linked to the loss of calcium and could be a warning sign of possible osteoporosis in the future?

It is estimated that about 1.5 million tonnes of DDT has ended up in the world's oceans. The algae in the world's waters provide more than 60% of the world's oxygen supply – converting carbon dioxide and limiting the "greenhouse effect"[143]. DDT appears to have killed off large amounts of these algae and may have reduced this oxygen production by up to 85%. The science of "Global

Warming" is extremely complex but it seems rational to assume that the destruction of the ocean plant life has contributed significantly to it. We know that toxification combined with a weak immune system can lead to cancer in mothers. It is the same with Mother Earth. It is as if we are toxifying it too much and destroying its immune system – Earth's wilderness places.

Rob has come back with some change from money that I gave to him to buy some sweets.

He says, "Dad, here's some change for you now that you are not working so much, in your situation you need all the cents you can get ..." Good advice however you spell it.

Trek – Day 5

Trekking Truism: There is a cowpat immediately after the one you have just managed to avoid.

1991: 28 November, Yakchuwa Village, The Himalaya

(See east Nepal side of the map[144])

I got up after an uneventful but unrestful night's sleep. I had left the recce until that day. It was bliss to tuck into a breakfast of fish and chips. Either the fish was getting better or my expectations were lowering.

I flicked through *TEMPLER* and came to the bit about a letter Field Marshal Montgomery sent to the then Colonial Secretary, Oliver Lyttelton, about the troubles brewing in Malaya in 1950:

"Dear Lyttelton,
[about] Malaya
We must have a plan.
Secondly we must have a man.
When we have a plan and a man,
We shall succeed: not otherwise.
Yours sincerely,
Montgomery (FM)[145]."

This could have been the motto for water supply up here in the hills.

I sent Subash off to fetch the village sponsor of the project. This was the person who had requested the survey. He was responsible for providing the village resources and co-ordinating the villagers' work. He was usually ex-British Army. Villages in the East Nepal are more spread out than in the West. In the West the houses are

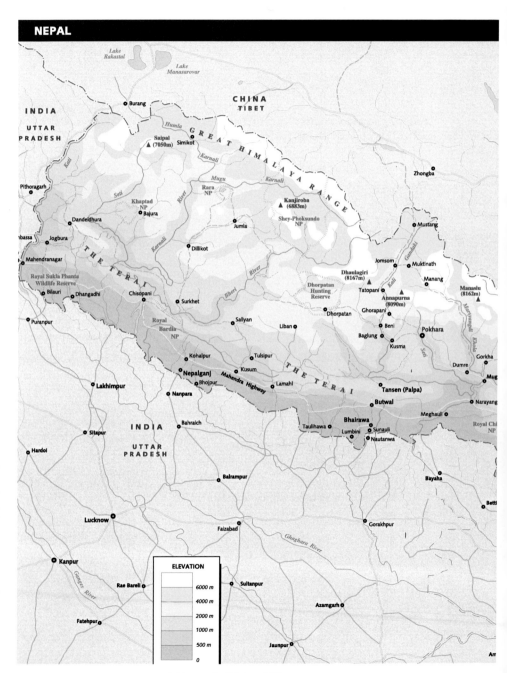

A House in Higher Hills

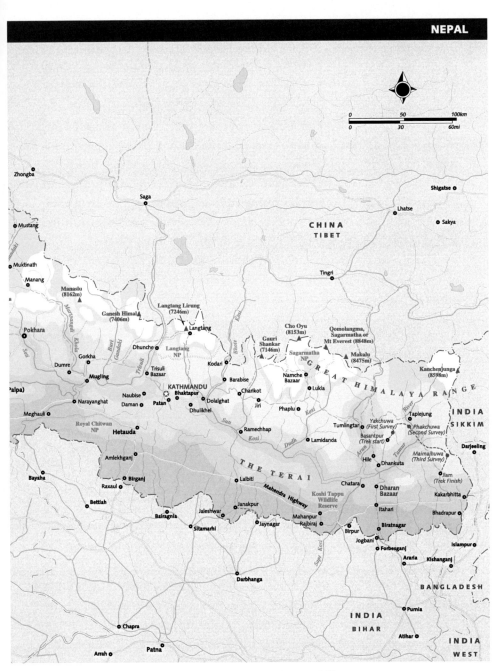

A House in Higher Hills

built close to each other and the land the villagers own is usually in plots surrounding the village. In the East the houses are built on the plots owned by the individual villagers and therefore houses may be hundreds of metres apart. Each close to their own rice paddies.

Some idea of the size of a village could be gauged by the four hours which it took Subash to walk to get the sponsor and return. I thought he had got lost but I should have known that only happens when he is with me! There was lots of work and not much time.

This was a relatively rich village. There was little sign of deforestation and they grew crops such as; potatoes, maize, millet, as well as apples, ginger, and lychees. Livestock was more limited as I did not see any livestock larger or smaller than chickens.

The Pradhan Panch, head of the village council, arrived in the afternoon with an entourage. They all filed up to me and saluted smartly. I thought it a sign of respect although unusual in the British Army as usually you only salute if wearing full uniform including headgear[146]. The Pradhan Panch looked relatively young, in his forties, but exuded a strong sense of presence combined with a gentle confidence. He had doleful dark brown eyes and the respect of the others. All four of them wore drab coloured jerkins and trousers with kukris tucked into cloth waistbands. The greys and greens of their clothes were contrasted by the bright yellow and reds of their Nepalese hats.

We sat around talking about the proposed plan for the water supply system. The water supply was clean and my calculations showed it would provide ample water all the year round. There were about 152 villagers living in 16 houses. Water is such an important commodity in the hills that it is bound to raise emotions and needs strong leadership to sort it out. He seemed to me to be the right man to do what was best for the village. The villagers agreed to dig and bury the pipeline but wanted all the materials provided for them. They also wanted six tap stands, excluding the one at the water source, and a faucet for a toilet. Most importantly they wanted one tap outside the Mukhiya's (village headman's) home. I replied that the water would only adequately supply five taps.

So the bargaining began … Dilba was the Mukhiya. He was small and lean, with an angular face and sharp features. He was adamant that the villagers would not do the digging or burying for anything less than six taps. He also wanted a tap near his house. Discussions got a bit heated and communication became more problematic. It was not so much because of the three languages being used, but was more because the communication emphasised talking more than listening!

I got closer to talking the number of taps down to five, saying, "I want this system built."

This was true, but I had "Shot myself in the foot" with these words as it limited my room for manoeuvre. But at least it stopped the bullet hitting a more critical area!

For them to give me the answer I wanted I needed to find the right question. I had stepped in a few cowpats as I trekked between villages and I now stepped in more, in these discussions. My porters did not understand Limbu as only about 1% of Nepalese speaks Limbu as opposed to some 50% speaking Nepalese. I finally got agreement for five taps when I asked the Mukhiya to sign a statement saying, he would not accept less than six taps and therefore agreed and understood that I would not be able to take the project further.

As we sat around the campfire I began to realize the extent of the work to be done if I was to keep on schedule. I thought about which of my porters were going to be most helpful in this task. Technically I needed Subash because he could translate for me, but he and Chandra also seemed the most detailed, concrete thinkers – and Subash also focussed more on the people element. All useful I thought in this case. Nadur and Ratna were more "big picture", creative thinkers. They would be good back at camp dreaming up some magnificent meal for our return.

The Journey Inside – Step 5 – Who Am I?

"If everybody is thinking alike, somebody isn't thinking!"
General Patton

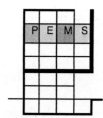 **Level of Wisdom – Decision Making**

A fundamental difference between intelligence and wisdom is in the focus of the decision-making. Wisdom is about an understanding and concern of others, whereas intelligence is more about learning and a concern for ourselves.

Hence the saying, "Too clever by half."

So wisdom has a "selfless" focus and intelligence a "selfish" one, although intelligence is often cleverly camouflaged to look like it includes others. Wisdom is of the 6th Chakra, whereas Intelligence is a manifestation of a 3th Chakra, a Level where the Mental Room is the main one.

The difference can be thought of as intelligence being about knowing the answers, and wisdom about realizing the questions

Life is a continuous series of decisions whether a small one such as "what drink to have", or a large one like "where to go in life". For any magnitude of decision, we gather information and ideas and then evaluate the pros and cons of the options (whether deliberately, or fleetingly in an instant) to arrive at a decision.

It sounds simple but "Most people take in less than one billionth of the stimuli that are present in their environment[147]."

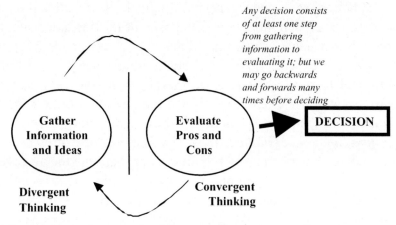

Any decision consists of at least one step from gathering information to evaluating it; but we may go backwards and forwards many times before deciding

All organisms have to do these two things to survive – but many do it in different ways, for instance snakes "see" in the infra-red spectrum. For humans there are only two ways to gather information/ideas and only two rational ways to evaluate the pros and cons.

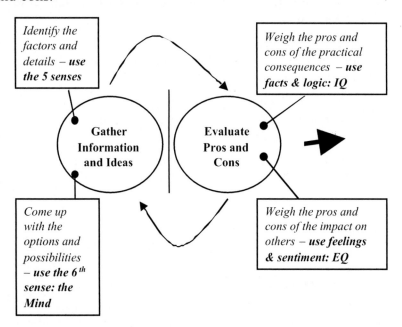

Although sentiment may be illogical, it is rational and is sometimes a much more powerful basis for making a decision than logic. For instance, sometimes a decision is best made by putting justice before mercy *(facts first)* but at other times it is much more powerful to base a decision on mercy *(focus on feeling)*. In the business world we tend to over-use logic (*use abilities related to Intelligence Quotient-IQ*) and under-use sentiment (*ignore abilities around Emotional Quotient-EQ*). The first mass use of IQ tests was in 1918 on American army recruits. Since that time the average IQ score has risen 24 points in America and other developed countries[148]. Comparable samples of American children were assessed in the mid-1970s and late 1980s. In thirteen years the children's EQ had noticeably worsened[149]. Although children from poorer families tend to start at a lower level, the rate of decline was the same across all economic groups.

The MBTI typology insightfully recognizes that intelligence is ultimately a combination of both how we gather information/ideas and how we evaluate them.

Floor Plan for Wisdom
(Where we make the right decision to get the best outcome for all others in the long term)

Look at the "floor plan" overleaf and turn to Annex A at the back of this Book and put a circle in the Room or Rooms that you tend to spend the most time in.

1   Look at the Styles in the floor plan on the next page.
2   Decide which one, or ones, you adopt significantly in your life.
3   Identify which of the four Rooms it is in.
4   Go to Annex A and look at the sixth Level.
5   Mark a circle in the corresponding Room(s) at that Level.
6   *As a guide – it is probably most accurate to circle one or two Rooms at this Level.*

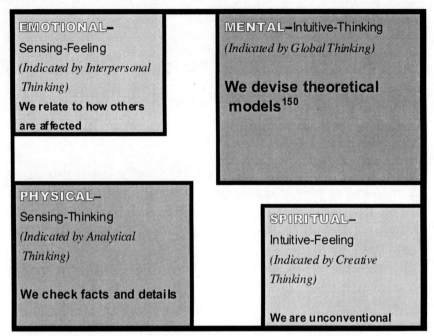

EMOTIONAL–
Sensing-Feeling
*(Indicated by Interpersonal
Thinking)*
**We relate to how others
are affected**

MENTAL–Intuitive-Thinking
(Indicated by Global Thinking)
**We devise theoretical
models**[150]

PHYSICAL–
Sensing-Thinking
*(Indicated by Analytical
Thinking)*

We check facts and details

SPIRITUAL–
Intuitive-Feeling
*(Indicated by Creative
Thinking)*

We are unconventional

The information from the diagram is adapted from *I'm Not Crazy I'm Just Not You*[151]. This book is a good source of more information on these types. (This typology can be applied to other Levels too.)

The different ways we may prefer to "mentally process" information has another major ramification. We tend to see others who prefer our method as more intelligent; they must be because they think like us!

We can do well to remember that "Half our mistakes in life arise from feeling where we ought to think, and thinking where we ought to feel[152]."

CHAPTER 10
Chemotherapy Number Three

1999: 17–18 August, Cabrini Hospital

This time the chemotherapy is started early, but I also get a migraine as part of the package. I ask Ruth and my Father to visit me later in the evening, as I want to have dinner and watch *Yes Minister*. There is nothing like a good laugh straight after chemotherapy!

I have brought Stephen Covey's book, *The 7 Habits of Highly Effective People*[153], to read again. His idea of three states – *dependence, independence and interdependence* align nicely to my model. *Dependence* (linked to immaturity, a childish approach) can be aligned at the bottom of this model – the Level of Survival. *Independence* (related to an adolescent approach to life – the transition from child to adult) is centred at the Levels of Pleasure and Power. At the top are the four ways to *Interdependence* (which is a characteristic of maturity and adulthood) which is when we are able to operate at the higher Levels of Compassion, Courage, Wisdom or Meaning. (The full relationship is set out at Annex C.)

The man next to me has oesophagus cancer of a type which gives him a 2% survival rate. He is 63 years of age and takes it all cheerily. I say I find meditation helps and he answers that it helps him too as he meditates by falling asleep.

A nurse arrives who is very friendly. She points out that I am older than most Hodgkin's patients;

"But I am only 23 years old!" I exclaim.

She gives me a look which suggests that I must have had a very hard life.

When my oncologist comes to see me I ask him about the reports saying that we all get cancers throughout our lives. Apparently we get them, on average, seven times per year but the immune system usually kills the cancer cells off.

He says he would be interested to know how they arrived at the figure "Seven times per year", but agrees that the evidence is that all of us get cancers throughout our lives, but the cancer is usually controlled by the immune system.

Doctor Virginia Livingston-Wheeler seems to support this idea. She has treated hundreds of people with cancer at her clinic with great success and says,

> "We all have cancer in our bodies; it's just that our immune system is keeping it in check … it's the breakdown of our immune system that allows cancer to grow … if you maintain a strong and healthy immune system, your chances of ever getting cancer are virtually nil[154]."

Lisa, a friend of ours, and fellow aerobics instructor of Ruth's, has given us some firewood, which was old wooden fencing in a past life. Lisa is a very bubbly person, with a zest for life. She is the sort of person you need to have at least one of, at parties! I pick the wood up from her garden. Somewhere along the line I end up cutting myself slightly and I am not sure whether it was on wood or a rusty bit of metal. My last tetanus was nine years ago and in Australia more than five years is considered out of date so I check to see if I could or should have a tetanus jab while on chemotherapy. The answer is a definite affirmative from my doctor, oncologist, and all other conventional sources I check[155]. The conventional line is that it is perfectly acceptable to have a tetanus vaccination during chemotherapy because it is not the actual virus. However, some types of vaccinations would be a big "no-no" in my situation. I remain a bit wary but I go to have one all the same.

My Father has not got out much while he has been over in Australia. So I drive him out to the surrounding hills to where some friends, Russ and Margaret, live. Their house is on a hill in Ferntree Gully – or at least one side of a gully. Their view gives my Father a picturesque perspective on the City.

Russ was in my company but subsequently left to set up his own consultancy. He and I have had a couple of discussions on God and whether She exists. He tends to believe that She does not, and I that She does, in some form. One night at a business conference dinner we had a particularly long discussion on the matter. The next morning there were a series of presentations and he was awarded a prize.

As he walked back from receiving it, he passed me and I whispered, "See, God does exist."

A bit later I too was awarded some prize, and Russ joked with me afterwards, "You know, I believed God existed for a moment, but then realized He didn't when you went up to receive your prize!"

We have an atheist's tea – God is not mentioned once. Instead we relax looking at Australians, cockatoos, possums and other animals which scurry past and around the house.

Afterwards, we return home where I look through some assessment work and think back to a best selling book Trevor recommended to me a few months back – *Built to Last: Successful Habits of Visionary Companies*[156]. In it the authors studied pairs of highly successful companies in the same field and same environment, for instance Pepsi and Coca-Cola Amatil. The world of business tends to focus on, and some would say it is stuck on, the lower three Chakras – the drives for survival, pleasure and power. In *Built to Last* one of each pair of the successful companies studied, did what most companies do, and focussed on the bottom line (survival) – at least breaking even. This makes sense because if they do not then they cannot do anything else. But the other of each of these pairs of companies has done much better over the long term, and these are ones focussed on higher Levels. This is what my model, *Mark's Mansion*, predicts as these higher Levels are more energised – have greater potential.

I am brought back to earth tonight when my sons watch *October Sky*, about a young American boy who is inspired by the launch of the Sputnik Satellite to build his own rocket. I do not watch the film but come in at the credits when it describes "what happened" to the young people portrayed in the film, later in their lives. I am just in time to see that one died from Hodgkin's disease at the age of 31...

Peter and I talk about life and the mountain climb we had prepared for the end of October (at the same time as my eighth chemotherapy). I still have it down in the diary. Peter reminds me that I have committed both of us to the Nevis Canyon Bungee Jump in Queenstown, New Zealand. It is 193 metres high and the jump is from a specially designed Gondola.

I tell him I can imagine my wife being approached at my funeral by someone saying, "I am sorry to see that the chemotherapy did not work."

"No, the chemotherapy worked fine, he fully recovered from the cancer but then killed himself doing a bungee jump."

I suggest to Peter that we start practising our smiling for the camera shots.

My Father and I take the boys to kick a soccer ball in the park before he leaves. It is a cold and bleak Australian afternoon, and it accentuates the way I am feeling. The boys shoot away while my Father and I try to keep up with them. After a couple of cold hours we walk back to the car. There is a lady playing Footie *(Australian Rules football)* with her young son.

The son is not too good and after watching the boy for a few minutes, Olly goes up to the lady and says, "He's doing really well kicking the ball."

He then starts by kicking the ball back and forth to the young boy.

Professor Wang commented some time ago, "[Olly] is very wise" after I had taken him for TCM treatment when conventional creams would not cure a severe rash all over his face. (Professor Wang used acupressure and herbs to treat him and he was cured within two days.)

Olly showed a compassion borne from this wisdom when he probably saved my younger son from serious injury despite being only four years old. I had put him in a large bath with Rob who was then about 12 months old. He was in a "bath chair" which had suckers fixing it to the bath floor. I rather foolishly left them unsupervised for a couple of minutes when I heard Olly calling out. The chair had given way and Rob was floating in the bath with Olly holding his head above the water.

I see another article in a sports/nutrition magazine arguing against food supplementation. Poor advice methinks... Eve Hillary[157] points out that,

> "Extensive testing of foods including conventionally grown fruits and vegetables confirms very low levels of essential nutrients and antioxidants. Organically grown foods are not only consistently higher in nutrients, but devoid of pesticide residues. In addition, over 3500 synthetic chemicals are used in processed foods as preservatives, colourings, flavourings, humectants, etc."

A 1991 Nobel Prize Nominee for medicine, Joel D Wallach B.S., D.V.M., N.D. believes that the genetic potential of human beings is to live to 120-140 years.

He warns against poor eating and said in 1994, "Every... human being who dies of natural causes dies from a nutritional deficiency."

Plants cannot make minerals, instead they have to get them from the soil. The US Senate document 264[158] states in part,

> "Do you know that most of us today are suffering from certain dangerous diet deficiencies which cannot be remedied until

depleted soils from which our food comes are brought into proper mineral balance... The alarming fact is that foods (fruits, vegetables and grains) now being raised on millions of acres of land that no longer contain enough of certain minerals, are starving us – no matter how much of them we eat."

That was published in 1936 and perhaps predicted that in the future people could be starving their bodies (of nutrition) while becoming fatter.

More recently a landmark US Department of Agriculture study on 21500 people discovered that only 3% actually ate healthy, balanced diets daily and of the people surveyed not one received the US RDA recommendation of the 10 most important vitamins and minerals on a daily basis.

I am not any more comforted by the use of NPK fertilizers as they provide only three of the 60 minerals we need. A number of studies are finding a massive decrease in the mineral content of food over the last fifty years and since the use of fertilizers. One indicates that you have to eat 75 bowls of spinach nowadays to get the same amount of iron as you got from one bowl of spinach fifty years ago[159]! The head of the British Food Standards Agency, John Krebs, has stated, in effect, that there is no evidence that organic food is any healthier than conventional produce. Conversely, a biochemist, John Paterson, has said that Krebs' statement is founded on little data. Paterson's team[160] has evidence that eating organic food may help to reduce the risk of cancer, heart attacks and strokes[161]. Farming without chemicals can produce more as Kenyan farmers have found when taking up the advice of World Vision and Australian experts. Workshops taught Makuyu farmers the use of composts, making of organic pesticides and care of vegetables and livestock. The results have impressed the most sceptical farmers and include increasing maize yields four fold and in some cases nine times! The *World Vision News* in January 2003 reported that, "Organically grown crops even out yielded those grown with expensive chemical fertilizers – by more than 60%" in Kenya.

It is going to be hard to prove the benefits of organic food. However, there are clues all around us. We have two young rabbits that were taken from their mother at a young age and have only been fed pet shop food. After a year we let them out into the garden and they seemed to know innately what they could eat and what they should not. It is likely that human individuals have evolved to know what to eat too. Confusingly, along come other people or society telling them that certain foods are good for these individuals because these people or society find them to be good. Unfortunately that does not follow logically.

A homoeopath[162]/natural therapist was recommended to me by a friend at work, John. John is an actor with whom I have worked on role-plays as part of the process of assessing managers. He is a capable actor. I try his recommendation out. It is interesting as I have had a bit of a craving for lentils for some time now, and I read a book the homoeopath suggested – *The Eat Right Diet*[163] – with interest. It basically says we need different things depending on our blood type. This makes sense to me as one-minute eggs are good for you, another minute they are not, and the list goes on. The authors believe that the common brown and green lentils can be considered an "anti-cancer" food for those of us with blood type A. That's me and perhaps the reason for my craving? It says that lentils should actually be avoided altogether by blood types O and B no matter what their state of health is. I find this more interesting as Ruth is a blood type O and lentils have never agreed with her. It predicts a whole lot else too. For example, I am allergic to shellfish and crustacean, food that the book says Type A's should avoid.

After reading this book I suggest Ruth go back to a high protein, low carbohydrate diet outlined in a book I got for her birthday last year, *Fat or Fiction: Are You Living a Fairy Tale*[164] by Donna

Aston. Donna was Australian Body Shaping Champion and ranked sixth in the 1999 Ms Universe Body Shaping Championships. Previously she had tried conventional diets, but felt lousy and put on weight. Yet with a high protein, low carbohydrate diet she lost weight and felt great. She has some very good advice about food and supplements too. Ruth does well on this diet but I have tried a high protein, low carbohydrate diet before and felt pretty average. I find *The Eat Right Diet's* advice good for both of us – a high carbohydrate/low fat diet for my A blood type, and a high protein, low carbohydrate diet for Ruth's blood type (while Type B's do best on a varied diet with a little of everything). The argument that a diet rich in meat is essential to build the human body up and make it strong is not very convincing. Humans are omnivores not carnivores, and have an intestinal structure more similar to herbivores. Everyone does not have to eat meat to be strong. Gorillas share 98% of our DNA[165] but are ten times as strong as the strongest man and they just eat plants, berries and leaves. Some of the very best athletes the world has seen were also vegetarian – such as Carl Lewis, who, as a great sprinter, still had to have lots of strength. Anyway Ruth's health improves very significantly; she is a lot less tired and appears more resistant to colds as long as she eats according to the diet outlined for her blood type[166]. (Interestingly, Ruth tries Valerian while I am using it but does not find it to be as effective as I have, as *The Eat Right Diet* predicts.)

Meanwhile I am religiously sticking to my diet although there is too much going on physically for me to know for sure what affect the vegetarian diet is having. That said, when I sit down for long periods I find myself leaning towards the light…

Trek – Day 6

Trekking Truism: Always check that the porters can say more than "yes" in English.

1991: 29 November, Yakchuwa Village, The Himalaya

We started early. I was helped a great deal by the villagers although was a bit confused by the body language. The Nepalese shake their head for "yes" as we in the West say "no", which left me feeling strangely sceptical of their "yes's". Of course it is the unsaid part of the communication, the body language, which was misleading me so much. The shake of the head for "no" in most other cultures is thought to come from the habit of refusing breast milk as a baby by turning one's head to one side. I was not sure where this cultural misleader comes from in Nepal. Perhaps there is such deprivation in Nepal that when a baby wants milk it must look for it!

I finished the survey at dark and had an exact estimate of the requirements. We were kindly offered a cup of tea at Dilba's. His wife served it with her head bowed, as she scuttled backwards and forwards from the kitchen. The kitchen fire is sacred in Nepal and off limits to strangers, so we stayed well out of it. Even a campsite fire is considered sacred and rubbish should not be thrown into it. However, our practice of burning rubbish before leaving camp was a generally accepted necessity.

The Limbu tradition values gold and many seemed to me to over-do it. Most women wore a nose ring which looked like a large "ear ring", which had to take some getting used to. I added a puritab to my tea as I was not sure about the water source or how long it had been boiled. I toyed with the cup as the tabs took fifteen minutes to take effect. My tea was a bit like flavoured swimming pool water, but at least it was decaffeinated … The body really can get used to anything – I was just finding out whether my mind could too.

We talked about their hopes for the water system. Life in the mountains meant that you could not forget that there was one season for sowing and one for reaping. A reality that we seem too often to try to ignore in western society. Either we try to reap straight after we have sowed, or sow just before we want to reap. I could not guarantee that the water system would be built but felt that their chances were high. It is well known that water supply design is like sexual relations, better between consenting parties, and I enjoyed a chance to joke and drink. After an hour we headed back to our tents stopping on the way to buy rather expensive eggs for 3 rupees each.

I took a multivitamin before lying down as I thought it was probably a good idea on the limited and unvaried diet I was having. As usual I got the two man bright orange tent, Subash the one-man one, and the three porters huddled under a single ground sheet. It was pretty cold and rained intermittently throughout the night. It all seemed a very unfair, but standard, trek sleeping arrangement. My porters would not have dreamt of having it any other way, fortunately for me!

Nadur had been explaining the caste system to me. Although the caste system is ignored to a certain extent in the big towns, it is obviously abided to up here in the hills. There are four basic castes, which can be largely identified by their tribal name. The Bauns, or priestly caste, are the most privileged and officiate at child naming, marriages, and horoscope readings. The Nepali Royal family comes from this caste. Then there is the Warrior caste that provides the bulk of the soldiers in the Nepalese and Indian Armies. Thirdly there is the Farmer/ peasant caste that provides many of the soldiers in the British Army. The smaller and lesser tribes form the lowest caste and are linked to occupations thought to be more menial in Hinduism. These include the Damai tribe, who tailor clothes and a musician caste, which provides music at weddings and funerals.

I talked with the porters about social duty and that having self-respect helped us to help others. For Ratna this came from a sense of "good will", whereas for Chandra it came from doing "good deeds". Subash took a completely different perspective on it, feeling it was about a graceful approach to life, while Nadur thought it arose from independence. Something that he had hoped the money from this trek would bring. From our discussion I saw a bit more of the coming together of ideas from "west and east". Starting with Hippocrates and Plato around 450-340 BC and their *Four Temperaments,* people and cultures in the West have noticed four main, and pretty distinct, personality "types". They seem to line up to the four Hindu goals in life that Ratna had told me about.

- Liberation = *Idealist*
- Success = *Rational*
- Pleasure = *Artisan*
- Duty = *Guardian*

Perhaps I was making a bit too much of the connection and as the fire's embers died, I crawled back to my tent only to be accompanied by a mosquito which proved you do not need to be big to make a difference, as he kept me awake for a few hours. I had heard that if you put out a cut tomato it drives mosquitoes away. Unfortunately I did not have the tomato, and would not have had the strength of will to resist it even if I had.

The Journey Inside –Who Am I?

"A coward is incapable of exhibiting love;
It is the prerogative of the brave"
Mohandas Karamchand Gandhi; known as "Mahatma"
which means "great soul"

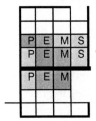 **Transition Levels – Temperament Theory**

The Transition Levels are the key point when we move from a focus on self to focus on others. In other words as we go from Power through to Courage. In this model there is a difference between being "stuck" or "showing a preference" even in these higher energies. Being stuck limits us, limits our choices, and conditions our lives. It is as if we go around trying each door on the one floor, thinking it is a complete life – the whole House. This is different from preferring to operate in a particular Room across all Levels which still gives us real choices in our own lives.

There are three questions below, adapted from David Keirsey's work on typologies, which may give an insight into what your own preferred style might be at these Levels. Choose one answer for each question. Think what your answer would be in terms of what you would prefer to do in your "own" environment, an environment in which you are very relaxed, being who you naturally are and doing what you would naturally want to do, with no external commitments to anyone or anything. This environment may be your home. Think if given the best of all possible worlds, what would you prefer to do, how would you prefer to act. Remember that there is no right or wrong way, nor better or worse way to answer. Imagine that you are free to choose what you want to and are not limited by any current situation.

1. What is your main source of self-esteem? This is one part of the Level of Power, where you derive your feeling of self-worth. It may also be your source of self-pride:

   a) Artistry – *feeling graceful and beautiful.*
   b) Respectability – *gaining recognition and respect*[167].
   c) Ingenuity – *showing inventiveness and innovation.*
   d) Empathy – *experiencing the feeling of understanding.*

2. What is your main source of self-respect? This is one part of the Level of Compassion; how you "put the emotional needs of others before yourself", It is an aspect of your ability to "love" and a pre-requisite for this is often loving or respecting yourself:

   a) Adaptability – *feeling spontaneous*[168].
   b) Beneficence – *doing good deeds.*
   c) Autonomy – *having independent thoughts.*
   d) Benevolence – *being of good will.*

3. What is your main source of self-confidence? This is one part of the Level of Courage, where "courage" is best defined as acting for the sake of others. How you "knowingly risk yourself physically, emotionally or mentally for the sake of someone or something else"- (when it is for our own sake, we tend to be acting out of a desire to control our lives or surroundings, and this is a part of the Level of Power):

   a) Audacity – *experiencing bravery.*
   b) Dependability – *taking accountability.*
   c) Resoluteness – *demonstrating resolve.*
   d) Authenticity – *living genuinely.*

Note your answers for each question by ticking in the relevant box below:

	(a)	(b)	(c)	(d)
Question 1 –				
Question 2 –				
Question 3 –				

(The definitions of the four styles – artistry, respectability and so on – are taken from David Keirsey's very complete guide on Temperament, *Please Understand Me II*[169] and a much more complete test, *The Keirsey Temperament Sorter II,* is in his book.)

Remember, typologies do not tell the whole story. If you are an *H* type, then in some ways you are like all other *H's*, in some ways you are like some other *H's* and in other ways you are like no other *H's*. On the next page is the Temperament style indicated by your results…

In terms of Temperament Theory we are probably:

- An Artisan if we answered mostly (b)'s =>
  We prefer to feel.
- A Guardian if we answered mostly (c)'s =>
  We prefer to act.
- A Rational if we answered mostly (d)'s =>
  We prefer to think.
- An Idealist if we answered mostly (a)'s =>
  We prefer to move beyond action, feeling or thought – to "be".

We may still be unclear about which Temperament style we are for a range of reasons, noting that this three-question test is, of course, a very simple one and is only a beginning. Keirsey's Temperament Sorter II gives a much better idea. Other reasons this test may not be clear include:

1 The questions are not clear to us, or we are not clear about our own preferences.
2 The environment has conditioned us in a way that is very different from our natural preferences.
3 We are trying to be someone different from who we are naturally.
4 We are in our thirties or older, and are therefore going through our natural stages of development where we become more interested in other preferences.

We can think of typologies offering us insights into who we are. This may be thought to cause stereotyping. However, in a way, it liberates us for we can intentionally be who we are not, only when we know who we are!

CHAPTER 11

"It is better to light one candle
Than to curse the darkness"

Anonymous

1999: 19–26 August

We have a family dinner for my Father's last night. Olly is merrily chatting away while eating at the dinner table.

So I tell him sternly, "Do not eat with your mouth full."

He starts laughing before anyone else, and, knowing what I meant, says, "How am I supposed to eat?"

Chemotherapy seems to be a good excuse for my confusion.

I give my Father his 70th birthday present – six bottles of fine red wine – as at 70 years of age it is probably worth receiving something that you can experience fully rather than a memento you keep for the rest of your life. But then that is sometimes true for a 37-year-old.

One of the first things I did, when I joined my company two and a half years ago, was to check that I was covered by sickness and disability insurance. Which I was. However, in February this year I felt compelled to check again, even insisting that a copy of the policy be sent down to me so I could check in detail. Did I know something then at some level? I talk with the insurance company rep about my insurance cover on the way to work. He is very considerate, and it looks like he will be able to ensure that I am covered despite the fact that, according to the letter of the policy, I may not be. Chemotherapy, as a day or overnight procedure, is not actually covered by this policy. We talk about his personal situation and he has lost a number of family and friends to cancer. He empathises with my situation and I thank him while still feeling stress at not knowing for sure whether I am going to be covered.

Saturday night I have the most incredible flatulence all night. It is not great fun for Ruth who tries on my Army gas mask but it does not fit. I have never experienced anything quite like this and clearly something is not quite right? By Sunday my left eye is beginning to hurt more, redden and swell up. Not a good sign. I go to see Doctor Soosay. He is professional and attentive as always. It looks like an eye infection and he thinks there is some pus, so he gives me a prescription for antibiotic eye ointment and cream.

It turns out to do very little for me. I am in increasing pain. I try to work at the computer and do some gardening by keeping my left eye closed. On a scale of *0* to *10* for determination I am a *12*. A level better described as "stubbornness".

I see the homoeopath again today. He identifies one possible factor in getting Hodgkin's was that two years ago I had three large amalgams removed, and it seems that quite a lot of mercury was left in my system. Is this a coincidence with what my dentist friend said a few weeks back? It is all the more strange because about three months after I had had these fillings taken out I had got an unusual and severe headache. I had likened it to having cool molten metal droplets falling onto my brain! At the time I did not link it to mercury as I had had it all removed from my teeth … so I supposed. He also demonstrated an uncanny ability, with his Mora machine, to identify other chemicals I have ingested, and picks up the tin poisoning. I rationalize this as having pushed my body over a toxicity "threshold" causing me to becoming ill. The homoeopath uses electronic acupuncture, which prompts the body to eliminate certain toxins and he recommends I take a microalgae to help move the mercury out of my system. It is Chlorella, produced by a Japanese company[170].

> "The Chlorophyll in Chlorella is one of the most powerful cleansing agents found in nature. It feeds the friendly bowel

flora and soothes the irritated tissue along the bowel wall. Microalgae also help suppressed immune systems."

Chlorella is a single celled fresh water plant believed to be one of the earliest forms of life on earth, existing some 2 billion years ago. It is also one of the richest natural sources of RNA and DNA[171].

The adverse effects of mercury can be very diverse. My homoeopath had a woman bring her young child in. The child wet her bed every night and the mother had tried conventional medicine and other therapies unsuccessfully for years. My homoeopath thought laterally when the mother mentioned she was going to have her mercury fillings out. Although the child did not have any fillings, some people believe that mercury from the mother can cross into the foetus during pregnancy/birth. Sure enough when he tested the child it indicated significant mercury toxicity. So he carried out a detox process with the Mora machine and a week later the mother contacted him ecstatically. For the first time the child did not nightly wet the bed – for six out of seven nights that week†!

Wendy is a close friend of ours, and fellow aerobics instructor of Ruth's, and she often sends me humorous emails. I chuckle as I read a biblically based one that she has forwarded.

> Apparently Adam was feeling unhappy and God asked him, "What is wrong with you?"
>
> Adam said, "I don't have anyone to talk to."
>
> God said that He was going to make Adam a companion and that it would be a woman.
>
> He added, "This person will gather food for you, cook for you, and when you discover clothing she'll wash it for you. She will always agree with every decision you make. She will

---

† Caution: Removing amalgam fillings can potentially release mercury so must be done very carefully. It may then be worth following it with a procedure, such as using the Mora machine, which can reduce any residue remaining.

bear your children and never ask you to get up in the middle of the night to take care of them. She will not nag you and will always be the first to admit she was wrong when you've had a disagreement. She will never have a headache and will be passionate whenever you want her to be."

Adam asked God, "What will a woman like this cost?"

God replied, "An arm and a leg."

To which Adam enquired, "What can I get for a rib?"

The rest is history.

By Wednesday I am not feeling fantastic. I keep having the strong feeling that my left eye is being squeezed and stretched, as if it were in some form of vice. This bit is not painful and I optimistically assume that my left eye is correcting its short-sightedness. I go to my Chinese doctor. He recognises the pain I am in and instead of a normal treatment just puts his hands on my abdomen for several minutes. It is strange to say, but the pain goes completely with no other treatment! However, after three hours it starts coming back again with growing intensity. I try a number of other pain relief methods, including singing too loudly to myself. I have chucked my teddy bear well into the corner by now. I stay at home wearing sunglasses or a patch over my left eye, while Ruth prefers to call me "Stevie Wonder" rather than "Nelson". I am getting very pissed off at the situation and also feel sure that the tetanus vaccination is directly linked to my current situation.

Thursday morning I get up at 04.30 am in much more pain and phone my Mother in England. It is probably an instinctive reaction, what a child does when in pain. But I do not tell her about the pain. I just talk for a bit. I phone Doctor Soosay and tell him how bad I feel and he tells me to go immediately to an eye specialist.

I drive there in a lot of pain and say loudly to myself, "Oh dear, this is all rather tiresome; it is a trifle painful."

Well those are not my exact words, but they capture the gist of what I say. When Doctor Joe Reich[172(address)] comes in, I mumble something about my left eye and pain. He whips out a little bottle and squeezes a couple of drops into my eye. The pain disappears instantly.

He says; "How's that feel?"

I say "Pretty bloody good" and only just resist the temptation to kiss him!

It was a bottle of anaesthetic drops and he quickly diagnoses shingles in the eye.

Shingles is the Chicken pox virus (a herpes virus) coming out to play when your immune is down. It can come out anywhere on the body. I have a large ulcer at the back of my left eye. There is a drug to treat it called Zovirax[173]. It is so expensive at A$30 per pill that my specialist has to get permission to use it.

In the instructions it lists possible side effects and then states "A small number of patients have had other unwanted effects after taking Zovirax."

I just hope I get some of the "wanted" ones; things like "an intense feeling of euphoria"…

Before this drug was around you had to grin and bear it and risk some more unpleasant side effects such as permanent blindness. Doctor Reich says my case is apparently moderate and he has seen worse. All I can say is that they must have been in absolute agony. This has been my nadir so far. I hope things do not get any lower.

I look up the reasoning for shingles in *You Can Heal Your Life*[174]. Interestingly it says: "Waiting for the other shoe to drop. Fear and tension. Too sensitive."

I don't know if others would agree that "too sensitive" applies, but the part about fear and tension might well. I am waiting for the Hodgkin's to disappear completely after each chemotherapy. Each morning I am very aware of the lump on my neck. I am conscious of it being there and anxious of any changes or pain. For instance it seems to harden up overnight and it was also for the first time painful to touch recently. What does that mean? Is it now a sign that my nerves can now detect it?

The mind is an important factor. Ian Gawler was diagnosed with osteogenic sarcoma in January 1975 and his right leg was amputated. His cancer reappeared in November 1975 and most people die within 3 to 6 months of developing secondary growths. But he recovered and was declared free of active cancer in June 1978. He now runs a Cancer Foundation and has publishes a very helpful book *You Can Conquer Cancer*. It is very useful reading.

He notes that "There is a typical psychological profile which occurs in 95% of all the many cancer patients with whom I have discussed the disease ... (the number exceeds one thousand)[175]." This profile was first put forward by Doctor E. Evans in 1926. It has gained increasing attention over the last few years, especially from the work of Doctor Lawrence. It is outlined in *You Can Fight For Your Life*[176]. Le Shan's work has been criticised as retrospective but the findings of Doctor Caroline Thomas, a psychologist at Johns Hopkins University, Baltimore, found the same result prospectively. Doctor Thomas was more interested in cardiovascular disease than cancer. But in interviewing medical students and tracking their history of illness, from a study of 1300 subjects she found that those who developed cancer had distinct psychological profiles. This included, during the patient's youth, feelings of isolation and despair and then the loss of a meaningful relationship (with a person, animal or work) which led to greater despair, reactivating a childhood sense of loneliness or aggravation.

> "They were often spoken of as: 'She was such a good, sweet person', or as 'such a saint'. The benign quality of goodness of these people was, in fact, a sign of failure to believe in themselves sufficiently, and of their lack of hope[177]."

At last, proof of something I keep telling Ruth: I am an angel!

It is true that some of this applies to many healthy people too. But their "House" is probably supported in other ways. At eleven years of age, I went to a good English boarding school with a healthy religious ethos *(the spiritual)*. Ardingly College helped me greatly both academically *(the mental)* and in sport (*the physical*); however, I encountered there a bit of psychological bullying which resulted in occasional feelings of despondency (*the emotional*). I think this was a factor linked to my temporarily having Hodgkin's. The door to illness was opened slightly further by changing my diet about 18 months ago. Up until then I always had lots of fruit for breakfast, and hence a high vitamin C intake. A study by Doctor A.W. Greene studied the psychological and social experiences of patients who developed leukaemia and lymphoma over a period of fifteen years. He too observed that the loss of an important relationship was a significant element in the life history of the patient. For men and women the greatest loss was the death, or threatened death, of a mother.

My Mother went to boarding school at six years of age and found it lonely and unpleasant. Her earlier years fit this "model" too. Not that everyone who has had this experience will get cancer – just that they may be more pre-disposed to it. Other research suggests that childhood physical conditions may also predispose us to illness. Mounting evidence shows that a child's diet is linked to the occurrence of adult prostate cancer, breast cancer and colon cancer[178]. In fact 30-35 per cent of all cancers are diet related[179]. A factor in the high rates of breast and prostate cancer in the USA has been linked to the high intake of dairy foods. The USA and the Netherlands (which also has a large dairy industry) lead the way for breast cancer deaths, and the USA has the highest rate of prostate cancer. Countries like Thailand, whose people eat very little meat or dairy products, largely depending on rice and vegetables, have almost negligible deaths from these two cancers.

Another important childhood experience is your family situation and the relationships. I am re-reading *Learned Optimism* by Doctor Martin E.P. Seligman and he says:

> "It seems ... separation or fighting in response to an unhappy marriage is likely to harm your children in lasting ways. If ... parents' unhappiness rather than overt fighting is the culprit, I would suggest marital counselling aimed at coming to terms with the shortcomings of the marriage[180]."

It is easy to divorce in our modern society and that may mean that we divorce too quickly. This is certainly not to say that single parents cannot bring up their children very well, of course they can. As a simile, some one-legged athletes can sprint 100 metres incredibly fast although it is usually easier with two.

Also separating is important when there is physical, emotional or mental abuse involved. In a study of bad parenting which was defined to include verbal or physical abuse and exposure to arguing parents (as well as neglect, lack of affection and discipline), children were shown to be more at risk from a host of behavioural problems, including depression, anxiety disorders, substance addictions and disruptive behaviour[181]. Lack of discipline adversely affects other animals too. I heard recently that a South African game park was having problems with juvenile male elephants which were going out of their way to be violent, "mugging" other animals and in some case trying to "rape" female rhinoceroses. Someone realized that the problem might be due to a lack of discipline – there were no fully mature elephants in the park to maintain order. Sure enough, they shipped in a couple of fully grown bull elephants and the problems stopped! The novel, *Lord of the Flies*[182], by William Golding describes how humans are no different.

A close friend, Nola, sends Ruth a card. Nola is the aerobics' coordinator at Ruth's Gym, and they hit it off immediately. They have very similar personalities – both have a contagious enthusiasm, natural creativity and tremendous empathy for others. Nola has written:

"No hesitation should be thought
Of calling us to come
It's only when we hold on tight
That friends can feel as one

Just take the time to look at things
And keep a balanced mind
There's clarity in doing this
And miracles you'll find… "

I was wondering if there might be the miracle of guardian angels but in that case mine seems to be on a coffee break.

Trek – Day 7

Trekking Truism: If you arrive at a village which corresponds to where you think you are on the map, you are not where you think you are.

1991: 30 November, Tehrathum, the Himalaya

I finished the survey that afternoon. Dilba and Ratnabahadur were evidently the major influencers in the village and they were aware of all the planned pipe and tap locations. They also greatly helped me with the survey. I kept Dilba's tap to the last which made sure that I got the maximum village resources all the way to the very end. It was useful considering my tight schedule.

As I had weaved my merry way down the hillside I had passed a myriad of houses with vegetable gardens and with marrows here and fruit trees there. I could almost have been in England barring the mangoes and the small houses. While it was true that houses back in England were generally bigger, more of them tended to end up as broken homes.

The villagers' day is never finished. Some were repairing or extending their houses, some building fences and retaining walls, and others preparing the land.

A villager walked up to me. I prepared myself to be ruined by the praise for doing the survey and helping the village take another step towards building a water supply system. It therefore took some time for me to realize that he was not happy. Apparently there was the feeling that an adjacent district with a school in it should be a higher priority. Could I have just surveyed the wrong village? My confidence in my map reading took a bit of a dive. The villager was a teacher called Netradahal.

There was no Mukhiya for this part of the village because of the recent changes in the Nepal's democratic system. He did not explain why this was but he told me that Nepal had a pyramidal, three-tier system of panchayats, or councils, below the national level and that they were all still trying to come to grips with the implications of these changes. In ascending order of importance were the village, district, and then zonal panchayats. Village panchayats were directly elected, and members of councils at the two higher levels were predominantly chosen by the panchayat at the next lower tier. The King retained executive power as he directly chose 16 members of the 35 member National Panchayat. The ban on political parties had just been lifted in 9 April 1990 and the opposition were leading an interim government.

I arranged to meet up with a group of eight representatives from this Ward and they had a good case. I promised to put their case forward and later found out that another officer from the Regiment, Lieutenant Andy, recced both areas the year before. He was only tasked to do the Ward with the school in, but the villagers requested that he do the other Ward too – the one I have now done – and he had surveyed it as well. I never clarified whether he did it because he did not know where he was either!

Back at my first survey Dilba agreed that they would have to do a lot of the digging and cover some of the cost. I told them to make arrangements through the AWO in Silsiliwar. It was then off for the final signing and a celebratory drink at Dilba's house. It turned out to be quite a little ceremony but had an informality which was so natural in the hills. I had a long talk there, with an ex-Queen's Gurkha Captain. He was a man of influence and obvious capability, and had done very well to reach this rank as all Gurkhas had to start from the rank of Private.

Dilba offered to show us the short cut to our next destination, Chuwan Danra. I thought it a kind offer but almost refused as I thought it would not save us much time. Almost one hour out of the village we passed a memorial standing in some splendour and isolation. It was built in memory of Dilba's only son, killed in his twenties. His son was involved in a vehicle accident in a Nepalese city. Dilba had built it on his own as a pilgrimage of love for his son. It was hard for me to really understand the loss of an only son for a Nepalese father. Not only was it a cultural divide which I was unable to bridge but it was also an experience I had only half of. I had a son who was still alive, so did not have that "experiential wisdom". However, it left me more confident that Dilba was the right man to lead building the water supply system — no small job.

I found it hard not to be content wandering these hills. We walked along tracks which weaved their way steadily uphill, then climbed steep rocky paths and dropped down to streams crossed by simple bridges. The bridges often comprised of felled trees and with one side planed to give a flat surface. Where we were crossing large rivers the bridges were of heavier logs, with simple bamboo railings, cantilevered out over the headwaters. They were always temporary as the bridges might not survive the flash floods of the Wet Monsoon. These bridges were a lesson in perception. It was easy to walk across a log bridge a metre or so above the river. When we came to a similar one about six metres above the dry river bed, Subash and the younger porters still galloped across it with gay abandon. Conversely Ratna and I crossed it like older, perhaps wiser, men. *Fear* is all in the mind and if fear is "*F*alse *E*xpectations *A*ssumed *R*eal" then perhaps death is an illusion too.

It was two and a half hours straight, and up, before we completed the "short cut". We stood on a resting platform built into the side of the hill in the middle of no particular place. These stone platforms were built by travellers, for travellers, so they could rest

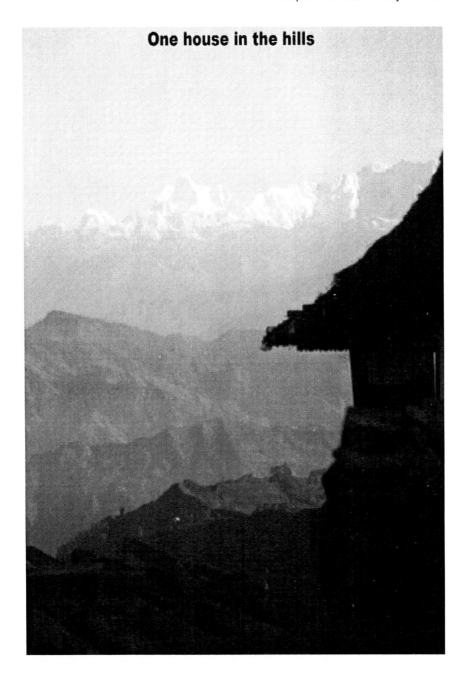

A House in Higher Hills

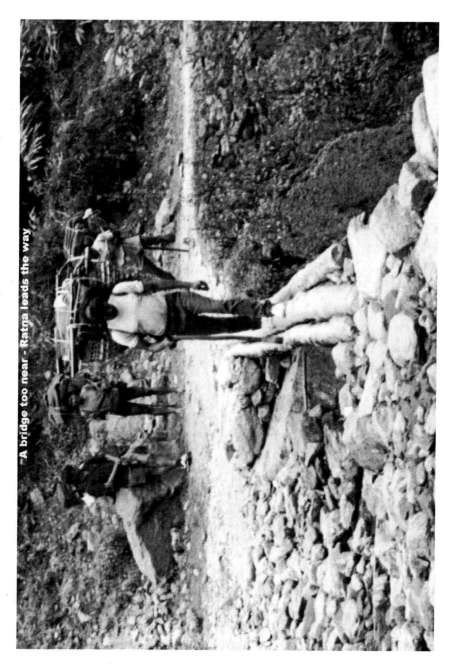

A House in Higher Hills

their heavy loads in secure upright positions. They marked the generosity of spirit here in the hills.

The valley's features were briefly accentuated before dying in the darkness as dusk kicked in. We bade farewell to Dilba and marched on. I could not smell it then but I guessed we walked with the "smell of travellers" that I had noticed at the start of my trek. The combination of heating fluids, flowers, food and fleeces which gave that distinct smell of trekking. While the grunts, gasps and group whistles which porters used to keep order, gave it its distinct sound. Two hours later it was time to pitch camp at a place called Hang Pang.

Ratna told me that he had had children when very young and it must have been tough, but good things came out of it. In the West women generally have far more opportunities than women in Nepal and other eastern cultures, which has been one of the major advances in Western society. But life is a combination of pros and cons, and the increased number of opportunities can mean that we may not realize the choices that are most meaningful to us each personally – until too late.

The porters seemed to differ in the way they saw the parenting role. Chandra believed that children must be civilised and fully support the community, whereas Subash saw things very differently. He believed children should test the boundaries of their environment for them to become free spirits. Nadur felt the parenting role was to help children to learn and become progressively self-reliant in handling life's many challenges. While Ratna simply strove for his children to have a positive self-image. Overall, both Ratna and Chandra saw the parent to child relationship as more of a "senior" to a "junior", in contrast to Subash and Nadur who saw it as one of equals, more like a brotherly or sisterly relationship.

I was beginning to believe that it was important to combine their different approaches. Early in a child's life it was Ratna's building of self-esteem, then Subash's testing of the boundaries, next Nadur's self reliance (*taking responsibility for oneself*) and finally Chandra's civilisation (*taking responsibility for others*). The difficulty appears to be that as parents we favour one of these approaches most of all and too easily use the same approach throughout our children's life. If there is "compassion with a purpose" then it is parenting, and nature has a funny habit of making sure that the children favour a different Room to the one that their parent prefers.

The Journey Inside – Step 6 – What Is My Purpose?

"You can't live a perfect day without doing something for someone who will never be able to repay you"

John Wooden

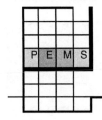 **Level of Compassion – Temperament Theory**

This is one of the levels of *L*ove, not *l*ove with a little *"l"*, which is often another word for lust or sexual passion, and is characteristic of the Level of Pleasure.

Being at the Level of Compassion can be defined as "putting others' emotional well-being before our own". In other words it is one form of love. The Main Room at this Level is therefore the Emotional one. To move to the Level of Compassion we must have self-respect. We have to believe in our own rights as well as others'.

As the saying goes, "To be able to love others we must first love ourselves."

Although the risk is that we love ourselves too much so that there is no room left for anyone else.

The diagram below is derived from Temperament Theory and is a way that we can answer Question 2: "What is my Purpose?" At this Level.

Floor plan for Compassion

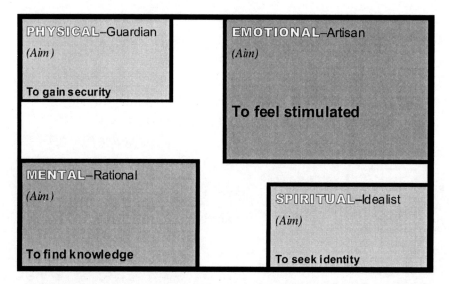

The purposes above are derived from the book on Temperament Theory, *Please Understand Me II*[183]. This book is a good source for finding out more about these types. (And this typology can be applied to other Levels too.)

Turn to Annex A at the back of this Book again remembering that you are looking at how Purpose is defined for you at this Level.

1   Look at the Purposes in the floor plan above.
2   Decide which one means the most to you.
3   Identify which of the four Rooms it is in.
4   Go to Annex A and look at the fourth Level.
5   Mark an "→" in the corresponding Room at that Level.
6   *Mark only one room with an arrow at this Level.*

Although Temperament Theory broadly identifies the nature of our purpose this may well change as we get into our thirties and beyond. Then the "purposes" representative of other Temperaments may become important to us.

The commitment of monks in any religion is to "put God first". It is a succinct way to "act out of love", for love *is* "selflessness". It is "putting others first". If we put a compassionate God first then we are likely to start whatever we are doing in some state of "*Love*". The House framework describes the two fundamental, and opposite, emotions. The ground and first floors are based on "*Fear*", and the top four floors are based on "*Love*". They are completely different parts of the House.

In the end the measure of compassion is how widely we love, as much as how deeply.

CHAPTER 12

If We Are Not In the Same Room Then We Must Be Talking Through At Least One Wall

1999: 27 August–1 September

I go to see my oncologist who takes one look at my eye and says he will delay the chemotherapy one week. Ruth is with me and she asks if this will adversely affect my treatment. The oncologist reassures us that it will not.

Lisa and Sue, another close friend of ours, come around to visit. Sue is a self-reliant person who has travelled throughout Australia. She worked on a cattle station in the Outback before representing Australia at rowing. She now coaches crews helped by her good eye for detail and great understanding of the sport. We start talking about marriage, and I input my male philosophy for what it is worth.

The romantic image advertised so heavily in the Western world creates high expectations. Ruth, Sue and Lisa don't think much of the idea of arranged marriages or the polygamous nature of Hinduism. This is despite the fact that our western society is also now pretty polygamous; our high divorce rate suggesting we are practising a form of polygamy – serial monogamy. I suggest that perhaps this is not surprising when we consider the basis on which we choose partners. We think that we have unlimited choice, but the choice may be made on relatively few options and little information. Research suggests we get to know well, on average, about 2000 people during our lives – which gives us about 1000 to choose from if we limit ourselves to the opposite sex. But then we should take out our relatives, people already "taken" – depending on our personal code of ethics – and people outside the "target age" to give us what is left. And that assumes we are going to wait until we reach the end of our lives before we marry. Of course we could choose someone we do not know that well but then are we any more likely to make the right choice than someone who chooses for us?

If both partners prefer the same Room they will be similar, but not identical, in some critical ways. Very good relationships can come out of any combination. However, research has found the most common pairings are between those who prefer the Physical and Emotional Rooms, and those who prefer the Mental and Spiritual Rooms[184].

There are other factors which affect our choice of partner, such as men looking for someone like their Mother, and women looking for someone like their Father. In modern society we emphasise the physical aspect of attraction of beauty or "good looks", too easily thinking that it is our unaffected judgement without realizing how much it is conditioned by society. "Beauty" has changed though the ages, as can be seen by looking at past photos and pictures[185]. In reality, a key aspect of attraction is the mental/emotional one of looking for someone who is in a different Room to us.

I say to them that "The western idea of 'romantic' love is a nice but poor model of reality. There are many people out there for each of us, not just one[186]."

So if one partner spends more time in the Emotional Room than the Physical Room, then the other partner tends to spend most time in the Physical Room.

Freedom		*Responsibility*
Emotional Room	▲	**Physical Room**

The other common pairing is on the other scale. Between those who spend most of their time in the Mental Room and those who spend most of their time in the Spiritual Room.

Objective Truth		*Subjective Truth*
Mental Room	▲	**Spiritual Room**

A House in Higher Hills

These pairings have a commonality in how they communicate. Those who prefer the Physical and Emotional Rooms tend to use concrete words when communicating. They tend to mean just what they say, with little in the way of implication. They prefer the factual, literal and specific. Those who prefer the Mental and Spiritual Rooms tend to use abstract words which communicate more than just what is said. They prefer the fictional, implied and more general.

This difference is highlighted for me when I hear the confusion between my two sons. Olly tends to be an abstract communicator, while Rob tends to be a concrete one.

Rob had already played *Star Wars – Episode I – Racer* on another friend's Nintendo, and had told Olly, "Cebula [one of the racers] cannot throw things."

Now they are playing this game together on their new Nintendo, and Olly could not get other racers to throw things.

He asked his brother, "How do you get other racers to throw things?"

Rob, still intently racing his "pod," replied, "You can't."

"What do you mean 'you can't', why then did you tell me Cebula can't throw things?"

"Because he can't!"

"But then why didn't you tell me that none of the racers can?" Said Olly looking at me as if to say "What planet is he on?"

Rob replied, "Because I was telling you Cebula can't!"

Both were right but their different communication styles led to both of them to appear wrong to the other. Sometimes mis-communication is just a mistaken belief of a shared understanding.

A few years ago while walking along St Kilda Road in Melbourne a friend mentioned that, "These skivvies[187] don't half cause a rash on my neck."

My immediate thought was, "I am not surprised if that's where you wear your underpants." Only to find out that skivvies in Australia are polar neck sweaters.

I think the preference for pairing with opposites is an evolutionary drive, as partners paired in this way have their strengths covering the other's weaknesses and they are therefore better able to protect their young. Evolution gives us the hint by the strong sense of sexual attraction it provokes. We may not know the other's preferences consciously, but our sub-conscious picks it up immediately. When we are in opposite "Rooms" it initiates a strong sexual attraction towards the other person. Lisa talks about being attracted by the "mystery" in others – a good word to describe this situation. We do not know much of the people we are attracted to as they are in a Room we rarely visit. However, this means that the very thing that attracts us initially is likely to annoy the hell out of us some time later in the relationship!

Close friends of ours, Sherry and Michael, visit us on their way back from skiing in Falls Creek. Sherry is Olly's American Godmother and while working with her I have often experienced first hand her very good interpersonal skills and sense of humour. She had promised to get me a suitable hat to cover my balding head and she arrives with cap in hand.

It is a pretty outrageous hat and I almost remark, "I would not be seen dead wearing it" but say instead, "This looks very suitable to wear on dark nights when no one else is around ... "

My Mother arrives the next night. I do not feel well enough to pick her up at the airport so Ruth meets her and brings her home. It is very good to see her. She is pleasantly surprised at how well I look despite my eye. I am taking the normal combination of four drugs for Hodgkin's. One of the drugs, Vinblastine, is made from the same Madagascar plant, the rosy periwinkle, which is the base for the chemotherapy drug which has raised the long-term survival rate of childhood leukaemia from about zero, to 90%. Lance

Armstrong had been started on the standard based treatment for testicular cancer but ended up changing treatments to one without Bleomycin as it is extremely toxic to the liver and lungs. Prolonged exposure to Bleomycin was likely to halt any chance of a cycling career post chemo because of damage to his lungs. New news, but not good news for me as I want to keep doing sport too…

My Mother is being a star helping around the house. She has reduced the "Annapurna 1" pile of ironing to a hillock in no time. Something which Ruth greatly appreciates as I think she would agree with Erma Bombeck who said, "My second favourite household chore is ironing. My first being hitting my head on the top bunk bed until I faint."

Sunday is Father's Day and Rob gives me a teddy with movable arms. An ideal gift for when things get rough as it gives me another one to throw into the corner. Olly gives me a leather key ring with the words *"WORLD'S GREATEST DAD"* although people may need more convincing.

At work I talk with a thirty-year-old friend who had quite a major operation to correct a problem only a few months ago without success. I had advised her to start taking vitamin C and within days her problem disappeared completely. "There are some great possibilities in nutrition."

I have invited a Qigong Master of Feng Shui, Doctor Clif Sanderson[188(website)], and Galina, his wife, to our house. He has an angular beard, and with his slightly greying hair would look in his fifties, except for his eyes which twinkle with the enthusiasm of a forty year old. Clif has published three books, and has a number of awards, including the *Albert Schweitzer Prize for Humanitarian Medicine* in 1992.

Schweitzer was the man who said, "Witchdoctors and I do the same thing – we both liberate the natural doctor within each patient."

Clif's work has frequently been published in medical journals around the world and more details are at his website[189].

He describes Feng Shui in very practical terms[190]. In Mandarin, "Feng" means Wind, and "Shui" means Water. When water is blown by wind, an energy field is formed. Basically it seems Feng Shui tries to minimize the small stresses that may occur in a house when things are in certain positions or orientations. For instance, if mirrors "cut you off at the head" and are not high enough then you will continuously have to push your body down to see yourself, consciously or unconsciously. Although this only slightly stresses the body, done every day several times a day this unnecessary stress may build up. I use four mirrors in the house, the one in the bathroom is the right height, but the one in the bedroom cuts me off at the chest – the location of my first tumour – a second mirror cuts me off at my neck – the location of my second tumour, and one we put up six months ago cuts me off at the eye – where my shingles was.

Mirrors are important in Feng Shui because they create what does not exist.

Now this is all probably coincidental but: "There are more things in heaven and earth, Horatio, than are dreamt of in your philosophy,[191]" and I decide to raise the mirrors anyway.

Ruth has a feeling for whether certain things are right or wrong. She points out many of the issues before Clif mentions them, such as the skylight in the kitchen. Apparently skylights under which you work or stand for long periods should be partially screened by something natural, such as a plant. It goes back to our evolution where we evolved using caves for protection which gave us security all around and above us. An opening above is associated with potential vulnerability and can cause slight tensions unconsciously. Much of Feng Shui is about common sense and to release these very minor stresses which otherwise might build up over time. Despite all this there seems little point in having your house Feng Shui'd unless it is by a very knowledgeable practitioner, and I find Clif to be insightful.

Feng Shui all sounds a bit weird to the Western mind. In Hong Kong, after my trek to Nepal, Ruth and I went to an old Chinese fortune teller. Being a sceptic I arranged it so that I would see him without Ruth. She was arriving later and would then go straight away to see him, alone. This was so he could not link the pair of us in any way. This was made easier as it was at the Queen's Gurkha Engineers' Regimental Ball with hundreds of people attending and a significant number of the partygoers went to see him sporadically throughout the night.

He looked at my palm and said through a translator that I had one son (no daughters), not a bad guess as I do not wear a wedding ring. His credibility could have been blown straight away. He then said I would have another son in two years' time, which has turned out to be correct. He looked like he would stop there but mentioned two other things when I asked him how long I would live. He indicated that I would suffer from a serious disease but then added I would have a "long life" and earn a lot of money. But then all things are relative. A long life for Nepalese is comparatively short being two-thirds that of Australians[192] and the average income in Nepal is A$350 per year[193].

When he looked at Ruth's palm he said the same thing. What was strange was that he confidently said she had a son and would have a son in two years' time. He got it right twice, suggesting he is a good guesser or ...? Other people there were surprised by the accuracy of his statements too[194].

I go to my barber, David Selby. It is a quick appointment as I am rather "hair challenged" although showing little signs of further hair loss. David is always cheerful and loves talking about his passions – trout and salmon fishing – which he educates me about with his easy sense of humour. Both types of fish are the same genus as the Northern Hemisphere fish which have been translocated to Australia and New Zealand. The difference is that trout live and breed in fresh water, whereas salmon live in salt water moving into spawn where they were born. This information is genetically encoded so strongly that they do not naturally breed in Australia, as it is not the "place of birth". Salmon in a couple of rivers near Queenstown, New Zealand, being exceptions.

He explains that what happens to most salmon in Australia is that they swim back up the river at breeding time, but swim around the river as if to say "What am I doing here?"

I answer, "Just like a lot of humans!"

So there are trout people and salmon people. David asks me if I know that married people live longer than single or divorced ones.

I reply, "Yes, I've heard about that research."

"Well, new research shows that this is wrong, it's just married people feel like they live longer ..."

Martin Seligman, Ph.D. asserts that optimism is an important part of a treatment in its own right. This seems reasonable to me, as optimism is a positive emotion, which helps with mind/body health, but is often easier described than done. The question is are people optimistic because good things happen to them, or do good things happen when people are optimistic? Seligman has devised some clever experiments to show it is the latter. He has identified three attributes to optimism;

1 *"Permanence*[195]*"* – will the events, good or bad, which happen to you, persist? For instance, "I have cancer" and "I have cancer temporarily", respectively. Highly optimistic people tend to assume that good things will persist and bad things won't.

2 *"Pervasiveness"* – do you make universal or specific explanations for the events that happen? For instance, "everything around me caused me to get cancer" and "the cause was a once off event which will not happen again", respectively. Highly optimistic people tend to make

universal explanations for good events and specific ones for bad occurrences.

3   *"Personalisation"* – do you blame or credit yourself, or other people/events for what happens to you? For instance, "I have cancer because of what I have done" and "I was just unlucky to get cancer", respectively. Highly optimistic people tend to blame others for anything bad that happens to them and credit themselves for anything good that occurs!

I think this analysis suggests that I am moderately optimistic? I am trying hard to find a way to get over this cancer because it is my way of avoiding "helplessness", whether in the Physical, Emotional or Mental Room. A habit that is too easily learned. It becomes most damaging when it becomes "hopelessness" in the Spiritual Room, which "learned helplessness" can lead to.

I phone our Sydney office as I drive in to work. I get through to Lorayne, who ends up thanking me for not making her, and others, feel awkward at my situation. I feel touched that she has the compassion to express herself so honestly, although I do not feel I have done much to merit these generous remarks. I do not know what to say in reply. Instead I enjoy a sincere and lengthy conversation about other things.

That night Peter phones me from New Zealand. He is now just about over the loss of the All Blacks (rugby team). I have been considering doing some art and he says he has been doing some still life drawings of naked figures; in fact he assures me his cupboard is full of nude women. Lucky him.

Trek – Day 8

Trekking Truism: The first three locals asked will give different directions for you to follow.

1991: 1 December, Tehrathum, the Himalaya

It was cold when I woke to a noise which turned out to be my teeth chattering. The porters were already up and greeted me as I got out of the tent. They then continued to cheerfully prepare breakfast.

I was surprised by the magnificence of a swing next to us. It was similar to ones at funfairs in England and seemed oddly out of place next to the ramshackle home that it dwarfed. It was almost as if some giant's toy has been accidentally dropped into the middle of nowhere. In fact these swings are built during the major Hindu festival of Dasain for anyone to enjoy. Dasain is in October and it is a similar celebration to Christmas in the West. There was no sign of life in the house and the swing was on a fast moving path to disrepair. However, a small point like this did not stop us from climbing the swing to see who could get the highest. I came about fifth.

We set off in beautiful weather but the clouds soon rolled over us. I was out of sterilized water so I boiled and added sterilised tablets to the water. It was the royal "I"; Ratna got the preferable job of boiling it, and I the lesser one of drinking it.

It still felt like an adventure; defined as, "What you want to be doing when you are sitting at home watching television and which, when you are doing it, you wish you were back by the television."

We went via Sunsari on market day. It was a sea of colour in stark contrast to what I had seen so far. I was definitely the main attraction – I felt like Madonna but would have settled for someone else …

If I had washed properly that morning then mine would have been the first white face the locals had seen in years. The town looked like an embryonic form of a modern town. Perhaps what life was like a hundred years ago? Heavily laden travellers were resting their loads while looking at the goods on sale. Children ran around their parents playing and tugging at their clothing. Older men bargained for the best prices while various youths gazed at all that was on offer. This mountain village bazaar was probably held bi-weekly, and, as is typical for this sort of bazaar, it allowed people to trade while taking opportunities for the *"4M's"* – mail, messages, meetings and marriages.

As I wandered around I came across a courtyard where some ceremony was in progress. There were Limbu drummers beating large drums made from what looked like bark and hide, and decorated with red flowers, similar to rhododendrons. There was also a procession of about ten male drummers rhythmically beating their drums as they moved around the courtyard. I guessed it to be a marriage.

I had been surprised to find out that Ratna had married his wife when she was just 13 years old, and I was even more surprised to hear that he was 13 years old too! Ratna felt a key to a good marriage as acknowledging the other's uniqueness in the relationship. Chandra had objected saying he liked the idea of the certainty and predictability that married life offers. For Subash it needed to be both pleasurable and exciting, while Nadur wanted a marriage to provide someone with whom he could share intellectual ideas.

I asked them, "What do you think about there being one ideal person in this world for us to marry?"

Ratna replied rather opaquely, "The extent to which we are limited in the number of people we love indicates the extent to which our mind is conditioned. That is all!"

I tended to agree that a good marriage or good anything depended as much on the 2E's as the 1C – the Expectations we brought to it and Effort we put in, as much as the Choice we made.

I wanted to buy a kukri[196]. The porters told me to find one I liked, then to put it back and go far away! They would do the rest otherwise I would be charged an exorbitant price. Every village has its blacksmith, usually from the Kamis. They are from the lowest caste but vital to the community as they forge scrap metal into the implements needed for farming.

The blacksmith had a randomly organized collection of kukris. I avoided the one that looked like a genuine imitation and pointed out another to my porters. My porters then bargained this traditional kukri down to £3.00 rather than the £12.00 I was asked for, yet all's fair in love and war. The kukri is the large curved fighting knife that a Gurkha always carries into battle. Carried on a wooden sheath covered with leather, it has two smaller knives. Chandra explained that the "karda" is a very sharp knife used for a range of things, anything from skinning animals, to splitting bamboo into long strips prior to plaiting them into baskets or mats. The other tool is a "chakmak", a blunt knife shaped implement which is used in making fire. Behind these two small knives the porters carried a leather purse with the essentials for fire making; quartz stone, fine dry tinder and some cotton wool. The quartz stone is struck against the "chakmak", and the resulting sparks caught up in the cotton wool are blown into a fire. It all looked very easy.

This kukri itself is razor sharp, and symbolizes the Gurkha as a fighting man. Originally an agricultural implement of eastern Nepal, it was adopted as a fighting weapon over the centuries. Ratna showed me the cutting edge of his kukri just above the handle where there is a notch – a Hindu fertility symbol. This also acts to stop blood dripping down the handle and onto the hands. However, the former appears more important than the latter as the kukri I bought has a fertility symbol that does not form a "break" in the cutting edge of the blade. Subash assured me it is all a handy myth that once a Gurkha has drawn a kukri he must use it to draw blood before returning it to its scabbard.

Chandra's gym shoes had eventually given up on him, so I gave him an advance of £4.00 for a new pair. I had not heard of the brand he came back with but they looked like *Unnikes*.

It was by now a habit greeting fellow travellers as we passed by, with "Namaste". This greeting is given by putting two hands together as if praying and bowing one's head slightly. It means "The God in me greets the God in you."

Coming down one path I met a fellow Englishman with his two porters. He spoke fluent Nepalese and turned out to be a vet who had worked for eight months there with the VSO (Voluntary Service Overseas). We talked for a bit about his experiences. He had that relaxed, yet serious manner, which a year in these hills gives. Approximately my age, he seemed to have gained some of the maturity that life in the hills offers to all. He was travelling to work in the next village and had some months before he would return to England. We wished each other good luck and moved off on our separate ways.

The way a water supply system changes the life of the villagers was impressed upon me as I watched the womenfolk. The village women fetch all the water for the household; for cooking, drinking, washing and cleaning. A pretty big chore as the nearest water source in this village turned out to be half an hour away, each way. But that was the good news – in the dry season the closest source frequently dried up. I tried to talk to a woman returning from picking up water. She giggled in embarrassment even though Subash translated. It had taken her over two hours as the source she had to use was almost one hour way. She was now carrying a traditional metal water pot of about ten litres on her head.

We had arrived at the second project site, Phakchuwa, and after setting up camp we ate daal. The meal's look was best conveyed by my momentary hesitation as to whether it was for eating or had already been eaten. At least my stomach was not going to have to do much. I shared my bottle of Bailey's Irish Cream with Subash and the porters, who tried it out of curiosity and politeness. As is customary in these hills they poured it into their mouths without letting their lips touch the bottle. It is a cultural habit born out of the poor standard of sanitation. So it was to save me as much as them. However, the Baileys was not really to their liking. Ratna and Subash pulled out cigarettes. Nadur only occasionally lit up and Chandra smoked like a yeti – which was not much at all? Ratna wore his cheery smile as he squatted next to the fire and cooked. Ratna had been a cook in the Indian Army for a number of years and it showed, as there was soon a delicious meal awaiting us all.

The Journey Inside – Step 7 – Who Am I?

"Where love reigns, there is no will to power: and where the will to power is paramount, love is lacking"

CG Jung

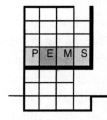 **Level of Compassion – Temperament Theory**

This Level is at the 4th Chakra and lies on the important transition point between the first three and last three Chakras, where we go from dealing with the world as an independent being to dealing with it interdependently. The Austrian physician, Eric Fromm[197], looked at the negative and positive sides of personality and in a way highlighted this transition point in his work. Fromm was part of a group, which included Maslow and Carl Rogers, which set up a different psychological methodology to psychoanalysis. In a different belief system, Christianity, this Level is symbolised by the sacrament of Marriage.

We cannot go beyond the 4th Chakra while our focus is on the ego rather than being egoless – while our energy is focussed on ourselves rather than others. The most significant Rooms at this Level are the Emotional and Mental ones, which is the same as at the Level of Power. Only the order of significance is reversed. Hence when moving from "selfishness" to "selflessness", a critical factor is our feelings and thoughts – in other words our "Mind".

Compassion is more about love than logic. As we make the transition upwards we need to subordinate logic for sentiment – put more emphasis on feelings than facts. However, that does not mean we forget logic. The Dalai Lama summed it up when he said, "We must forgive [*the emotional*] but not forget [*the mental*]."

Floor Plan for Compassion
(Where we put others' emotional needs before our own)

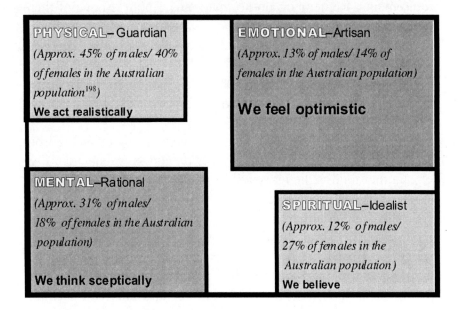

The purposes above are derived from the book on Temperament Theory, *Please Understand Me II*[199].

Turn to Annex A at the back of this Book and put a circle in the Room or Rooms that you tend to spend the most time in.

1   Look at the Styles in the floor plan above.
2   Decide which one, or ones, you adopt significantly in your life.
3   Identify which of the four Rooms it is in.

4   Go to Annex A and look at the fourth Level.

5   Mark a circle in the corresponding Room(s) at that Level.

6   *As a guide – it is probably most accurate to circle one or two Rooms at this Level.*

You do not have to like the Room(s) you have circled but they should be the ones that you spend time in significantly. For instance you may have circled two Rooms; one you are naturally in/like spending time in, the other where you spend time because of work requirements. Remember; do not mark any Room if none of them is relevant.

There is still the great debate about whether a human can ever act selflessly.

The argument against says that we are solely selfish beings – that "Everything we do is for personal gain, no matter how indirect or shallow this may be."

Part of this is definitional. This argument seems to spring from the bottom three levels of *Mark's Mansion* and says that even if we help another totally, then it is still selfish because we did it because we wanted to do it, at some level.

However, it could also be that it came from a different and innate drive, beyond "wanting". Worker ants forgo their own chances of reproduction and instead help raise their sisters. It is a common feature of species that live in colonies, such as ants, bees and wasps. Is this a "selfish" act? If not and ants can act non-selfishly, then surely we can sometimes too[200]? Recent research is not only questioning whether humans are innately aggressive[201] but also whether they are instinctively selfish and egotistical. Studies carried out, such as those at Arizona State University[202], show that humans have a tendency towards altruistic behaviour. In fact it makes perfect evolutionary sense – what better way to ensure the survival of the species than relying on the continuation of the genes rather than necessarily the individual. It is then likely to follow that altruism is in our very nature. In other words the more self-aware we are the more selfless we will tend to be.†

This fits with *Mark's Mansion* which shows "It just depends at what Level they are operating!"

It is my impression that those who argue adamantly that everyone is solely driven by selfish motivations have not themselves visited the selfless Levels.

But we do not need to get worked up about this philosophical debate. It is enough to know that even if humans can only ever be selfish, then we can be "selfish" to one degree or another. In this case there is a continuum of "selfishness" – high to low – and the less selfish the motivation then the higher the Level at which we are operating.

---

†Note: *New Scientist*: 15 March 2003: Inside Science 159. Together we are stronger. "*Was Darwin wrong? Wherever you look, it's cooperation not selfishness that reigns supreme. James Randerson explains how team spirit evolved.*"

CHAPTER 13

Not my Adventure of Choice

1999: 2–5 September

I am feeling the fear of the loss of the control of my life I thought I had! Yet that was only ever illusory. I have not even made the half way mark yet I have a definite sense of "unwellness" and wake up several times through the night. Apparently tests have been done at an American university on sleeping couples by playing sounds softly of a baby crying, and those of a tiger growling softly. Women woke up in the first case, men in the second. Perhaps my waking has something to do with a meta-physical tiger stalking my corridors?

I am feeling increasingly certain that the tetanus vaccination was a major factor in my shingles through its effect of lowering my immune system. Despite it being recognised as a safe procedure to give to patients on chemotherapy, it does not mean the vaccination was not directly linked to my "shingles" experience.

I ask my oncologist why with lymphoma I had not been ill for some eighteen months before my diagnosis. He replies that this is common because when the body has Hodgkin's then the immune system is kept in a high state of readiness as it recognises there is a problem. So how come I got shingles? Apparently although Hodgkin's boosts the immune system in some ways it also depletes it in other ways. The immune system is known to be a very complicated set of systems and processes.

My unstated question is, "So why then can't vaccinations do exactly the same thing – boost the immune system in some ways and deplete it in others?"

I believe the flatulence was a further sign of a low immune system, as it is the immune system which helps keep the gut's bacteria in check. Getting flatulence and shingles might be a coincidence, but just because the link is not known does not mean that there is not one.

There are, at least, two schools of thought on vaccinations. The conventional view is that modern vaccinations are safe and have done much to reduce the terrible effects of disease in the world. The ravages of smallpox have been largely eradicated by vaccination. Smallpox has a very high mortality rate of about 30%, but the risks and benefits always need to be weighed in life. Routine smallpox vaccinations were halted in the United States in the 1970s because the risks from the vaccine became higher than the risk of catching the disease. Two studies in the 1960s found that 1-2 people out of every million vaccinated with the smallpox vaccination will die directly from it and the death rate will now probably be significantly higher. In addition, people can infect others for up to 3 weeks after being vaccinated[203]. Also it is unlikely that people will either die or be totally unaffected in the long term. It is much more likely that there is some form of normal distribution of effects with vaccinations. If a few people die at one end of the spectrum then the distribution would predict that significantly more will be physically handicapped or seriously damaged by the vaccination, and many more will suffer significant permanent damage. At the other end of the spectrum are the people whose health is completely unimpaired. This suggests that most people will suffer some form of definite, but possibly small, health impairment, although it may not be easily linked to the vaccination.

A close friend, Kim, comes around. Ruth got to know Kim when she came to her aerobics class at the local Gym, and I later got to know her friendliness and sincerity. Kim is a member of the AVN[204] and suggests I contact them. I soon receive some information confirming that vaccinations are, like many other things, a matter of balancing risk and reward.

Professor George Dick at London University said: "Every vaccine carries certain hazards and can produce inward reactions in some people … in general, there are more vaccine complications than is generally appreciated."

Some vaccines carry a significantly greater risk than others. Hepatitis B vaccine was developed in 1987, so it is relatively new. However, a report 7 years later from the Institute of Medicine stated a causal link between this vaccine and Guillian-Barre Syndrome, Demyelinating Disease of the Central Nervous System, Arthritis and SIDS[205]. The Australian Government reported recently that the rate of teenage diabetes has doubled in the last 5 years (1993-1998), and some specialists believe that vaccinations are a significant factor in this increase. We may be dealing with sacred cows here but even sacred cows may have BSE[206] – Mad Cow's Disease. Good decisions in life require us to balance risks and rewards, but to do that you have to know what they are.

I think that I largely have the tetanus vaccination to thank for my experience with shingles but it was my choice in the end. How often do you think you are practising prudently only to find out you are performing perilously? It is not even certain how much credit to give vaccinations, rather than improved lifestyle, for reducing the frequency of disease. Despite there being no mass vaccinations for scarlet fever, its death rate has declined at the same rate as diseases which were vaccinated for, such as whooping cough, measles and diphtheria. A lot of credit for this should go to those people who worked selflessly to improve slums, bad ventilation, poor water, unacceptable sewerage, dangerous work, slack food inspection processes and ignorance about sexually transmitted diseases. Even antibiotics may not be as beneficial as changes in lifestyle. For instance, in Britain deaths from tuberculosis fell 86 per cent before the age of antibiotics, and only 9 per cent after that[207]. Why wouldn't lifestyle changes not significantly impact cancer too?

John phones up and listens to my criticisms of vaccinations and my perception of their link to shingles. I am feeling the need to be more critical of things – I am operating out of the Mental Room and I find I am more readily critical than when I am in the Emotional Room. John is very supportive and says he will confirm they give the same advice in England[†].

John says he was talking to a friend in Switzerland who said he was taking his 30-year-old son to hospital because he had broken his leg competing at moto-cross. Surprisingly it was not for the broken leg but because he was diagnosed with Hodgkin's "five years ago" when a very fit ski instructor. He was going for his five-year check to confirm he was still free of the disease, which he was. John adds that a female British athlete has just won an event at the 1999 World Athletics Championship at Seville in Spain. She had breast cancer and had just finished her chemotherapy course two weeks before competing. I find it emotionally helpful to hear how people have regained their fitness and it helps me maintain a sense of optimism.

Rob is really into soccer and I go out to play with both my sons – or at least stand in one spot and try to reach the ball. It is piggy in the middle with the person in the middle trying to get the ball from the other two. When they are successful the person who lost it goes into the middle. Olly almost kicks the soccer ball through the large glass window at the back of the house.

I tell him, "You must not do that. You must be more careful."

---

† Note: John found out that the United Kingdom's National Health's advice is exactly the same as in Australia. It sees no problem at all with certain vaccinations, such as tetanus, during chemotherapy. However, I do, and wonder how many other people have had significant reactions from vaccinations when their immune system has been down?

Rob reinforces my words, "Yes, you mustn't do that otherwise you'll go straight into the middle."

Not exactly my reasoning!

My Mother talks about how "coincidental" it is for her and me to have lymphomas within a year of each other, as the oncologists have told both of us that lymphomas are not hereditary. She reminds me how, in 1995, I was hospitalised here in Australia with severe stomach pains one night and kept in for 36 hours. Despite numerous tests no reason was diagnosed. About five days later I learnt that my Mother, while in the UK, had been hospitalised with exactly the same pains at exactly the same time and no reason could be found for her either. Now here I am having a lymphoma at around the same time as my Mother.

John phones up to talk with my Mother and, although he does not mention it, he also phones to keep me positive. He does this well although he is still not keen about the "alternatives" I am taking. I say that we really cannot intellectually understand everything and must go with our "intuition" at times. He agrees but not quite in the way that I mean. I remind him of the very strange experience he had in December 1997. His sister-in-law dragged him in to see a Swedish clairvoyant to try and get some guidance on how to handle a family problem involving one of their relatives. John was reluctant believing it would be a complete waste of time. Anyway, they produced a photograph and the clairvoyant said that this person loved them dearly but was being strongly influenced by someone else. The clairvoyant then told them that she could see a very serious health problem developing unless immediate action was taken. That prompted John to phone a member of his family afterwards only to discover that the problem was not with her, but with her daughter, who, when taken to the doctor, was diagnosed with leukaemia. Fortunately it was caught early enough to treat it.

After making this comment, the clairvoyant turned to John and said that she had something personal to tell him and, in spite of his protestations, she insisted that his sister-in-law leave them. The clairvoyant asked him to confirm that he was in a steady relationship. Then she drew a simple figure of an abdomen representing his partner and made a strong blob with the pen on the left side of the navel of the drawing – exactly where my Mother's primary tumour was diagnosed two months later.

John has dismissed this as all one big coincidence. However, it seems a bigger leap of faith to believe that it is a coincidence rather than the clairvoyant, like all of us, being able to glimpse into the future at times. Some are better than others, but we all have this ability, even if somewhat dimly, to the extent that we can get our logical minds out of the way†. (John kept the drawing.)

Mark, a friend of John's, said to him several weeks before my Mother was diagnosed, "John, I don't want to frighten you but there is something seriously wrong with Isobel, I can see it in her eyes", after meeting my Mother briefly.

My Mother had been checked frequently over the preceding nine months by her doctor, and after that too, and the doctor insisted she was fine. Perhaps Mark's job as a farmer and gamekeeper keeps him more in touch with nature and harmony?

We change the subject to shooting. John is a keen wild fowl shot and a first-rate clay pigeon shot, having won the 1992 British Open Helice[208] Championship. He tells me he has just enjoyed a few hours' shooting on a very wealthy English man's estate. He was told it takes the estate owner eight hours to drive around in his Landrover.

I reply, "Yes, I once had an Army Landrover like that too!"

---

† Note: I do not necessarily recommend going to see clairvoyants or fortune-tellers. If you do then bear in mind that even the very best are human and therefore presumably make mistakes. My impression is that there are also many who cannot usefully predict the future for others.

Trek – Day 9

Trekking Truism: Up in the hills you will invariably go the wrong way if you do either of two things: go the way you think you should go, or go the way you are told to go.

1991: 2 December, Phakchuwa Village, The Himalaya

I got up before breakfast to go to the toilet and was joined by a handful of spectators. It might have just indicated the level of excitement in their lives but I was now the inelegant main attraction as they glimpsed my technique. I needed practice for this sort of fame. I was using toilet paper which was unusual in the hills, where local people carry a little container of water for the same purpose. The latter is both cheaper and environmentally friendlier.

It was breakfast with a difference that day, fish and no chips, and I ate as the locals do – right-handed – for reasons linked to the aforementioned containers of water.

After checking the water supply with Captain (Retired) Bir, the village Mukhiya, and Corporal (Retired) Ananda, the sponsor for this project, I confirmed the not so good news. Unfortunately the water source was too small to provide the number of taps wanted. Only a limited number of supply systems could be built, therefore they had to be prioritized like all things in life. I told them that I did not think that this one had a good chance of being put forward for construction. Understandably it was not something that they wished to hear and they tried to persuade me to recommend it. I remained frank, but resisted, thinking that there was probably more chance of the village being hit by a tidal wave than the water source providing the number of taps needed. They left deep in thought.

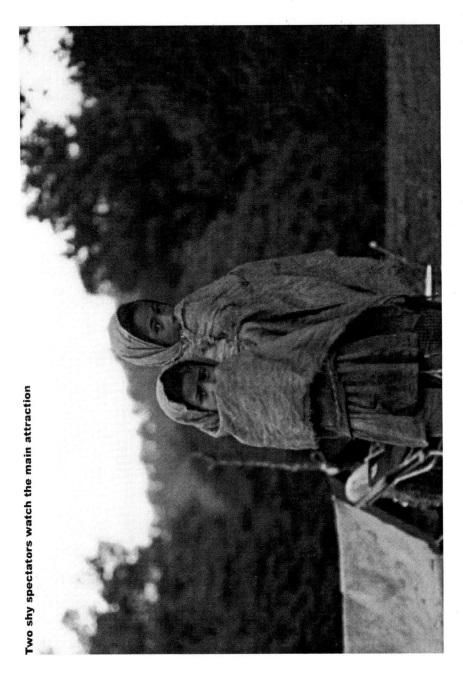

Two shy spectators watch the main attraction

A House in Higher Hills

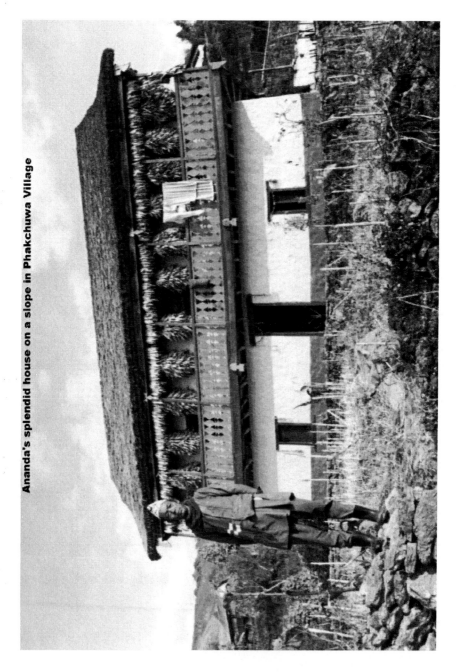

Ananda's splendid house on a slope in Phakchuwa Village

A House in Higher Hills

For lunch we had rice, vegetables, fish and no chips. The vegetables were the type that are fed to pigs in Hong Kong. No different here I think as I wolf them down. I was reminded again that life was hard for everyone here in Nepal as I watched more village women carrying water up from the river. Perhaps an open partial system could aid them but such a system did not bring the benefits of a closed water supply system in terms of durability and effectiveness. Therefore it was unlikely to be a high priority in terms of funding.

My knee had been giving me hassles as I climbed up and down the hills, so I strapped it up. It got me thinking that this short-term remedy is a simile for many medical interventions. In the short term it protected my knee, something necessary at the time. But if I had kept it on in the long term, then it would have caused my knee muscles to deteriorate, and made me more at risk from injury later on. This balance of risk and rewards in the short and long term is the same for most medical interventions. Vaccinations may protect the body from one disease but they weaken the immune system in the process – making it more at risk from other diseases ("falls"). Vaccinating for a whole range of non-life threatening diseases seems about as sensible as strapping the whole body up. It may just increase the risk of weakening the immune system so that it cannot handle more severe threats (of falling over and permanently damaging ourselves).

I enjoyed my last bit of Bailey's Irish Cream which had by now curdled into Bailey's Sour Cream. It still tasted remarkably palatable but then "all things are relative". The porters were not so sure and politely turned down my offer of a sip as I passed it around.

Bir and Ananda came back after lunch with a new plan to influence me. They would cut down the number of taps to three. Their plan was to co-locate some of the taps which was certainly not the best use of the system.

If "Necessity is the mother of invention" then "Desperation" was looking like the father of poor ideas.

After dinner we sat by the firelight as it slowly died, but not so my general frustration at the villagers' ideas; Subash and the porters sense this. Ratna understood my irritation at my lack of power to get what I wanted. Chandra sympathized but found disobedience most frustrating, while Subash coped least well with the boredom on this trek. Nadur empathized and seemed closest to my position as he found intellectual incompetence hardest to stomach. They all had their remedies. This ranged from Subash's advice to throw myself into all aspects of building the system, to Chandra's suggestion that I look for a new group of villagers to work with. Instead Nadur recommended that I start thinking about the next design project.

Interestingly, Ratna raised a caution about too much information, saying something that reminded me it was a mistake to think, "Knowledge is power" because when combined with "Power corrupts", it suggests knowledge is not always that helpful.

The Journey Inside – Step 8 – Who Am I?

"Power tends to corrupt, and absolute power corrupts absolutely. Great men are almost always bad men" [!]

Lord Acton

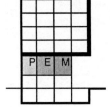

Level of Power – Movement Types

Frustration is a lack of control and is commonly caused by a blockage at the Level of Power. In Christian tradition this Level is symbolised by the sacrament of Confirmation, an expression which cements our individuality and self-esteem. Alfred Adler's[209] psychoanalytical approach focussed on understanding personality at this Level which described it in terms of a need for power.

Frustration is basically not getting what we want and we can address it in two ways. Either,

• We get the power to get it, or
• We ignore our craving for it.

Both achieve the end result – eliminating the frustration but only temporarily, because we are not dealing with the root cause. The Level of Power is the highest of the "selfish" drives but still not a place to be stuck.

Lord Acton's words apply to being stuck at any of the selfish levels; so "Pleasure tends to corrupt, and absolute pleasure corrupts absolutely. Hedonists are almost always base people."

Floor Plan for Power
(Where we control others, and our environment, for our own sake)

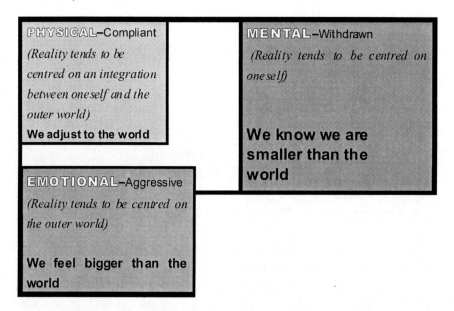

PHYSICAL–Compliant

(Reality tends to be centred on an integration between oneself and the outer world)

We adjust to the world

MENTAL–Withdrawn

(Reality tends to be centred on oneself)

We know we are smaller than the world

EMOTIONAL–Aggressive

(Reality tends to be centred on the outer world)

We feel bigger than the world

The styles above are adapted from *Our Inner Conflicts*[210] which describes the Level of Power, and is linked to how we see our reality. This book is a good source for finding out more about these types. (And this typology may be applied to other Levels too.)

Turn to Annex A at the back of this Book and put a circle in the Room or Rooms that you tend to spend the most time in.

1   Look at the Styles in the floor plan above.
2   Decide which one, or ones, you adopt significantly in your life.
3   Identify which of the three Rooms it is in.
4   Go to Annex A and look at the third Level.
5   Mark a circle in the corresponding Room(s) at that Level.
6   *As a guide* – it is probably most accurate to circle one or two Rooms.

Power gives us the ability to go where we want to, but it may be worth remembering that, "The darkness of the soul is not lighted by moving the body to another place.[211]"

CHAPTER 14

Chemotherapy Number Four

1999: 6–10 September

A m I looking forward to my fourth chemotherapy or what? No. It is half way through the planned eight and I'm feeling like things are going much more slowly than I would like.

Margaret is my chemotherapy nurse today again and she tells me that if the nausea is really bad then I can use a stemetil suppository. "You must use a water based lubricant with it, like KY Jelly, as substances like Vaseline will stop the absorption of the suppository and cause irritation."

This is continuous learning and I reply, "I don't think I will need it for now but I'll be sure to use it just for fun later … "

It is feeling like a long climb. As I am lying in bed Julie, the hospital counsellor, comes to see me. Ruth asked the hospital about some counselling for Rob as he is continuing to be very emotional at home and in school. He has been getting quite tearful at times, although he is always very caring towards me.

His teacher told Ruth that Rob, who is just six years old, had burst into tears in the middle of class and, when she asked what was wrong, he had said: "Nothing, I am just having a bad day."

Julie suggests that Ruth and I sit the boys down independently to read a booklet called, *My Dad Has Cancer.* It sounds like great reading! She then asks me how I am feeling. Instead I tell her my belief that this stage in life is where my experiences and thoughts have brought me to, with perhaps a few previous lives thrown in! I feel it is very important to take responsibility for what is happening to me, but at the same time to walk the fine line of avoiding blaming oneself. I tell her that I am from a Christian background but now feel that Buddhist ideas provide more clarity on my life. I have gone from a group who make up some 33% of the world's population to one that makes up just 6%. Buddhist philosophy is mistakenly thought to be about accepting passively what is happening.

However, it is about accepting "The reality as it is now", for if you don't accept where you are then you cannot know which direction will get you to where you want to go.

Buddhism accepts the need for force too, at times. But force motivated by the love for the person you act against. It is behaviour to stop the offender hurting themselves by the evil they are trying to commit. It is best done without attachment, but with a clear focus. Julie listens, carrying out the role of pastoral nurse quite beautifully.

Jennifer, the pharmaceutical nurse, comes up to see me as usual to check my drug situation.

She goes through my cabinet counting them all up and says, "It's fine."

I agree but add "You did not spot that I have run out of the cocaine."

Margaret has told me that cancer wards sometimes supply cocaine solution to patients in cases where their tongue and throat are very badly infected. I start feigning swallowing difficulties … Another nurse goes through the usual checklist to see how I have been.

"Any trouble with your sense of touch?"

"No."

"Any trouble with your sight?"

"Nope."

"Any trouble with your hearing?"

"Pardon … "

She asks about how I am finding my chemotherapy generally and I answer, "I'd recommend it to anyone."

At about 4.00 pm the oncology nurse tries to put the drip in but it is not her day. Despite being very experienced she fails with her first two attempts – probably because my veins are disappearing. She says that if the third does not work, she will go and get another nurse to do it. I tell her that it is going to be harder as she is now under a lot of pressure to perform. A fresh nurse comes in and manages to put it in first time.

My first three drugs are injected within 45 minutes then the fourth drug is dripped in, intravenously. It usually takes one or two hours but has to be slowed down for me as it is causing me quite some discomfort. In the end it takes four hours and my sense of humour has definitely left the building.

Ruth has looked after me tremendously throughout this time but I prefer to be on my own while all this is happening and so ask my Mother and Ruth not to come to see me. I am riding the rollercoaster and not sure whether I am at the top or bottom.

The next morning my oncologist comes to see me. He is as prompt as ever. I ask him if he thinks I might not need radiotherapy after the chemotherapy. He seems to be doubtful that I will avoid it and this depresses me more than I want to admit. He wants to increase the amount of one of my chemotherapy drugs as he says I am taking it so well. I make a mental note to contact that acting school.

I feel the lump on my throat from fear and the tumour. It seems more solid than usual, I don't know whether it is scar tissue or a sign of the tumour growing. Either way I am feeling pessimistic.

A couple of days later I talk with a friend at work. Ian is one of the master trainers in the organisation. He is a trainer of trainers. He tells me his father died of liver cancer a few years ago and empathizes with me as we talk about "experience" and its insights. When I was first diagnosed he came to me to suggest that I investigate Ian Gawler. My experience is that many of us know people who have died or been close to dying, and we have put ourselves in their shoes albeit intellectually, but you just cannot get the same insights that you get from actually going through the experience of a life threatening illness. There is too much which is beyond words, beyond intellect. Ian concurs that we cannot intellectually appreciate feelings we have not experienced. I mention Doctor Meares and the "banana story", and add that it is no less a truth even if we do not like the taste.

That night I start hiccupping. One or both the anti nausea drugs I take for two days after the chemotherapy give me the hiccups continuously. I think it is the Dexamethasone. Anyway, I am not a good sleeping partner and so Ruth sleeps with my Mother in the double bed in the spare room, again.

My Mother, like my wife, is a beautiful woman both physically and emotionally. Both have a tremendous sense of humour and a great ability to laugh at themselves – which is perhaps one of the greater signs of spirituality. My Mother has always looked much younger than she is and she was awarded a London Diploma in Modelling after having my brother and me. Even into my late teens I was frequently asked what my "sister's" name was! However, my Mother has always been rather flat chested, and she tells Ruth how she was at the hospital waiting for a session of chemotherapy a few months ago. There she got chatting with the woman in the next bed. This woman had just been diagnosed with breast cancer and had recently had a mastectomy. After explaining this to my Mother, the woman said how sorry she was to see that my Mother had had a double mastectomy! I can hear Ruth and my Mother laughing deep into the night.

Since my Father left I have been writing the rules of the game about the power play that sometimes happens between father and son. It is my attempt to highlight the lighter side of fathering…

MALE ORDER

A Game For Any Boy Who Has Ever Had A Father

Male Order is a game of skill played between teams selected from two groups of players. The first team, called Sons, may comprise any male person. The second team is formally entitled Fathers but also referred to as "Dad" for short or "MOM" (standing for My Old Man) for confusion. It is often, but not always, selected from the older male section of society. The game is played on a four-dimensional board, called "Parenthood" (which is to be purchased separately) and involves the second team trying to get from one end of the board to the other. Progress across the board will be subject to a number of handicaps (from now on called "Expenses") suitably provided by the first team.

Play is initiated at the start by an external agency called "Mother", sometimes assisted by a range of other external agencies, such as "Midwife", "Doctor", "Nurse", "Ambulance Man", "Passer By" … etc. Sons' job is to surprise Fathers by presenting them with the most difficult and unlikely Expenses when they are least expected and on the most inconvenient occasions, something which comes quite naturally to the Sons' team. Timing is important and experienced players will wait for Fathers to have just bought a house, married off the last of "Daughters" (usually an avid "Spectator" agency), or made some other major payment. Holidays are another high scoring opportunity.

Following the signal of "Play", each team endeavours to score as many points off the other side as possible until Fathers have reached the end, Sons leave home or either

Team decides to call in the Third Party Umpires by "Declaring Bankruptcy".

Points are awarded at each development of play as follows:

Sons get 1 point for every pound they can borrow from Fathers without returning any money which they have borrowed previously. They get a bonus of 20 points if they can persuade the external agency called "Sister" to give them the money to pay Father back, a difficult but quite rewarding play.

Fathers are awarded 2 points for every bit of advice that they can get Sons to accept, and a bonus of 100 points if their Son is four years or older at the time. This eventuality is of course quite exceptional.

Sons get 20 points for every large purchase they make using Fathers' money. Fathers may nevertheless claim 50 points if they tell Sons that the purchase is only worth half of what they paid for it. Their score is tripled if this is in fact true.

Fathers are credited an automatic 100 points if Sons are distracted by a particular form of the external agency, "Girlfriend". This version is often called "She's Loaded". However, Sons are usually more interested in winning the game and make sure they are ditched, which means that Father automatically loses any points gained.

Sons can increase their score in a number of ways:
- 20 points if they borrow any of Fathers' clothes,
- 40 points if Fathers don't notice, and
- 60 points if anyone compliments them on their dress sense.

These unlikely point credits are matched by corresponding losses of 80 points if they are seen by their friends with these clothes on, and 100 points if they fit!

Fathers are awarded 150 points for every year below the age of 20 that they are able to get Sons to leave the home. Fathers are unlikely to gain any points with this move although it is a geographically affected play – for instance in Australia the average age for leaving home is 28 years of age and increasing!

However, *Sons* usually make a bluff move at about 10 years of age, packing their bags, insisting on leaving and saying something like the words of Captain John Oates, who died with Scott of the Antarctica, "I am just going outside, and may be some time" for 200/x points, where x is the actual number of words used. Fathers are quick to spot the chance to keep a stack of points; however, this move can be guaranteed to be blocked by Mother.

Sons lose 10 points if they remember Fathers' birthday, and 50 points if they do anything about it. Experienced Fathers will realize that the move, when played, is only a tactical move to gain a high scoring opportunity later.

Fathers can make a quick 25 points by reciting quotes in general support of their team such as Charles Wadsworth's quote, "By the time a man realises that maybe his father was right, he usually has a son who thinks he's wrong" or Mark Twain's quote: "When I was a boy of fourteen, my father was so ignorant I could hardly stand to have the old man around. But when I got to be twenty-one, I was astonished at how much he had learned in seven years."

However, Sons can finesse this move for 40 points by

walking off at the word "father". Very experienced players will score 80 points by leaving on the word "a".

Sons may make a common scoring play for 10 points by leaving an expense unresolved for so long that it becomes an emergency and the external agency, "Creditors", tries to contact Fathers directly. However, skilled Fathers will trump this move by being away at lunch … (irrespective of the time of day). It is at this stage of play that Creditors may use their special move and call in the player "Private Detective". If Private Detective finds the team player then Sons are deducted 200 points and their player may have to be retired from the game prematurely.

Fathers earn 50 points every time they reprimand Sons for putting their elbows on the dining room table, saying, "don't put your elbows on the table at mealtimes, you can only do that when you're 16." Fathers get 110 points if they have their own elbows on the table while they are saying this, which of course will be a normal play.

Sons lose 10 points for gaining the status to join Fathers; however, they gain an extra one point a week for every week before Fathers find out that Sons have in fact joined their team, up to a maximum of 946 points. Fathers get a bonus score of 1500 points if they tell Sons of Sons' change of status before Sons realize it themselves! This is a particularly tricky play and usually involves moves such as "DNA Testing", "Paternity Suits" and the like.

Finally, *Fathers* receive 5000 points for reaching the square "three score years and ten".

Trek – Day 10

Nepalese Proverb: Never solve a small problem if by leaving it a little longer you can precipitate a crisis.

1991: 3 December, Phakchuwa Village, The Himalaya

It was up to cocks crowing and the earthy smell of life close to animals. That morning Bir and Ananda were punctual for the recce. We had agreed to go with a more limited design, and they had mobilised a small force to give me a hand.

The survey went well downhill and before I knew it, it was lunchtime and noodles, pig vegetables and rice. It also marked the rapid demise of my "villager rich" environment.

The number of water sources seemed to have increased to five. This could have been good news but they were in line and seemed to me to be the same source appearing five times above the ground. I could have tested it by dropping a dye into the top source but unfortunately I had nothing suitable. It was probably fortunate as turning their water orange was unlikely to have gone down well.

It is hard to overstate the importance of water in the communities up in the hills and these sources could always be a source of friction. As I was doing my survey there were some heated discussions in the local dialect. None of my group understood, but the body language gave me a good idea. Unanimous villager support was a prerequisite for a successful build and I talked with Bir about how they could ensure they got this. Without it there was always the risk of passive resistance, or even sabotage. The situation was made more difficult because out of the 55 houses in the village, each with an average of about 8 people per house, only 22 houses would be helped by the planned water supply system. However, the village also had much going for it. It was well irrigated with significant areas devoted to rice growing, and other small water sources providing localised and effective irrigation.

The houses in this village were simple block designs. Ananda proudly pointed his out. It had its walls brightly decorated with red and white clays. The upper storey had a veranda running along it with blue balustrade and maize hung up to dry along its length. The roof was immaculately thatched. It was a simple symbol of the self-reliance of these hill people.

The survey finished at 3.00 pm and when we got back to the village I was invited to the local hostelry, back in Sunsari. Once there I found it had a similarity to western pubs, it had walls! I sat on a bench only to be asked not to sit on the table. An old stereo system was cranked up, but not quite well enough to tell what language the lyrics were in. We drank tongba and some imported beer called "Iceberg" and laughed for about four hours in a tri-language of Nepali, Limbu and English. The hostelry had a convivial atmosphere and I relaxed as the evening drew in. Bir told me how tongba was made in case I wanted to taste a bit of the Himalaya when I got home. First boil two kilograms of millet for several hours in a container. The millet expands considerably so I would have to keep it topped up with plenty of water so that it did not stick. The resulting product is blended and put it into a 25 litre fermenting container, before adding a bit of burgundy yeast and the juice of a lemon. It is then left for a couple of months to ferment. Finally, I would have to strain the final product through a cloth to remove any remaining yeast. It is then drunk from a tongba. It was that simple…

We left late and as we left the hostelry, Bir and Ananda each grabbed one of my hands. I was quite taken aback and at first thought it might be the drink. However, the reason was soon apparent as we navigated the forty-five minutes back to the tents. The track became very rough and we stumbled frequently in the dark, no doubt helped slightly by the alcohol. I created the appropriate drinking song as we went along:

> "One Tongba
> Two Tongba
> Three Tongba
> Floor"

The threesome worked well and we never got to "floor". Back at the tents I joked with Subash and the porters about holding hands. But they seemed to find it strange that I had the self-esteem to feel awkward about such a thing. Probably because theirs was more robust although it came from different sources. For Chandra it was from his reliability, Subash's from his flair, and Nadur arose from his ingenuity.

Meanwhile Bir had gone off and returned with a gun! I wondered whether he particularly disliked my song or my water supply design that much; or was I just suffering euphobia[212]? I started regretting not buying that bullet-proof tent, but we just discussed the finer points of life in the hills and the porters joined in, in a rather animated fashion.

The Journey Inside – Step 9 – What Is My Purpose?

"There are two types of people in the world; those who want to break in, and those who want to break out"

PK Shaw

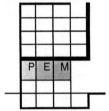

Level of Power – Movement Types

S elf-esteem is about personal power – believing in our own worth. The Mental Room is the Main Room at this Level but there is a significant Emotional component too. We can relate this awareness (which has been defined as the time between naps!) to the "House" model:

- Rooms we are in and which are lit = *consciousness*
- Rooms which we find difficult to see in because they are dark or poorly lit = *sub-consciousness*
- Rooms we have not yet entered = *unconsciousness*

At this Level and the Level of Pleasure there is no Spiritual Room. It may not therefore be a surprise that the Level of Power is also a characteristic Level of one of the other *Po's* – politics.

If we do not believe in, or see, a "spiritual" aspect of life then it can be a sign that we are operating solely out of either of two Levels (Pleasure or Power). It is easy to do this in our modern society because these two Levels are emphasised so strongly.

Floor Plan for Power

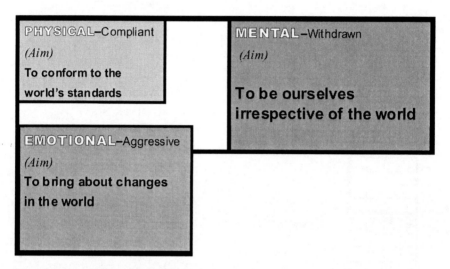

The styles above are adapted from *Our Inner Conflicts*[213] which describes the Level of Power.

Turn to Annex A at the back of this Book again remembering that you are looking at how Purpose is defined for you at this Level.

1   Look at the Purposes in the floor plan above.
2   Decide which one means the most to you.
3   Identify which of the three Rooms it is in.
4   Go to Annex A and look at the third Level.
5   Mark an "→" in the corresponding Room at that Level.
6   *Mark only one room with an arrow at this Level.*

We can start to see the weakness in the Freudian idea that pain and pleasure drives all behaviour. To the degree we are operating at the Level of Pleasure this is true, but it loses its significance and any meaning to the extent that we are operating at higher levels.

CHAPTER 15

"True Cynea, we cannot fly – But do not excuse your hesitation for lack of wings"

Clavidicus, Roman writer

1999: 11–20 September

I go to the Theosophical Society bookshop[214], a world-wide non-sectarian organisation, on the way back from work. I like the Theosophical Society's motto, "There is no religion higher than truth." There I pick up a book about the journey of conquering fear.

The book is about the "Enneagram" whose name is derived from the Greek word for "nine", so Enneagram roughly translates as "a nine diagram". Its origins are unclear and it has been speculated that it was first devised around 2500 BC in the Middle East. It is generally agreed that the Islamic Mystics, the Sufis, used it in its present form before the fifteenth century. It was brought to the West by George Ivanovitch Gurdjieff early in the twentieth century. In the early 1970s several American Jesuit priests adapted the Enneagram for their counselling needs and it has now spread to many other circles.

So a personality descriptor from the Islamic tradition is being used in the Christian tradition, and beyond. I think it is good to see the coming together of world religions, as truth is surely the commonality in them. The Christian "Seven Deadly Sins" which the poet, Dante listed in the Purgatorio Section of *The Divine Comedy,* relate directly to seven of the nine Enneagram types, while the three Buddhist "primary" personality types are described in the *Abhidhamma.* This classic work on Buddhist psychology, relates the Enneagram Types Three, Six and Nine to the Buddhist types. These three Buddhist types are "Greed", "Hate" and "Delusion". The "Greed" type is motivated by gain, the "Hate" type sees life as a battle, and the "Delusional" type tries to function without paying attention. Buddhist philosophy advises that these states are countered by cultivating non-attachment, compassion and mindfulness, respectively.

It shows how hate is not *the* opposite of love. Hate is a second order negative emotion; generally an expression of the primary negative emotion, anger, which itself is a form of the fundamental emotion – fear. The same applies to the other secondary negative emotions, such as greed, envy, laziness, and so forth. They are as much "opposites" of love, as hate.

When low points happen for me they tend to happen in the middle of the night. In the day I have other things to think about, and things are pretty easy. I wake up in the night sweating, and with my right foot hurting at my lung's acupuncture point – on the middle of the sole, just below the three middle toes. I also have stabbing pains at the end of my left heel. This corresponds to the glands' acupuncture point. I ignore Professor Wang's advice and feel fearful. Is this a bad sign that things are getting worse or good sign that the body is doing something about the cancer? I think you basically have three choices when dealing with fears. You can either be controlled by them, suppress them or try to face them. I have often tried to do the last of these. Therefore, although anxious about heights, I have abseiled, jumped out of a plane, bungee-jumped from a bridge, and rock-climbed. I have looked at fear in other ways, fighting the very experienced and then current Australian middle weight champion at Taekwondo[215]. In games like tennis, if you are much worse than your opponent, then you lose six games to love. In full contact Taekwondo losing tends to be a bit more dramatic. But I am finding this experience now a more difficult fear to deal with.

It is to homoeopathy next, a natural holistic therapy which views the patient and their illness in a fundamentally different way from conventional medicine. Extremely small doses of natural drugs are prescribed which can be safely administered to the youngest infant. Both double blind statistical studies and experience indicate that the concept of the infinitesimal doses works. However, the idea of lower doses having more effect is in direct contradiction to current medical knowledge in pharmacology[216], and homoepathy has largely been dismissed because there is no scientific rationale that can fit into the current scientific model. A case of not letting reality spoil a good theory! However, a study on mice into the safety of weedkillers found that the adverse effects of a common herbicide were greatest at the lowest doses[217]! In the case of one herbicide it was at one-seventh the US Environmental Protection Agency's recommended limit for drinking water. The conclusion of the researchers was that there is a specific, very low level at which chemicals have the most effect, and, at higher doses, an unknown protective response kicks in and overrides the effect of the chemicals.

This could explain the effectiveness of homoeopathics and raise questions about arguments such as, "That pesticide, or chemical, is in such small doses that it will not have any effect on you."

Hippocrates, the Father of modern medicine, wrote of symptoms as the expression of Nature's healing powers; "Through the like, disease is produced and through the application of the like, it is cured."

Homoeopathy sees the symptoms of disease as the manifestation of the body's fight against that disease, which is, therefore, an expression of the body's curative mechanism. A homoeopathic doctor will treat the ailment by stimulating these symptoms. In contrast, conventional medicine sees the symptoms as a manifestation of the illness and therefore treatment of the disease involves suppressing the symptoms.

Homoeopathy was used extensively throughout the modern world until the "miracle drug" revolution in the 1930s, whereupon its use declined significantly. However, it has seen a large growth in the US and Europe as the side effects of conventional drugs, and the treatment of patients as whole people, have become more highlighted. Homoeopathic medicines are developed under two principles; "like cures like" and "the more dilute the medicine the greater its effect" (as long as it is diluted in a certain way). The dilution obviates any poisonous or undesirable side effects.

My homoeopath uses a "Mora" therapy, using a "Mora" (pronounced "more-a") machine. The Mora machine is like a Vega machine but much more complex and expensive[218]. It is pretty strange but the therapy is helping me feel better, even if it is all in the mind. That said the argument that it only works because of the "placebo" effect is much more damaging for modern medicine. How much do pharmaceuticals work because of people's conditioned belief in their effectiveness[219]?

The British NHS now has four homoeopathic hospitals, and homoeopathy has been part of the National Health Scheme since 1948. It has also emerged that Queen Elizabeth II uses homoeopathic medicines, for instance she fortifies herself before speeches with a cup of arsenic and onions in water, a homoeopathic remedy to prevent sneezing.

I mention this to my homoeopath who replies that it is interesting that the Royal Family "who have access to the best medicine in the world, use homoeopathics!"

In the evening I see my Mother using fluoridated toothpaste. I advise her not to as I have read in *The Joy of Perfect Health*[220];

"In 1990-91 forty US dentists sued the American Dentist Association for misinforming the public and the dental profession about the effects and extent of amalgam and fluoride poisoning[221]."

I repeat Doctor Dean Burk's comment, from the National Cancer Institute, "Fluoride causes more human cancer death, and causes it faster than any other chemical[222]." It is the long term use that is the problem, just as no one is going to die from smoking one cigarette, no one is going to die from drinking one glass of fluoridated water. I think that adding fluoride probably helps reduce dental decay but at what cost to human health...? My Mother is not convinced, as it seems to be such a widely accepted practice. Phillip Day states in his book, *Cancer-Why We're Still Dying to Know the Truth*[223],

> "In May 1992, Doctor William Marcus, the senior science adviser and chief toxicologist with the United States Environmental Protection Agency, was fired from his post after publicly disclosing his frank comments concerning mass medicating the public [with fluoride]... after a long fight, Doctor Marcus was reinstated on 28th February 1995." Doctor Marcus commented, 'If this were any other chemical but fluoride there would be a call for the immediate cessation of its use. It shows potential for great harm[224]'."

I end by saying to my Mother,

> "Fluoride is a poison. According to the 1984 issue of Clinical Toxicology of Commercial Products (Williams & Wilkins), it is more poisonous than lead and just slightly less poisonous than arsenic[225]."

As if to highlight the point, Ruth comes back from shopping at *Great Earth Health Shops* with toothpaste called Natural, by a New Zealand company called Red Seal[226]. It seems to be a good product and has a natural sweetener – the Stevia herb (which is 150 to 400 times sweeter than sugar – without the calories, and which actually helps sugar metabolism with some reports indicating that it has a number of beneficial effects on the body and that it may be tolerated by diabetics).

The toothpaste does not have any added fluoride stating on its packaging "Many people get all the fluoride they need from their usual dietary sources (tea, seafood, processed food, soft drinks, etc[227]).'' Nor does it have the detergent, sodium lauryl sulphate (*abbreviated to SLS or SLES*), which is a foaming agent used extensively in toothpastes, liquid soaps, and many shampoos. SLS happens to be an industrial degreasant and garage floor cleaner, so somehow it does not seem appropriate to be putting it into your mouth twice a day. The Journal of American Toxicology describes how this SLS can damage eyes permanently, adversely affect the immune system and irritate the skin[228]. The next day I go to see John at Bionic Clean Air and Water[229] (address). He has a wide range of health equipment and I get a filter which takes out much of what the water authorities put in!

When talking with John in UK about the evidence that free radicals are a contributory factor in cancer, I explain that oxidation can cause free radicals but there does not need to be any oxygen present for oxidation to occur. Some substances are much more powerful oxidisers than oxygen – for instance fluorine will even oxidise oxygen. He does not seem to be fully in agreement with this but gets me thinking again why fluorides may be such a problem in our diet.

On Sunday I go for a lunch with 80 other Taekwondo black belts to celebrate Jack Rozinszky reaching 8th Dan Jidokwan. It is the highest Dan you can earn in Taekwondo and it takes 28 years as an absolute minimum to reach this Dan after first gaining a black belt. Jack is the Chief Instructor and founding member of the Melbourne Taekwondo Centre[230] (website). In 1967, he became the first Australian to gain a Taekwondo black belt. In the early seventies he used to go down to the ships in port and invite anyone who could fight up to the club, so that they could learn the latest ideas. Things were a bit rough then and the mythology is that in those times it was not unheard of to start competition bouts in the club which concluded out on the street. Throughout his time Jack has inspired thousands of people through his courage and dedication, and Greg steps up to present him with his new belt. Greg is a close friend and a 5th Dan black belt in Taekwondo as well as a very good instructor. He and his wife, Bronwyn, are both 5th Dans in Taekwondo (and she is also a 1st Dan in Judo!) Greg has spent many hours with me over the years coaching me on the finer points of the Taekwondo technique and has helped me to improve markedly.

As he hands Jack the belt Bernie shouts out words to the effect, "Look he's wearing a zebra!"

It is one long series of black and white lines.

The facilitator for the day gets people to come forward to describe the difference Jack has made in their lives. I am not one of the planned speakers but feel the urge to talk a bit about my experiences, and the facilitator adapts his schedule to accommodate me. I stand up to talk. The audience listens in rapt silence, possibly because they think it might be their last chance to hear me!

I thank Jack for his guidance in the art that is Taekwondo. I also thank the other club head instructors who work for Jack. Alfie was ten times a Taekwondo National Champion and also won a World Championship medal. I give special thanks to him for his fight coaching which I liken to having a third leg in the ring.

I end the talk by saying I do not know how things will turn out for me but,

> "There are both pros and cons in my situation. The cons are pretty obvious, but there are definite pros too. One is getting a better insight into life of the sort which you cannot get without experiencing something like I am experiencing now. And please remember one thing; if you see only bad or only good in a situation, you aren't seeing the whole picture."

As I sit down I feel that I have not somehow bridged the gap between me and my young audience. With hindsight – which is usually 20/20 – I could have better communicated by recounting the story by the Taoist writer, Liu An:

"An old man and his son lived in an abandoned fortress on the side of a hill. Their only possession of value was a horse. One day the horse ran away. The neighbours came by to offer their sympathy. "That's really bad luck!" They said. "How do you know?" Replied the old man. The next day the horse returned, bringing with it several wild horses. The old man and his son shut them all inside the gate. "That's good fortune!" The neighbours said. "How do you know?" Asked the old man. The following day, the son tried to ride one of the wild horses and fell off. In doing so he badly broke his leg. The neighbours came around as soon as they heard the news. "That's really unfortunate!" They said. "How do you know?" Answered the old man. The day after that, the Army came through, forcing all the local young men into service to fight a distant battle against northern barbarians. But the son was not pressed into service because he could not walk. This Army was annihilated."

In other words you cannot begin to evaluate whether experiences are good or bad in your life until you reach the end of it, and that assumes you only have the one.

As the French Philosopher, Voltaire[231], commented, "It is no more surprising to be born twice than once."

There is a group photo and then lunch. I am physically up to the former but not the latter. I say my farewells to Jack personally before leaving.

Wendy is at home with Ruth when I arrive. Wendy is an experienced personal trainer and one of this world's gracious people. She greets me in her typically compassionate manner. Ruth and Wendy are planning their "walking groups" which they intend to set up. I hear them also talk about "cross-training" which I find out is not only when the aerobics instructor gets particularly pissed off with her class.

That evening we watch the film *Lorenzo's Oil* again. In it Doctor Nikolei is hesitant about the "cure" Lorenzo's parents have discovered. Neither parent has a medical background and they seem to have found an answer that has eluded medical experts.

He supports his indecision by saying, "This science of medicine, you know, it is not like physics. There is no mathematical certainty."

Doctor Nikolei remains hesitant about publicly supporting the parents' attempts to get the mixture of oils which they think will help their son because of concerns of possible damage to his prestigious medical institute.

Lorenzo's mother replies, "We are asking for your courage."

This is their request to show the true meaning of courage, which I hope I too am up to, although I do not need quite that much bravery for my scheduled X-ray. However, I feel that I have had quite enough radiation so do not need the standard "two" shots, just the one as it is only the "front" X-ray that seems to be of interest. The specialist is professional and wants to take two. I insist that she saves the hospital money in this case, as my oncologist won't need both, and nor does my body.

When I see my oncologist he confirms that I am looking much better and is sorry I suffered the discomfort of shingles. I tell him that's life and I don't really mind.

What is more, "I would not want to go through chemotherapy without feeling really shitty otherwise I would not be getting the full experience!"

He understandably gives me a look that suggests the chemotherapy must be affecting my brain.

Trek – Day 11

Trekking Truism: If you are making good time you are on the wrong route.

1991: 4 December, Tehrathum, the Himalaya

I got up to meet Bir and Ananda at 0700 hours. Time did not mean quite what it does in the West and I went and checked another water source sprung on me the night before. It turned out to be too small and too far from the other water source to be useful. Bir and Ananda arrived as I returned from this short recce and we signed the final agreement. I said my farewells to my hosts, thanked them for their hospitality, and departed.

We soon passed through Ishibu Panchayat, which they told me had a water supply system built by the Canadians. They seemed to be confusing the source of funding with the builders. During one of the World Wars, Canadian soldiers fought with the Gurkhas and came to admire them enough for their Government to fund some of the cost of building these systems. We in the Gurkha Brigade take the opportunity to do the work and suffer the fun.

I was asked by Loknath, a local villager, if I could repair it. Unfortunately I did not have the equipment and told him he would have to put the request through the formal channel – the AWO at Phidim. I also thought I lacked the time to do this. However, I realized later that I really meant it was not a high enough priority for me. If I had been offered, say, one million pounds to fix it, then I would have found the time to try without any other change to my circumstance!

We stopped at 11.00 am and a slick routine went into action. My porters collected firewood and started a fire. In no time we were eating a tasty meal of rice and split lentil soup. I noticed that Ratna put some grains of rice aside as an offering of food to the gods, while I munched away looking down the side of a large valley which dropped away to the River Tamur and then rose sharply on the other side. It was just one of many spectacular views on this trek. The sun's rays danced over us while a cool breeze swirled around. It all seemed a bit colonial. The porters fortunately took offence if I tried to do anything. Instead, they had sat me down on the deckchair, which they carried for me, and then had brought me lemon tea and lunch when it was ready. It was a rough life, but then someone had to do it.

When we reached the Tamur River we found out that it was wide, and flowed surprisingly fast and cold. The only way to cross was by swimming, not a great option, or by using a dugout canoe. The canoe was made from a single tree and skilfully paddled by two enterprising young Gurkhas. They were from one of the lowest castes, ferrymen, and were, unusually for hill people, expert swimmers. I imagined that these young entrepreneurs would have had some thriving computer business by now, if born in the West.

The canoe looked pretty unsafe from the outside and did not even seem that secure once inside. I was not reassured to see my porters bless the boat quickly as they got in, and hoped their blessing included me. It had no keel but was pretty stable as long as we remained low and statuesque. I took off my back pack in case this turned into the "not a great option".

We made the other side and paid our toll to the ferry boys. They smiled and happily took the next customers back across. On the other side we could see a relative metropolis, a site of scenic shops and eating house.

Now we made a much more civilised crossing over the second branch of the river. It was via a pretty modern steel suspension bridge, in "strong" contrast to the first crossing. The bridge played a doleful tune as our feet drummed upon it. Many of these suspension bridges were originally built by Scottish engineers in the late nineteenth century. The bridge swayed a little, and my confidence was swayed a bit too. It is not so much because I knew the Scots like their whisky, more that from my degree, I knew the definition of engineering,

> "The art of modelling materials that are not fully understood, into shapes that cannot be precisely analysed, so as to withstand forces that cannot be properly assessed, in such a way that those around have no reason to suspect the extent of the ignorance![232]"

I wanted to set up camp away from foot-bound traffic, although thefts were extremely rare and almost always non-violent in this part of Nepal. When stealing did occur, the thieves usually slit open tents with knives in the middle of the night and ran off with whatever they could snatch. With that in mind I decided not to sleep with my head too close to the tent's side.

We set up camp in a small re-entrant, a mile past the village. It was next to a semi-permanent fish trap in the middle of the fast flowing river. We had covered a lot of ground and I looked for a marker to reassure me that we had also travelled in the right direction. A habit useful in life.

With the calming sound of the river coursing its way in the background I read some more *TEMPLER*. I came to one of the many stories of Gurkha bravery – of Rifleman Ganju Lama of the 1st/7th Gurkha Rifles. He won a VC (Victoria Cross) as a young soldier. The citation for the medal reads:

> "In an action South of Imphal in 1943, Rifleman Ganju Lama MM[233] went forward on his own with a PIAT (Projector Infantry Anti-Tank) and promptly attracted withering enemy fire which smashed his left wrist and hit his arms and legs. Despite his wounds, he crawled to within thirty yards of the leading enemy tank and knocked it out with a single well-aimed shot. He did the same to a second tank, returned for more anti-tank rounds, and went forward again to do the same to the third tank, killing its crew."

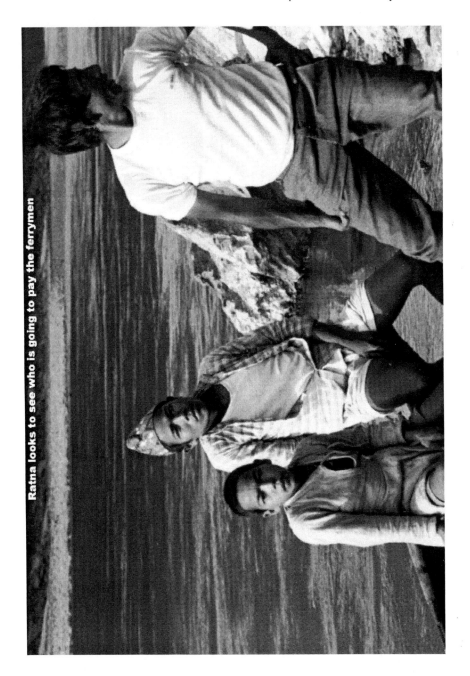

Ratna looks to see who is going to pay the ferrymen

A House in Higher Hills

A high street in Phidim

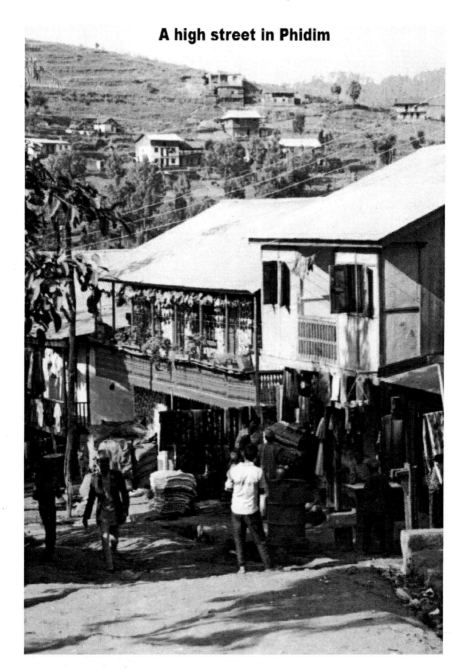

A House in Higher Hills

The PIAT was a fine example of British World War innovation, rather than invention. It was an awkward weapon and hurled a hollow-charge projectile with a reliable range of about 70 metres. Apparently, it had the veritable "kick like a mule" and it is unclear whether he got the Victoria Cross for destroying three tanks or firing the PIAT three times in succession from the shouldered position!

Only a month before winning the VC, he had crawled out into the open when under intense 37mm shellfire to within 55 metres of some Japanese tanks. He had destroyed two tanks while covering his comrades' withdrawal from their exposed position, before he finally crawled back to safety.

This action gained him the Military Medal (MM), "For his resourcefulness, coolness and disregard for his personal safety."

Ganju ended up being so badly wounded in winning his Victoria Cross that he had to stay in hospital for 22 months. More than twenty years later his leg swelled up so he applied a poultice to it and ended up drawing out a bullet that had lodged there during these encounters[234].

His actions were what I would describe as courage – "risking himself physically and emotionally *for the sake of others*."

The Journey Inside – Step 10 – Who Am I?

"Courage is resistance to fear, mastery of fear – not absence of fear"

Mark Twain, Writer

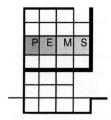 **Level of Courage – The Enneagram**

It may seem surprising that the Level of Courage is a higher energy than Level of Compassion. "Courage" is defined in numerous ways, but it is most meaningful if it is about selflessness. When we operate at the Level of Courage we are actually demonstrating a form of love.

Lord Moran, who had experience as a British Army medical officer in the trenches of the Western Front, formulated the idea of a "well of courage". Everyone has a well or reservoir of courage. They may differ in size but, no matter how big or small, everyone has courage and everyone will run out of courage if put in a very difficult situation long enough.

He wrote, "A man's courage is his capital and he is always spending. The call on the bank may be only the daily drain of the front line or it may be a sudden draft which threatens to close the account.[235]"

Doctor Richard Holmes in his excellent book about courage and battle shock, *Firing Line*[236], wrote, "A man's bravery may fluctuate from day to day... The rifleman who turned and ran on Monte Grillo, next day held fast and fought like lions."

(In the future we may find science will help us to understand this more; apparently geneticists have already found the gene for shyness – it is hiding behind the one for bravery!)

The Enneagram is a typology that identifies patterns of behaviour in the human population based on our "fears". Each type is defined by a physical, mental or emotional fear. No one type is better or worse than another per se, but every one's fears have consequences. Courage is about how we deal with these personal fears so that we can help others.

Floor Plan for Courage

(Where we knowingly risk ourselves physically, emotionally or mentally, for the sake of others)

MENTAL–The Thinker, Loyalist & Generalist *(Two of the "Seven Deadly Sins"–Avarice and Gluttony–characterize the negatives)* **We think perceptively, co-operatively or productively**	**PHYSICAL**–The Leader, Peacemaker & Reformer *(Three of the "Seven Deadly Sins"–Anger, Lust and Sloth–characterize the negative aspects)* **We act authoritatively, reassuringly or ethically**
EMOTIONAL–The Helper, Status Seeker & Artist *(Two of the "Seven Deadly Sins"–Pride and Envy–characterize the negative aspects)* **We feel altruistic, self-assured or self-aware**	**SPIRITUAL**– Any of the Nine Types **We are ethical, altruistic, self-assured, self-aware, perceptive, co-operative, productive, authoritative or reassuring**

A House in Higher Hills

The styles are taken from *Personality Types*[237]. This book is a good source for finding out more about these types. (And this typology can be applied to other Levels too).

Turn to Annex A at the back of this Book and put a circle in the Room or Rooms that you tend to spend the most time in.

1 Look at the Styles in the floor plan above.
2 Decide which one, or ones, you adopt significantly in your life.
3 Identify which of the four Rooms it is in – noting there is the choice between two Rooms for each Type at this Level – the Spiritual Room for a passive descriptor and one of the other three Rooms for the more active form. Choose either or both as appropriate.
4 Go to Annex A and look at the fifth Level.
5 Mark a circle in the corresponding Room(s) at that Level.
6 *As a guide – if you identify more than one of the Enneagram Types as describing yourself then at least two of the Types should be adjacent to each other as shown below:*

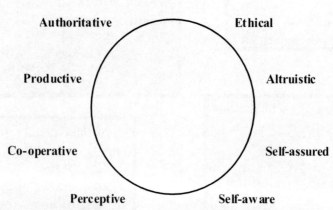

Experiential Wisdom is much more powerful than *Intellectual Wisdom*. Very few people suffer PTSD from reading about a stressful situation!

CHAPTER 16
Chemotherapy Number Five

1999: 21–27 September

My Mother and I watch a wonderful documentary in the afternoon before she leaves. It is by the National Geographic Society called *Lions and Hyenas – Eternal Enemies*. Dereck and Beverly Joubert spent many months in northern Botswana filming one group of lions and one of hyenas, and showing how much of an even battle it is between these two warring clans. Even this battle is mirrored by the battles between clans of lions versus lions, and hyenas against hyenas. It is an animal tale describing our human story in many ways. How we can be conditioned to behave outside our essential nature, in conflict with our world. The film closes with:

> "It was not always easy for us to witness these struggles for life. But, at the end of it all perhaps, we came to know more about ourselves and the struggles that rage within our own savage souls."

I am planning to take my family to visit Shamwari Game Reserve near Port Elizabeth in South Africa next year. There you drive around in open top landrovers amongst the wild game. I have been told that as long as you are driving in the vehicle you are safe from the animals such as wild lions, but if you climb out of the vehicle then you are liable to be attacked. It seems that the animals do not realize that the person in the vehicle is a separate entity to it. I think it symbolizes the mistake of atheism. To explain this we can see what the following interpretation might explain:

- Landrover = *the physical body (where the engine is the brain)*,
- Steering System = *the mind*,
- Driver = *the spirit.*

Fuel is the food in this metaphor and deep ruts in the road are like mental conditioning. If you fall into them then the road decides the direction, and once in them it is hard to get out. The mind is linked to the "brain" but extends throughout the vehicle. A physical addiction is symbolized by putting additives into the fuel. It may help initially, but in the long run this damages the vehicle and stops it from being able to drive over life's hills. It seems to me that the atheists' view is that of the lions'. They think the vehicle is driving itself[238].

This odd bit of reasoning is partly prompted by the highly insightful book I am reading called *The Monk and the Philosopher*. Written by a father, Jean-François Revel, a highly regarded French agnostic thinker and philosopher, and his son, Matthieu Ricard, who left his doctoral work at the Institut Pasteur in Paris 25 years ago and became a Tibetan Buddhist monk. This book records their ten days of discussions in Nepal and formulates the wisdom of the East in a way that the western mind can comprehend.

We all have the idea of "I". Western philosophy follows that with the assumption that there is a separate "self" that makes up a separate identity for the individual. Whereas in Buddhist philosophy,

> "That idea's just the mind's own fabrication... If you look for that 'me' somewhere in the stream of consciousness or in a body, or even in the combination of the two... you'll never succeed in identifying any entity, mental or physical, that corresponds to an individual self[239]."

So both western and eastern philosophy start with different possible but unprovable assumptions and then applying rational thought to each one takes you to very different conclusions.

My Mother adds to the wisdom that day in her own way saying, "People will remember you less for what you tell them and much more for how you made them feel."

I arrive at Cabrini Hospital for my fifth chemotherapy. Up at the ward I am directed to a single room, a little bit of luxury. On the wall next to the door as you go in, is a plaque with a poem which seems to be in memory of a lady called Diane who, I think, died in these wards.

The clock of life is wound but once
And no man has the power
To tell just when the hands will stop
At late or early hour...
The present only is our own
Live, love, toil with a will
Place no faith in tomorrow, for
The clock may then be still.[240]

As usual, I get very professional treatment from the very professional nurses. Margaret is my oncology nurse for today and she is excellent as always.

The nurse helping her gets slightly confused with some of the drugs and Margaret, who is a brunette, smiles and asks the nurse if "She is having a 'blonde' day!"

My mouth ulcers hurt a bit and the nurse confirms they are quite bad. So she gets me some Mouthwash powder from the Peter McCallum Cancer Institute[241]. It's good stuff – much better than the simple things like champagne and fine cognac … She also offers ice or an icy pole to chew on. I take the ice while the chemotherapy is dripped in. Apparently this closes the blood vessels to the surface of the mouth limiting the amount of chemotherapy that gets there, and so reducing ulcers later on. Either that or she doesn't care for my conversation.

After she puts the drip in she says she will go and get the chemotherapy drugs and that I can sit up and be a "free man". I reply, "Great! I'll go home then."

The phone rings once I am on the drip and it is Rob to tell me that the bread I put in the bread machine last night is an unleavened lump. I must have forgotten to put the yeast in. He finds it hilarious. Unfortunately, I am having a hard time finding much funny as the chemicals drip in.

At 7.00 pm an oncologist who is standing in for mine comes round. He is very upbeat about my outlook, so positive I almost feel quite good about being here in hospital! He has read of my interest in Taekwondo and jokes that, with my fighting successes, they will be very keen to take good care of me. I mention to him that I understand patients using combined conventional cancer treatment and alternative therapies, such as Chinese Medicine, do better than those who just use conventional ones. He tells me that just the opposite has occurred with studies he has seen on breast cancer patients; those using combined therapies have in fact done worse. I think that might be to do with the use of Tamoxifen in the treatment as the WHO formally designated Tamoxifen as a human carcinogen in 1996, grouping this substance with around seventy other chemicals – approximately a quarter of them were pharmaceuticals[242].

After an average sleep the nurse comes in to dole out my drugs. She gets out the tablets for uric acid build up and the nausea, and she gives them to me saying, "We don't want you feeling chucky." I agree saying, "Chucky wouldn't like it."

Back home, I have that glow that can only come from good steroids. The food is pretty fair at Cabrini but it is good to be back to Ruth's home cooking. Several people ask me why I look so well. I guess people are surprised that you can look healthy on chemotherapy. Even Ruth wakes up a couple of mornings later, looks at me and asks me how come I am looking so well! All things are relative but my Mother says it is the steroids that give that ruddy complexion. Conversely my oncologist reckons it might be the relatively high dose of beta-carotene that I am taking. Another possibility, the particularly sunny weather, is definitely not a factor.

I read a bit more of *Stalingrad* at a time that another tragedy of war is occurring, Kosovo. I am saddened to watch the news about it, or perhaps it is the reflection on my situation. Racism or ethnicism is clearly both fear based and irrational. To think that all of a certain group of people are better or worse than all of another group of people is so obviously ludicrous, as to be almost funny – if it was not so destructive. The differences within groups are often greater than between groups as race is one of the least significant distinctions between people[243].

I am feeling pretty drained despite sleeping 10 hours a day and meditating for one and a half. I wholeheartedly agree with both my doctor and TCM's advice to conserve your energy when seriously ill. In this situation TCM recommends avoiding any vigorous activity, including sex – not a big problem at present.

My Mother, not believing much in alternative medicines, comes with me to see Professor Wang. She accompanies me in part to check what he does and ends up feeling pretty good after her acupuncture treatment. The Chinese philosophy on health believes that energy from the acupuncture, and the doctor, helps to fortify the body.

It may sound a bit wacko in conventional scientific terms but then beliefs can blind western medicine to effective treatments. In the early 1980s Doctor Barry J Marshall at the Royal Perth Hospital, Australia, teamed up with a Doctor Robin Warren who had found some bacteria which appeared to be in the human gut. Doctor Marshall did not come from the field of pathology and this gave him an advantage. He was not hampered by the conventional paradigm of people operating in this area that bacteria could not survive in this part of the human body. He found that 90% of patients with this certain bacteria had ulcers. Over the next two years he gained more evidence that this bacteria was a major factor in some ulcers. He pioneered a simple and inexpensive four week treatment with antibiotics, which could replace more costly and less effective treatments.

Based on his experience with 200 trials he went to an international conference and gave his evidence that many ulcers were in fact caused by bacteria and could be cured by inexpensive antibiotics rather than expensive pharmaceutical drugs. His findings were dismissed by experts and pharmaceutical companies. It was only in February 1994 that he finally got endorsement from a major health organisation, a decade after his discovery[244].

A close friend, Narelle, comes up to me in the office to ask how I am. Narelle joined my company just before I arrived, but was quickly promoted to the position of IT specialist after showing both a motivation and capability to deal with more technical issues. She somehow always manages to bring a sense of appropriateness and camaraderie to the office. However, it is flu time and most people have sniffles and colds, so I ask her to stay back and refrain from showing me too much camaraderie at the moment! I think cancer is enough for now.

The boys are on their school holidays and have the energy to meet a small city's electricity requirements for a couple of days. Ruth watches while Rob jumps from ever higher steps on the stairs. Finally she says, "Don't jump any higher otherwise you'll kill yourself."

He eyes her with a quizzical yet comical gaze then replies, "Don't be silly – I'm too new to die."

It is a useful philosophy to keep to, at any age.

By Friday the boys are desperate for a McDonald's, which I do not like them having regularly. I am not questioning the quality, I question the composition. Robert Vogel MD[245] has reported that the sharp constriction of the blood vessels can injure the inner lining of the blood vessels which is indicative of a heightened risk of developing hardening of the arteries. He confirmed that after volunteers ate a "Big Mac with fries" their blood flow dropped by 34%.

Fast food may also provide excessive fat. Doctor Timothy Lobstein[246], who had joined the "fast food panel" of the British Government's Nutrition Task Force, commented on the eight meal combinations published by McDonald's.

One of his examples is something Rob would like, "A Big Mac, Large French Fries, Apple Pie and a Regular McDonald's Cola."

For a child taking in 2000 Kilo calories a day, a 35% fat allowance[247] would mean 700 kcal or 78 grams of fat was recommended, yet this combination provided 64.4 g, or over 80% of the daily quota. Melanie Polk, the director of nutrition education at the American Institute for Cancer Research says;

> "We… also know that obesity can increase cancer risk… Most people have learned that obesity can be associated with high cholesterol, diabetes, high blood pressure, but many don't recognize that obesity is also a risk factor for several types of cancer."

I believe "fast food" of today will be considered in the future as smoking is now – although I do not imagine "passive eating" will ever be a problem[248]!

There is also a link between "food and mood". Our nerve cells communicate by releasing chemicals called neurotransmitters, and these regulate our appetites and moods. They are turned on and off by what we eat.

> "Eat all the wrong foods at the wrong times, which is what most of us do, and we upset this chemistry leading to depression, stress, fatigue, insomnia, PMS symptoms etc[249]."

Is it any surprise that 25% of children and 8% of adolescents are estimated by doctors in the USA to have depression[250]? However, my sons are deriving their emotional pressures from me rather than food. Olly has been getting stomach aches for no apparent reason. It could be the stress but Ruth and I are concerned in case lightning strikes thrice. We book him in to see Doctor Soosay. Walking up the stairs I find Rob writing something rather coyly.

"What are you doing?" I ask.

He answers that he has written something for Mum and me. It says in brightly alternating colours;

To mum and dad
I love you
a lot I like my
bedroom.
I know your
favurt color dad
it's blu. Mum
your favurt color
is purple
dad's favurt
sport is Tae kwon
do. Mum's
favurt is
Aerobics
the End

Trek – Day 12

Trekking Truism: When traversing a high ridge, don't look where you don't want to go.

1991: 5 December, Phidim Village, The Himalaya

We rose to scenic surroundings and climbed 1500 feet climb to the Phidim AWC. I was lost in thought and slipped, potentially falling some way before Chandra and Subash dive to make a fine catch.

Yes it is true "A good scare is worth more to a man than good advice[251]", and I began paying much more attention my steps and less to my thoughts.

The locals' directions were consistent in one respect. They always gave the same time to our destination no matter how far we had gone. We had to be walking in one large circle – quite possible with my map reading. It is like Sir Percy Fitzpatrick's experience in *Josh of the Bushveld.* He remarked how everyone has a tendency to walk to the left or the right when they follow a "straight line" naturally, without the aid of a compass or landmarks.

Along the way we passed a wayside effigy shrine. It differed from the Buddhist shrine I had seen as it was a half metre high wooden statue of a man grasping something around his neck with two hands. On his head and wrapped around a piece of wire strapped to his side were a mass of white, red and green tassels. These effigies are meant to appease departed spirits.

Phidim turned out to be a very quaint and surprisingly picturesque town.

I took a look around and used affirmations to improve my photography... "My name is David Bailey, my name is David Bailey."

It was not very effective as I ended up opening the back of his camera before rewinding the film. It felt like a mini-disaster but perhaps a few frames would survive[252].

Soon after arriving I checked the cash and medical equipment at the AWC. As was to be expected, it was all in very good order. I mentioned the Ishibu Panchayat's request to the assistant AWO. However, he said that the village lay in Taplejung's area of responsibility, not his, so he would have to pass it on.

I decided to take a wash and was shown a wash area camouflaged as an outhouse. After a bracingly cold shower I went clean into town. I wanted to take a few repeat photos in case I had ruined the other film, so I took a picture of a rather splendid boarding school funded by the Brigade of Gurkhas. School attendance is required for all Nepalese between the ages of six and ten but many more boys than girls attend school in this patriarchal culture. Only about 20% of the Nepalese population aged 15 or more is literate. I was shown around the school by a master who spoke very good English and was clearly very proud of his school. I found it delightful to see the kids smiling merrily away, just enjoying themselves. They crowded around me in rapt curiosity, wearing a mixture of expressions – from serious confusion to smiling anticipation. The facilities were very good for this part of Nepal but obviously limited compared with what we are used to in the West.

I asked him about the school's philosophy on teaching and he described a "teacher" centred approach. I mentioned to him that in the West we were attempting to make it a more "learner" centred focus.

He seemed open to the idea saying something like; "Yes, schools are not really about teaching but learning. Even the best teacher can only teach students to teach themselves."

However, he personally preferred a more "project centred" approach which seemed to be in line with the Chinese saying, "I hear and I forget. I see and I remember. I do and I understand."

Neither Nadur nor Ratna had had the chance to go to school. As was typical from early days they were integrated into the routine of the home up in the hills. From about 10 years of age they were often alone with the animals in upland pens. They soon learnt the ways of life and the living, and death and the dying, as the young animals came into the world. They learnt the uses of trees and plants, which wood for houses and fencing, which trees for boats, and the myriad of uses for bamboo up here in the hills. In this way they developed the self-reliance to make things which my son (when old enough) would just buy from shops. Baskets made from split bamboo, rope from vines, bows from trees, and pellets to kill birds from the colourful white and red clays found in the soil. They told me how nothing is ever thrown away in the hills. Even a piece of wood had a myriad of uses.

Chandra was lucky to have had basic schooling but he still spent many days learning from his father how to plough the wet paddy and dry maize fields, and yoke the oxen. He also became expert at repairing paddy walls and irrigating the terraces. He learnt to hunt when necessary and how to play his part in bazaar business and the buying of land. All the same, Chandra clearly greatly appreciated the time he had had in school and worked hard at it, as so many children do in poorer societies.

The thing that struck me most in this school was the effervescent smiling of the children; it was quite infectious.

Walking on into town, I passed through the market and high street with its bright blue and white houses set on a steep incline. Vegetables hung from the verandas overlooking the material for sale below. I found a barber and had the haircut among haircuts. At £0.22 I might have been charged over the odds for the area but it was the first time since Sandhurst that my toenails had been longer than my hair. I also got by far the best massage I had ever had with a haircut. The barber started with my fingers, cracked them all, then my arms, my shoulders and finally clicked my neck. I generously tipped him one hundred per cent.

Not surprisingly in such a small town, I walked into Ratna and Chandra who were out buying provisions.

Lentils had featured prominently on our dinner menu and Ratna was now keen to try something else but Chandra said, "What if that food is worse?"

Ratna replied, "What if it is better?"

I was with Chandra on this one but left before they got to "Cogito ergo sum[253]".

TEMPLER was proving a heavy read but I read with interest how Templer recommended the Army Appreciation as a means to approaching all problems in life.

> "Gerald's success as leader was based, however, not only on his personal example and dynamism but on skilful organization, hard thought and careful staff work.
> 'Ever since my young days [he wrote in 1976] I have tried to tackle every problem which has presented itself to me – whether in soldiering or in private life – by thinking it out along what some people may think is an old-fashioned appreciation of the situation: the object, the factors, the courses open, and the plan. It pays an enormous dividend[254].'"

I had found the process useful to use on this trek when I remembered it, and as the night compressed around us I settled down to dinner and rum at the AWC. It was as close to fast food as you could get up here in the hills – it was mouse-hare meat. The mouse-hare (called "pika") is a type of quick moving guinea pig, although this one had not moved swiftly enough.

The Journey Inside – Step 11 – What Is My Purpose?

"How a piece of bread looks depends on whether you are hungry or not"

Arabic Saying

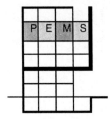

Level of Wisdom – The Appreciation

Although the Level of Wisdom is in the Mental Room, it is not just about the intellectual. Any of the Levels may be believed, understood or experienced – the three types of Wisdom.

As the alchemist said in Paulo Coelho's enchanting novel[255], "There is only one way to learn… It's through action."

It reflects the importance of the Physical Room. Real wisdom comes from "Experiential Wisdom".

In the psychological field, Jung's work typifies this Level, whereas in Christianity it is symbolized by the sacrament of Ordination. It is about knowing the path to "godliness" – knowing oneself.

Life is a continuous process of making decisions, every moment of the day we make decisions whether small such as what type of drink to have, to major ones like when to have children. Therefore, if we improve the quality of our decision making then we transform our lives. We can do this by using an "appreciation" methodology. A form of the Appreciation is shown diagrammatically on the next page, with four key Steps:

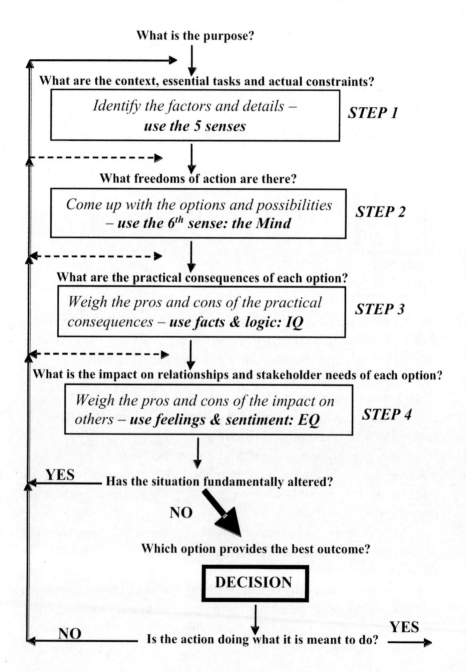

Research by George J Schemel and James A Bornbely[256] indicates that each of us will focus more on some Steps than others. We will naturally spend over 75% of our time and energy focussing on two Steps – Step 1 or 2 plus Step 3 or 4.

If we only consider the last two steps then we will tend to spend between 65-90% of our time and effort focussed on either Step 3 or Step 4. So our focus is up to nine times greater one way than another, yet we tend to think we cover each way equally.

Floor Plan for Wisdom

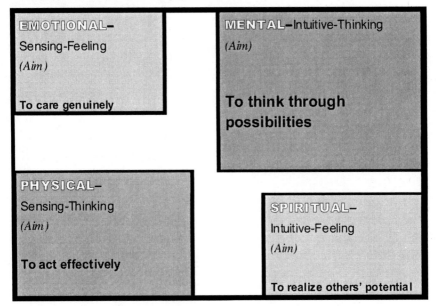

EMOTIONAL–
Sensing-Feeling
(Aim)

To care genuinely

MENTAL–Intuitive-Thinking
(Aim)

To think through possibilities

PHYSICAL–
Sensing-Thinking
(Aim)

To act effectively

SPIRITUAL–
Intuitive-Feeling
(Aim)

To realize others' potential

Turn to Annex A at the back of this Book again remembering that you are looking at how Purpose is defined for you at this Level.

1 Look at the Purposes in the floor plan above.
2 Decide which one means the most to you.
3 Identify which of the four Rooms it is in.
4 Go to Annex A and look at the sixth Level.
5 Mark an "→" in the corresponding Room at that Level.
6 *Mark only one room with an arrow at this Level.*

The Appreciation is used in the British, and British trained Armies worldwide. Steps 3 and 4 are combined into one Step in the Army Appreciation. Research on personality indicates that it is not as effective as separating them out as each of us naturally focus on one or the other. What may not be initially obvious is that *"others"* in Step 4 includes animals and plants!

It all starts with keeping the aim in mind. No matter how good a marksman we are, we are unlikely to do any better than a poor shot if we do not have the right target.

CHAPTER 17
Chemotherapy Number Six

1999: 28 September – 11 October

I find out my blood count is borderline but the oncologist still wants to up my dose to get a cure as quickly as possible. It seems reasonable but probably means that the roller coaster of treatment will be a bit more of a ride than usual. However, despite feeling hesitant, I agree.

My employer has been very supportive and I warn Kevin that I plan to work even more from home. Putting down the phone I am impressed by the sense of quiet humanity he shows. Particularly as he will have to shoulder some of the work I do not do, and he is already working at weekends on top of 07.00 am to 11.00 pm week days.

John phones me up and asks about my tumour. "Is it one swollen lesion or a series that have coalesced together? Is the one on my neck the primary or secondary?"

I thought I had answered these questions and start second-guessing why John is asking this now. My second-guessing dwells on the bad and the ugly rather than the good, and I find myself feeling pretty unsettled by it all.

The office is pretty quiet when I get in there mid-morning. I see Patricia who is as considerate as always. Patricia came to our company a couple of years back as a temp but quickly impressed with her maturity and quiet determination to get more than the job done. Another lady, Desiree, has just joined from South Africa, and I say I am surprised that she's not heard about me over there. She jokingly tells me she has, that is why she almost stayed there!

Patricia's twenty-four year old brother was diagnosed with Hodgkin's disease six months before me. The tumour in his chest was the size of a bowling ball when it was discovered! The chest has so much space in it that sometimes people are unaware until it has grown very large. It makes my tumour seem pretty small in the grand scheme of things. I tried to empathize with her as best as I could at the time, little knowing that I would be following the same track. She keeps me informed of her brother's recovery which I find helpful, especially as she says I seem to be doing much better than he did at equivalent stages. I have offered to talk with her brother about what I have found helpful in the way of nutrition but he does not come back to me.

Patricia ends by saying, "Don't worry, Mark you will be all right."

Mentally this may not count for much, but I find it very comforting emotionally.

At the end of the day another close friend, Shane, is working late again and is the only one left in the office when I leave. He was an Education Officer in the Royal Australian Air Force before going into civilian life as a trainer. He now focuses on developing business helped by his quiet maturity and patience. We laugh about our times in the Services and I remind him not to forget to go home.

My Mother has been a very great help to me, and given Ruth a well deserved break. She is now heading back to the UK. The kids and Ruth say good-bye to her before I take her to the airport. We don't say much to each other in the car. I want to park to see her off, but she is adamant that I must just drop her outside the terminal. She is worried that I may be too stressed or pick up a cold from people in the airport.

She is very upset when we say our goodbyes, and I say, "Don't worry."

Words which, it turns out, do not comfort her.

It is chemotherapy number six today and I do not feel out of the sticks – yet. The good news is that my oncologist reckons I have been taking the chemotherapy very well, the bad news is that he wants to up the dose of Bleomycin some 20%. I know Bleomycin is the drug that is most linked to hair loss not that that bothers me, it is that my high dose chemotherapy is just about to become a higher dose one. What I do not realise is that there is an increased risk of scarring my lungs under certain conditions. One of the four drugs is giving me pain and Robyne — a very cheerful and extremely experienced chemotherapy nurse — comes in to help.

Marissa, another chemotherapy nurse, gives me some very timely and useful advice. She advises when visualising the body eating up all the cancer cells to imagine it as a Pacman eating all the cancerous cells. It feels like a very powerful visualisation.

On the way back from the hospital I keep seeing things differently. I see the beauty of the trees in a new way and am reminded of Sergeant Joyce Kilmer's poem:

"I THINK that I shall never see
A poem lovely as a tree.

A tree whose hungry mouth is prest
Against the sweet earth's flowing breast;

A tree that looks at God all day,
And lifts her leafy arms to pray;

A tree that may in summer wear
A nest of robins in her hair;

Upon whose bosom snow has lain;
Who intimately lives with rain.

Poems are made by fools like me,
But only God can make a tree."[257]

A few days later John, a close friend of ours, phones me about a friend of his called Vito. Vito was diagnosed with Non-Hodgkin's disease at 38 years of age. He went through a full course of chemotherapy after which he seemed to be cleared. He then went back to work a month after it finished, but another lump appeared. It was recommended he go through another full course of chemotherapy and he did two sessions before deciding to try alternatives. John asks if I am prepared to give his friend advice.

I say, "Of course."

Ruth and I have been going to Qigong classes run by Clif Sanderson regularly in a veteran building which belongs to the Australian Unity Limited. Clif goes through a much more complete pattern of Qigong than Professor Wang showed me a few months back. Movements in Qigong are always meant to be simple, relaxed and light. Clif explains the movements and the benefits in a very common-sense way (a bit like his Feng-Shui). He emphasizes the importance of breathing, suggesting few people breathe properly. As others have highlighted, he indicates that poor breathing can contribute to illness, and identifies the three keys to Qigong;

- Breath,
- Intention,
- Movement.

We have some interesting discussions before the practice.

Ali is only twenty-six years old but says wisely, "I could not think of a better way to spend two hours and twenty dollars."

He has been thinking how words tell us so much. Why "We" is more meaningful than "Me". "W" is unlimited; infinite as it is an open character. When you put it upside down you get "M", which is a character with a finite space. He suggests that "We" is inclusive and "Me" exclusive!

I raise the question of how much "hands on healing" is in the mind? Pam is a middle aged nurse who comes regularly to the Qigong. She picks up on my question. She says a few years back her 15-year-old Labrador, Dell, started suffering from a badly ulcerated colon. She took him to a very good vet who said that unfortunately nothing could be done. Not satisfied with this she took him to a healer. The healer did one hands-on healing and the dog was immediately and completely symptom free. When she took Dell back to the vet, the vet agreed Dell was healed but was understandably sceptical about the reason.

Nine months later Pam came down in the morning to find Dell lying in her own urine and faeces, unable to move. She took her to the vet again, who diagnosed a stroke and said that Dell would have to be put down. Yet again she was not satisfied with that and took Dell to the same healer. The dog was in such a bad state that it could not even get out of the car. So the healer went to the car and laid hands on Dell. The dog immediately got up, wagged his tail, and jumped out of the car. The vet was quite amazed, to put it mildly, when he saw Dell again. The nice thing about this example is that the healing of the dog could not have been "in its mind".

I asked who the healer was and she said, "It was Clif. I have looked for a healer for twenty-five years and come across many people claiming to be able to heal before I finally found Clif."

Clif modestly adds, "Everyone is able to heal, you just have to get your logical mind out of the way."

It all impresses me more and more. I went to Qigong feeling pretty sick and after fifty minutes of doing the patterns I am feeling very well. There is something in this and it also fits in with my experience of Reike. I picked up Reike Level 2 on my travels and have experienced healing through it in ways not easy to rationalize. In 1996 I tore the ligaments in my right ankle during Taekwondo competition training. I phoned Carol who had taught me Reike, to do some "remote healing" which sounded pretty wacky. But on the one hand "wacky" is just the term to describe things which do not fit the normal way of seeing the world. On the other hand if your mind is too open perhaps your brain might just fall out!

Anyway, she said she would do it the next evening. The next morning I was sitting at my desk in the office when I got this strong sensation in my ankle, lasting for several minutes. I immediately wondered whether Carol had just started doing the Reike. It was 08.55 am and I resolved to contact her, which I did two days later. She said she had started the Reike at about 8.00 am. No match there I thought, but then she added that she had finished just before 9.00 am! All very strange but I saw later reported in TIME Magazine in 2000 that;

> "It is enough to make a sceptic squirm. After analysing the results of two dozen trials, researchers say there may be some merit in the alternative art of 'distance healing'… "

I comment that it seems to me that when any of us start accessing the ability to heal it becomes difficult not to let our ego come marching in. Once the conscious mind does that, it blocks our ability to heal. I am told the "trick", if there is one, is to remain humble and recognize it is not us doing it. Instead it must be a selfless act. Ian Gawler had severe cancer yet after going to the Filipino healers he experienced a remarkable and generalised healing process. The tumours kept growing, although much more slowly. He writes,

> "It was obvious to me I had not made the necessary changes in myself. Only after many more efforts, culminating in meeting Sai Baba, a Holy Man of India, was I really able to get free of my cancer problems[258]."

In 1987 Ian Gawler was awarded the Order of Australia Medal in recognition of his services to the community.

I want more vitamin C powder and arrange to see Edna. I stand behind the counter chatting with her for a while and she tells me more about what happened when her son was two years of age. Edna had felt that things were looking very uncertain and she ended up telephoning an astrologer. The astrologer asked why she would want to have a future chart drawn up for her two-year-old son.

Edna replied, "Because I have a very clever child."

She did not tell the astrologer about the diagnosis her son had just had. This was in 1976, and the astrologer went through the chart predicting a number of issues for her son. The astrologer immediately raised concerns that her son was born at the time of an eclipse when all the other planets were lined up "*against*" him. In his case, she predicted, that this would unfortunately lead to an adverse effect on his health. She went through 1977, 1978, 1979, 1980, and then stopped at 1981. The astrologer was not able to go on past this year, although she did not know why. It turned out that Edna's son's kidneys failed in 1981 and he went on a dialysis machine and then had a couple of kidney transplants. He is still well today as I write this.

Edna asks, "Was this coincidence or was the astrologer picking something up? I don't know."

Edna has kept the original chart with all the predictions.

John T., my best man at my wedding thirteen years ago, phones up. He trained and served in the Royal Engineers with me. He also served in the Queen's Gurkha Engineers, but left the Army a couple of years before me to study for an MBA and work in industry. He is highly competent and professional, yet can always see the funny side to life. We talk for a bit before he asks me how I am going and I tell him my news. He is a bit taken aback and I mention how quite a few people were in tears during my talk to my company in Sydney, a while back now. We both chuckle as I realize John is refraining from asking whether this was due to the moving content or poor presentation...

Trek – Day 13

Trekking Truism: Anything you do can get you lost, including nothing.

1991: 6 December, 11am, The Himalaya

I got up at 04.30 am feeling some effects of last night's rather pungent rum and water. It was alleviated slightly by Chandra who brought me tea in bed. He noticed I was feeling a bit hung over and offered to lighten my load by carrying *TEMPLER*.

We caught the 6 o'clock bus to Pouwa from where we began to walk to Maimajhuwa. It was "all aboard" again Nepalese style. Up in the hills it is a regulation free zone – there are no compulsory courses for anything.

The bus was going along merrily one moment then suddenly stopped the next in the middle of nowhere. I assumed that it was picking up some lost passengers, but started to wonder if this was a permanent premature stop. Several passengers and the driver got out and looked like they were trying to threaten the bus into action. After they gave it a good beating my initial bout of optimism faded. The engine had had it. Subash and my porters had sensed the reality of the situation better than I and were waiting on the roadside with all the bags, as I got off.

There were no connecting buses out there so our trek started sooner than planned. I was not sure at first where we were, so it was quite hard to decide in which direction to go – like life at times!

I had also thought that we might have had the last of the scenic views, but there were some more striking ones along our way. We were almost at 10 000 feet and had a majestic view of Kumbakarna and its surrounding mountains. The mountain air seemed to be entering lungs for the first time each breath we took and an entourage of birds followed us along the tree-lined route, one moment providing us with sweet twittering music, the next a cacophony of sound. There are more than 800 species of birds in Nepal; that is more than in Canada and USA combined, and it has nearly 10% of the world's species. In the background to this music I sensed a faint roar. Far in the distance I saw a faint movement of white across a white-capped mountain. Perhaps it was an avalanche rolling its way down.

I thought of these distant summits as a simile for my ideals – rarely reached but useful to help me to chart my course. They also confirmed at what stage I was at, at any one time, and when I would finally reach my destination – the taller the mountain, the greater the vision, and vice versa.

We sat in the shade of a line of tall trees. As we enjoyed the shade and comforting surroundings, we talked about experiences we had had, lives we had led or wished to lead. I asked my porters what they wanted from this trek, and primarily it was a job. With Subash making up for my inconsistent Nepali – which was now more flowing but no more fluent, they followed this up by selecting one of Aristotle's sources of pleasure. Chandra wanted to acquire more assets. Subash was more interested in the sensual pleasures that money could buy, while Nadur looked for greater knowledge from this trek. Ratna did not really answer this question. His reply was more about moral virtue, about "being". In a way it emphasized that we are human beings – not human doings!

I had read in Hong Kong Lao-Tzu's comments about being who we are, and they seemed to be well in line with Ratna's sentiments, "Rather abide at the centre of your being: for the more you leave it, the less you learn. … the way is to be."

Up there it seemed much easier to live in line with this.

Although I knew where I was I was not too sure where I was in relation to anything else. This might unfortunately scotch my chance of a trip to Darjeeling, India after this trek. We passed a lone family living high up in the mountains. They had a small pond and a couple of buildings, but lived several hours away from anyone else. Their young children came running out to look at us, dirty but glowing with health. They first gazed at us strangers in astonishment and then smiled as we passed. I wondered if they were a Sherpa family. The woman who watched us would have then been a Sherpani[259]. There might have been more males because the Sherpa practise polyandry – "female" polygamy. I resisted the temptation to photograph them as the Sherpas are generally camera shy. Only about 0.7% of the Nepalese speak the language of these people of trading and Buddhism.

Nepal has a Gross Domestic Product estimated to be only US$210[260] per person. Although this is somewhat misleading, as basically 90% of the population are subsistence farmers operating outside the cash system, it is still pretty bleak and showed there in the hills. However, these hill people seemed to accept the hand life deals them. I guess it was because their expectations matched their conditions. Happiness is a function of *opportunities* (self-created and otherwise), less some function of *expectations*. Where this function of expectation exceeds lifestyle it equals unhappiness. Up in the hills expectations were low enough for the villagers still to be constantly happy. It seemed to contrast with life in the West, where happiness is linked to success – defined as either getting what you want or what society expects you to want.

We were now one day behind schedule and we bivouacked that night. There was very little to eat as I had planned to reach the next village to buy dinner, proving a variation of an earlier *Trekking Truism*; if you cannot read a map of the way then your porters are going to fast!

The porters bought a scrawny looking chicken from an isolated household nearby. It looked like it must have died from starvation

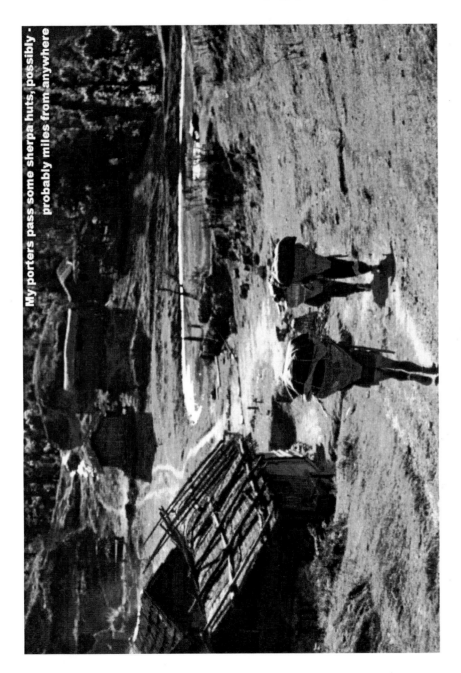

My porters pass some sherpa huts, possibly - probably miles from anywhere

A House in Higher Hills

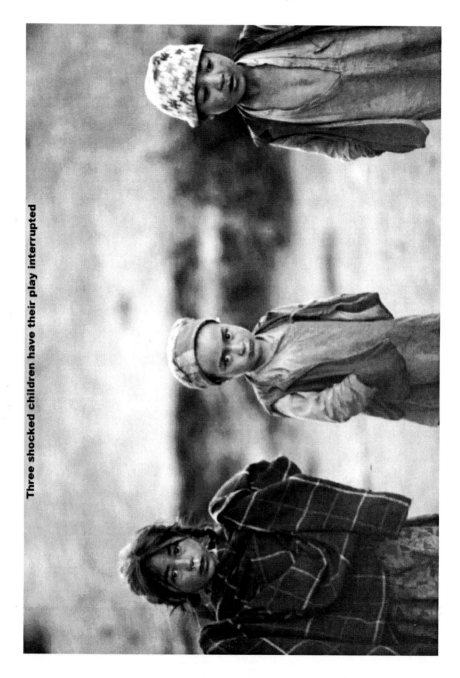

Three shocked children have their play interrupted

A House in Higher Hills

but chickens were still expensive up here and we paid through the beak for it.

Ratna, the cook as usual, had his ingenuity tested but rose to the occasion, adding a whole load of ghee[261] and producing something that I had never seen before.

I took one look at the chicken and decided to pass on this occasion despite it fitting the old colonial adage, "If you can cook it, boil it or peel it, you can eat it … otherwise forget it."

The other part of the meal did not half taste good.

The Journey Inside – Step 12 – What Is My Purpose?

"Many persons have the wrong idea about what constitutes true happiness. It is not attained through self-gratification but through fidelity to a worthy purpose"

Helen Keller

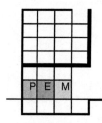   **Level of Pleasure – Physiognomy**

It is at this Level that the Freudian idea applies – that we do *everything* either to gain pleasure or avoid pain. This Level is about fun and passion. Anthony Robbins, one of the world's leading motivational speakers, emphasises "living with passion[262]" and this is largely about focusing on this Level, which can be very good for us. However, it will not necessarily take us to the other Levels and if we solely live on this floor then the other floors are going to get mighty dusty. Using the House simile again we can see that this is a very important Level, because it is at this Level (the Ground Floor) that we usually leave and enter any house. It is also the Level where we tend to spend much of our day depending on how old we are.

The link of character to physical type is not surprising. Appearance leads to experiences which lead to character. Physical ability tends to do likewise. Caroline Myss identifies this Level as being symbolized by the Christian sacrament of Communion – the receiving of the grace of God.

Floor Plan for Pleasure

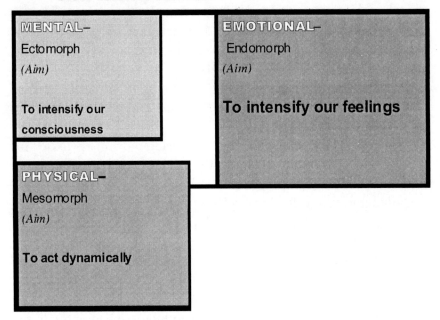

The styles above have been deduced by the author from information on *The Varieties of Temperament*[263].

Turn to Annex A at the back of this Book again remembering that you are looking at how Purpose is defined for you at this Level.

1. Look at the Purposes in the floor plan above.
2. Decide which one means the most to you.
3. Identify which of the three Rooms it is in.
4. Go to Annex A and look at the second Level.
5. Mark an "→" in the corresponding Room at that Level.
6. *Mark only one room with an arrow at this Level.*

In the mid-nineties scientific journals published about 100 studies on sadness for every one on happiness. However, more American studies are now focussing on the latter and

Doctor Martin E.P. Seligman, and other experts, are pin-pointing why some people are happy and others not. Findings so far suggest that the happiest people spend the least time alone, pursue personal growth and intimacy, and judge themselves by their own yardstick. However, these findings may be less relevant to other cultures. Seligman has concluded that everyone has a "set point" for happiness, just as they do for weight.

Ed Diener from the University of Illinois in USA has studied thousands of people over the last ten years and what makes them happy.

One of his conclusions is that, "Materialism is toxic for happiness... [although] People living in wealthy nations are happier than those in dire poverty[264]."

Although Diener does not believe that there is any "recipe" for happiness he has noticed that the "Happiest people all seem to have good friends."

Other important findings are that happiness is about 50% determined by genetics, marriage tends to make people happier and a close family protects children against despair.

There is evidence that altruism acts to increase happiness in the giver, and researchers have also found that gratitude for what one has and forgiveness are both strongly linked to happiness.

Christopher Peterson, a psychologist at the University of Michigan, has commented, "[Forgiveness] is the queen of all virtues, and probably the hardest to come by[265]."

CHAPTER 18

"A man with outward courage dares to die, A man with inward courage dares to live … "

Lao-Tzu

1999: 12–18 October

I read a touching story about courage going around the world on email. Whether it is true or not, it is a story which clearly illustrates courage. The author apparently worked as a volunteer at Stanford Hospital in the USA, and got to know a little girl called Liz who was suffering from a rare and serious disease. Her only chance of recovery appeared to be a blood transfusion from her 5-year-old brother who had miraculously survived the same disease and had developed the antibodies needed to combat the illness. The doctor explained the situation to her little brother, and asked the boy if he would willingly give his blood to his sister.

The boy hesitated for only a moment before taking a deep breath and saying, "Yes, I'll do it if it will save Liz."

As the transfusion progressed, he lay in the bed next to his sister and smiled as he saw the colour returning to her cheeks. Then his face grew pale and his smile faded.

He looked up at the doctor and asked with a trembling voice, "Will I start to die straight away?"

Being so young, the boy had misunderstood the doctor; he thought he was going to have to give to his sister *all* of his blood.

Courage is different from "guts". The first focuses on others, the second on oneself. I have parachuted once despite not caring for heights, but I decided to go "sport" parachuting. Unlike parachuting out of a burning plane, which would normally be acting out of the Level of Survival, this was an act of "pleasure".

Best summed up by the idea that, "You take risks not to escape life but to stop life escaping you."

We went up in a light plane and being the one officer with four Gurkha soldiers, I was expected to go first. No problems. I climbed out along the wing and jumped on the count of three: it would have taken more nerve to refuse!

However, my confidence had not been helped when the jump instructor had earlier gone through "What can go wrong …"

> "Firstly the static line may not release so you are left dangling out of the plane at 2500 feet. No problems. The jumpmaster will show you the axe. You put your hands on your head to signal that you have seen it and then he will cut you from the plane and you release the reserve.
>
> Secondly, sometimes people find this situation so uncomfortable that they black out. The jumpmaster slides down the static line using a karabiner, and earning his money, grabs the unconscious parachutist then cuts the static line. As both fall away the jump master releases the reserve of the unconscious parachutist then pulls his own. Finally, sometimes the parachute opens too soon and gets wrapped around the tail of the plane, doing an impression of a bloody great air brake. In that case you quickly press the quick-release pins of your main parachute and as you fall away you release your reserve."

There was a pregnant pause and I said, "Wait there, you've forgotten one eventuality. What if your parachute opens too early and wraps around the tail plane, and you black out?"

"Well funny you should mention that. It happened in America. In that case the pilot radioed down to the tower and asked for a lot of foam on the runway!"

(The parachutist apparently fully recovered from a lot of broken bones and a very sore head.)

I was reminded of the saying, "If at first you don't succeed, then parachuting is not for you!"

I am lying in the bath wishing this would be over, and I start thinking about suicide, about ending all this. It is difficult to relate exactly what I mean about this. The thought occurs to me of committing suicide, but it is not out of a desire to do so. It is just one of life's many thoughts, things which are not part of us. Yet I know if I start dwelling on this thought it is likely to become stronger and feel more a part of me. My aversion to it will make it more real. But I am comfortable for now accepting that we are neither our mind nor our thoughts. I ignore this thought and reflect simply that even when it is raining the sun is still shining above.

I do not think suicide is likely when we focus on others, by way of compassion, courage or wisdom. It seems to me to be most dangerous when we have a sense of despair because of hormonal or other physical reasons. Only ten months ago a very close friend of Ruth's, a thirty-seven year old mother of two young children, killed herself. It has been immensely difficult for the many people who cared about her and it seemed so pointless. But without being in her situation we cannot begin to understand the enormous amount of anguish she must have been going through.

I have decided to try Clif's hands-on healing. There is nothing like doing something different. This experience of cancer is difficult yet it is telling me in plain English that there is no way to totally control life. A message I don't like, but one I perhaps need. Clif has had many "experiences" with hands-on healing. In one case he was at a

> "… Hotel – far north of Amsterdam – and at the end of the evening… The owner of the Hotel/Motel, asked if I might treat his elderly friend. I seldom ever ask why a person has come and I simply invited him to lie on [the] bed while I applied the usual non-method. He stood up after twenty minutes or so with a strange look on his face. The disbelief on his face was comical. 'No, I don't believe it,' he kept repeating as he probed at his legs and waved his knees about. It seems he had had seriously painful legs and buttocks for so long that his

wife could not recall him ever getting out of the bed without a struggle. Next morning (and for three years now) he has had no recurrence and no pains. Later [the owner] told us he was one of the local multi-millionaires!"

As someone once said, for those who believe, no examples are necessary; for those who do not believe, no examples are sufficient. I feel happy to accept a former Minister of Israel, David Ben Gurion's, acute observation, "Anyone who does not believe in miracles is not a realist."

As a scientist by training I know that miracles happen. Miracles are simply events that science cannot explain, and therefore they must occur since scientific knowledge is finite.

An obvious question is, "Why don't healers heal for money?" The Filipino healers that Ian Gawler encountered asked for twenty-two dollars *in total.* It appears that those who become flushed with success and who start to charge larger amounts lost their powers. This is what makes it so difficult for us to heal.

When it starts working we can become focussed on "I'm doing it", the ego grows and our healing abilities diminish.

It also explains why it is so difficult to get it to work under laboratory conditions. The focus tends to change from helping others to proving "your abilities" or some other focus on self. It may not be an objective/ scientific truth as it is not reproducible at will, yet does that mean it is not real?

That said I believe it is important to keep hold of responsibility for your life whether you go to a doctor or a spiritual healer, or anyone in between. To hand over responsibility for your life is to me like treading on quicksand. It may seem all right, but it will start giving way when you come under pressure. Taking responsibility for our lives means responsibility for our sickness too. This is not to blame ourselves but to see more clearly that doctors and healers are there to assist us in living our lives, not to live them for us. My

Mother had spoken to me on the phone about how she let doctors have full responsibility for her recovery. I felt this was unwise†.

I suffered from persistent warts when I was about nine years old. I had over twenty on my hands (and two on my wrist). Doctors, parents and I tried a whole load of creams and ointments to get rid of them but nothing worked. So my Father asked his mother, who lived in South Africa, to do the "wart cure" she was taught by an African Medicine man. You rub a small piece of steak on each wart and bury the pieces at the time of the full moon. As they rot so do the warts as long as you have the correct incantations! All very mysterious; however, all my warts disappeared *on my hands* within a couple of weeks. We forgot to do the warts on my wrist and they only went some twenty years later. Coincidence? Maybe, but the same coincidence happened to my Father when he was a young boy. All in the mind? Perhaps; but then why did they not go with the conventional medicine creams – I would have believed in them a lot more? While we have to deal with the here and now, perhaps we must still be open to the "there and after".

Ruth's body language says "alleluia" when I tell her we are off to Keith and Margaret's for lunch. She cannot believe that we are going out, as basically we have not done this since I was diagnosed. All four of us have decided to become Australian citizens. Although we feel very British we have decided to make this lucky country more of a home.

He thought he was inviting someone around to his house with less hair than he!

He pretends to be a touch miffed when he sees me, exclaiming, "I can't believe it. You still have more hair than I."

During a very pleasant lunch we plan a little celebration party.

On Saturday I take Olly to soccer training and see a friend there. She mentions how her nine-year-old daughter had a lump in her breast so she rather anxiously took her to their doctor.

---

†Note: My Mother died two and a half years later from cancer.

He checked her and said, "Don't worry; it's just a breast bud."
"But isn't this a bit young to start getting breasts?"
He replied that he sees young girls of six years of age getting breasts. This doctor explained it was because of all the hormones given to cows to increase their dairy production. The hormones apparently remain in the dairy products and cause girls to reach puberty earlier, which has been linked to an increased risk of breast cancer later in life[266].

I tell her that recommending milk because it is rich in calcium is like recommending people eat steel bars because they have a lot of iron in them. It is the amount absorbed by the body which is important. Many green vegetables have calcium absorption rates of over 50%[267], compared with about 32% for milk[268].

I ask, "Have you ever thought where cows get *all* their calcium from?"

However, I add that it is probably best to play safe and to take calcium supplements if not eating dairy food.

I have found conventional nutritional advice pretty confusing and its general advice around health has not seemed much clearer to me during this time. My metaphor to explain health and sickness is as follows;

"We are born with a shield formed by our genetics to a certain shape, size and thickness. The environment fires various 'bullets' at us from the start of our lives, made up of bacteria, viruses, chemicals and other toxins, and some of these bullets are more like cannon balls! Our shield then deflects these bullets as they come whizzing by. Inevitably our shield rusts and degrades over time but good nutrition and a healthy lifestyle stops our shield from dissolving away too fast. The mind is another key factor in our protection and can either make sure that our shield is in position covering us well (e.g. positive feelings) or it can move it out of the way (e.g. adverse/ negative stress)!"

Another friend, Linda, stops over for a cup of tea. Linda is a mother of two young daughters and has proved to be a very reliable friend who has greatly helped. Several times she has readily looked after the boys at short notice when I have gone for treatment. While she and Ruth talk, I make some *"Mark's Mansion"* home-baked bread with the Panasonic bread maker we bought when I was diagnosed with cancer. It has seven ingredients or Levels, and *Mark's Mansion Bread* goes like this:

Bread Improver	1-2 tsps	*(Vitamin C)*
Filtered Water	410 ml	*(Non-fluoridated)*
Sea Salt	2 tsps	*(With KCl)*
Olive Oil	4 dtsps	*(Extra Virgin)*
Dry Yeast	$1/_3$ - 1 tsp	
Pure Honey	1 dtsp	
Organic Spelt Bread Flour	600 gm	*(White & Wholemeal)*

gm =grams

dtsp =dessert spoon

tsp =teaspoon

ml =milliliters

As I load up the bread maker today, I think of it symbolically as representing the Levels.

1   Bread Flour = Survival – *bread is both symbolically representative of the physical body in religion as well as practically the food that sustains many people who are on the breadline.*

2   Honey = Pleasure – *symbolized by the idea of the "land of milk and honey – (or use brown sugar).*

3   Yeast = Power – *in that yeast provides the power to lift the bread.*

A House in Higher Hills

4   Olive Oil = Compassion – *olive oil is food that provides the "Mediterranean effect" in lowering heart disease despite a fatty diet: olive gardens also feature as places of tranquillity in biblical stories.*

5   Sea Salt = Courage – *one way to interpret "salt of the earth": those who are hardworking and brave.*

6   Water = Wisdom – *the truth that is part of all living things: it is used in mythological stories to represent wisdom, for instance in the Wizard of Oz where Dorothy killed the witch by throwing water over her (the water symbolizing the wisdom that overcomes evil).*

7   Bread Improver = Meaning – *vitamin C is the main constituent of improver and its ability to physically detoxify symbolizes the detoxification at this Level which represents removing layers of mental conditioning.*

I mention the rationale for "my order" to Ruth over lunch. She is understandably far from convinced, "That is a bit far fetched – it could easily be a coincidence", and adds bread did not used to be made with these ingredients.

This is true, but not all mythological stories have all the ingredients of selflessness either. At the end of the day it does not matter if others find it meaningful.

It is a significant ritual for me, where "The art of ritual is really the magic of making use of energy to achieve a specific goal[269],"and so getting a good outcome which is probably the case because a number of friends tell me it is about the best bread that they have tasted.

The taste is undoubtedly helped by the bread flour we get from *Simply No Knead*[270]. It sells spelt[271] flour which is a low allergy and high energy flour. It was one of the first grains farmed[272] and is generically different from wheat.

Saint Hildegard[273] wrote about spelt: "The spelt is the best of grains… It produces a strong body and healthy blood to those who eat it and it makes the spirit of man light and cheerful!"

Spelt is not only high in B vitamins (including B_{17}) but also contains special carbohydrates (Mono-poly Saccharides) which stimulate the immune system. Which all sounds good, particularly if you have cancer. In contrast, wheat has negligible B_{17}.

Noel, another very good neighbour, comes over as I am going out to the car. He is originally from Ireland and came over in 1963 as a ten pound immigrant. I thought it was always by boat but he took the option to fly. He is a forthright individual with a typically sound Irish humour. He has had to face a few health issues in his life too, having had a quadruple bypass four years back and a kidney stone removed before that. His specialist had told him that his kidney stone was probably caused by drinking too much milk as a youngster. Another good reason to be careful with your dairy consumption!

He asks how things are going and seems to be surprised how well I am looking.

I tell him, "Fine," and he stresses, as he told Ruth when I was first diagnosed, "If you need any help you know where to come."

As I stand by my gate I see a large magpie eyeing me. I immediately think of the English rhyme – "one for sorrow… " – not very uplifting. But then I spot another in the garden across the street – "two for joy". It's a bit like life – there's always another magpie, always some good news, although you may have to look.

Ruth's making some boysenberries and custard for dinner tonight.

Rob comes up to me and asks, "Do you want to have some poisonberries."

He is either communicating courageously or erroneously, and if it is the former then I am getting quite enough of that intravenously for the moment!

Trek – Day 14

Trekking Truism: Directions in the Himalaya follow the law of inverse proportionality. The closer you get to your destination the more inaccurate they become.

1991: 7 December, Maimajhuwa (*I think*)

We left at 07.30 am after a quick breakfast and aimed to arrive at 10.00 hours. I chose a route decisively and it took four and a half hours, two hours longer than I expected. My GPS was not working too well again and the locals kept pointing in several different directions. I felt like I was on a dance through the mountains – "fox-trotting one way, two stepping another up the Himalaya."

For a while all news seemed to be good news. The views were terrific and we were making good time. We dropped more than fifteen hundred feet over rough terrain to the bottom of one hill.
The porters said something like, "See you at the bottom," then seemed to fall all the way to the base of the mountain.
I was not even half way down when I saw that Nadur and Chandra had reached the bottom, with their 40 kg loads and flip-flops. Even old Ratna arrived slightly ahead of me. I then realized the bad news – we were on the wrong path.

The Gurkhas apparently develop their knee muscles they have to an exceptional degree from walking in the hills. Although I had no trouble keeping up when going up hills and walked faster on the flat, they left me for dead going downhill. It was quite a sight to behold as they darted down like two legged mountain goats. In contrast, I was feeling like a bit of an old man – my knees hurt, possibly courtesy of cartilage operations I had had on both of them.

That said I happily ignored this pain, as in life I was finding that I generally got what I focussed on.

I stood bemused at one point as two locals stood side-by-side pointing in almost opposite directions when asked the way. Perhaps it was just a comment on life… several ways will get you to your goal? Fortunately an old man walked up and clarified the situation. He was an ex-Gurkha soldier who had been in the Gurkha Parachute Squadron raised after World War II. It no longer exists but there is a story about how it was raised.

> "Shortly after World War II it was decided to raise a parachute battalion from Gurkha volunteers and the Gurkha Regiment's Commanding Officer gathered the men on parade so that a Parachute Regimental Colonel could talk to them through a translator. The Colonel explained that they would first do some tough physical training, and then start with training jumps at 1200-1500 feet, reducing to 600-800 feet as they become more proficient. The Commanding Officer asked for volunteers to step forward, but not one did. He was livid, repeated in outline what the Parachute Colonel had said and demanded more volunteers. Out of a thousand soldiers only a couple stepped forward. He was irate at the lack of courage being shown when a Gurkha NCO put up his hand and asked if they could do the first jump from about 300 feet.
>
> 'Don't be silly,' he answered, 'the parachutes won't open.'
>
> 'Oh! We will we have parachutes' the NCO exclaimed, and the whole Regiment stepped forward.'"

When we stopped for lunch a passing old man greeted us graciously. I got a strong sense of sincerity and he turned out to be a holy man from southern India. With his grey hair and beard, he had the peaceful determination of someone who had thoroughly explored himself. He was going on a pilgrimage to a holy site in northern Nepal, a long way away. He was a fakir, an Eastern term for someone who reaches for God through the physical expression of intense determination and an iron will. In due course he bade us good-bye as he moved off towards his own destination. Ours turned out to be just around the corner – in Himalayan terms.

It had been worth the extra time. I lapped up the scenery although I was hardly moving cat-like. We were only a short seven hours' walk from the Indian border, as I had now realized that the border was just over the top of the mountains upon which we had camped the previous night.

We arrived at Maimajhuwa and I saw that the other two water points had been good preparation for this one. This was a very large one so I wanted to recce it straight away.

Fortunately the village teacher arrived and I paid heed to the old advice: "If communication is to change behaviour it must be grounded in the desires and interests of the receivers[274]."

I told him how I was here to design a water supply system for the village but only had a couple of days to do this big task. Could he therefore take me to the source? Without any hesitation he led me, Subash, Chandra and Nadur there. It took over two hours. The only feasible route for pumpless water supply system was to follow the sides of hills where the vulnerability of pipelines to landslides was all too evident.

These hillsides were steep and navigation was made more difficult because of stout bush growing on them. I told the village teacher that the bushes needed to be cut out of the way for me to do my survey first thing tomorrow morning. I knew it is going to be a tough job, but, of course, nothing is impossible for the one who does not have to do it. Perhaps it would happen by magic, and villagers up in the hills tended to have a definite belief in the supernatural. I had my doubts that it could be done otherwise in this time frame despite their kukri skills. I had tried cutting with the kukri I had bought at Sunsari market, but only made small nicks in thick wooden branches. Chandra, three-quarters my size and strength demonstrated the skill involved by effortlessly cutting the same wood in half. In the main religious festival in Nepal –

Dewali – adult buffaloes are sacrificed by cutting off their heads with large two-handed kukris. It is not for the faint hearted. The first buffalo usually comes into the sacrificial area willingly; any that follow are not nearly so amenable. It is a very poor omen if it requires more than one cut to sever the head from the body. Yet individual Gurkhas have even cut the heads off bulls with a single-handed kukri, with all the risk and the ignominy for failing. As for me, I would have been lucky to cut the head off a slow moving cauliflower.

Around us were some bulls being used for ploughing and I expressed my confusion to Ratna as I thought they were "holy". He explained that these were oxen, not bulls. Cows are "holy" and cannot be used to pull ploughs or do work of any nature. Villagers will only use them for milk and dung production. Bulls are also considered holy, but oxen, castrated bulls, can be used as beasts of burden. He clarified that it is oxen which are killed at religious ceremonies. I made a mental note to try and not be reincarnated as an ox. Not only are you castrated, but you are also eligible to do all the work and be executed.

Darkness fell … heavily, as I almost did when walking back. Stumbling across the ploughed fields with my feet sinking into the soft mud, I arrived to the welcome smell of cooked potatoes. Ratna had produced a rice and vegetable meal – a relative feast. We had small potatoes which were boiled and then peeled, and about 2 kilograms of green unripe tangerines. The total cost was 35 Pence. After having had them I broke Miss Piggy's Fourth Law of Eating; "Never eat more than you can lift," and crawled to my tent.

There I turned on my radio to listen to the crackles of the BBC World Service in my home from home.

The Journey Inside – Step 13 – What Is My Purpose?

"Fear not that thy life shall come to an end, but rather fear that it shall never have a beginning"

Cardinal John Henry Newman

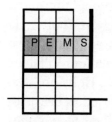

Level of Courage – The Enneagram

When self-confidence comes from a belief in our ability to intervene for others, then it is about courage. Courage is best defined as *"knowingly* risking ourselves physically, emotionally and/or mentally for the sake of others".

If the "5-year-old brother" had given blood to his sister without believing there was any risk he would be hurt, or die, then it would be hard to see his action as courageous – compassionate yes, but not courageous. The fact that he was never going to die is not the point. Courage is not necessarily the action – it is the perception that leads to the action! On a different matter our ability to recognise that nothing is all good or all bad is one way to assess our level of maturity and, to a certain extent, our courage.

The Emotional Room is large at this Level, and that is perhaps why Courage is so often identified with the "Heart". For instance

Richard I, a King of England, was noted for his bravery and given the name "*Coeur de Lion*[275]". In fact the French use the same word, 'coeur', to mean heart and courage. However, courage is mostly about the Physical Room, probably because, whatever its source, courage concludes with doing something. A form of purposeful action (as opposed to the "Reaction" where we are being controlled by someone or something else). In the Christian Tradition, this Level is symbolised by Confession where we act to cleanse our "spirit" of negative acts of will.

Gurkha officers do not usually think of Gurkha soldiers as mercenaries even though they fit the common definition in the sense that they are hired soldiers working for a foreign army. However, being paid for military service is not enough to be defined as a mercenary; otherwise it would include almost all soldiers and even conscripts. Nor is being a hired soldier in Foreign Service, as then all soldiers on attachments or working for coalition forces would be mercenaries. The motivation for serving gives better clarification around this point – if the soldiers serve primarily for money, in other words they are operating at the Level of Pleasure, then "mercenary" is an apt description. Gurkhas generally serve the British crown out of a sense of "honour", which is at a different Level – the Level of Courage (when it is a positive code of honour). This is borne out by the very high number of Gurkhas who have been awarded the very highest medals for valour. The result is that the Gurkhas strive more powerfully to achieve the purpose than mercenaries, and others who operate at lower Levels. In the Diagram below are the ways we may try to get into the Rooms at this Level.

Floor Plan for Courage

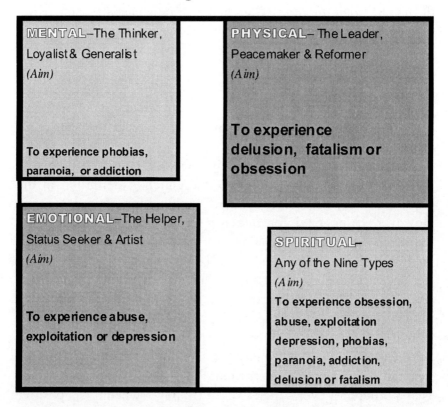

The purpose for each Role is derived from *Personality Types*[276].

Turn to Annex A at the back of this Book again remembering that you are looking at how Purpose is defined for you at this Level.

1 Look at the Purposes in the floor plan above.
2 Decide which one means the most to you.
3 Identify which of the four Rooms it is in, noting there is the choice between two rooms in each case at this Level.
4 Go to Annex A and look at the sixth Level.

5   Look back at the Rooms you have circled at this Level. If you have not circled the Room which corresponds to your choice of Room in this part, then mark an "→" in the Room. If there is a circle in this Room then mark an "→" in the Spiritual Room (whether or not there is a circle in the Spiritual Room at this Level).

6   *Mark only one room with an arrow at this Level*[277].

"Courage" is used generally to describe a range of types of bravery. Where our intent is selfish we are operating at other Levels. If we are bravely controlling our external surroundings for our own sake, then it is about Power. If we are showing the "guts" to stay alive, then it is about Survival.

For example there is no doubting Adolf Hitler's wickedness or bravery.

In respect to the latter, he "was a dedicated, courageous soldier[278]" and, as a runner in the German infantry in the trenches of World War I, was awarded the Iron Cross Class 2 for saving his Regimental commander's life under fire, in 1914.

Later, in 1918, he was awarded the Iron Cross Class 1 – a rare achievement for a corporal – for bravery shown in delivering an important dispatch through heavy fire. However, whether it was courage or not depends on whether his motive was selfless – purposefully risking his own life in order to save others' – or selfish – for recognition/power or survival.

CHAPTER 19

Chemotherapy Number Seven

1999: 19 – 24 October

I go to my usual Ward for my seventh chemotherapy wearing some clothes that used to be tight. I am met by blank faces at reception. I have not been booked into chemotherapy or the Ward. Sounds good! Anyway I resist the temptation to scarper and I am quickly booked into a general Ward on the next floor.

One of the nurses says, "A change is as good as a rest."

However, I'm not so sure.

I go to this ward and drop off my overnight bag. It is a four-bed ward and the Nursing Supervisor for the floor checks me in slowly as they do not usually deal with chemotherapy patients. She reads the paperwork carefully and finds a consent form for the treatment signed by me. I assure her it is a forgery.

Next to me is Dick, a 74-year-old man who had been diagnosed the night before with lung cancer. He seems as upset at someone my age having cancer as in his own predicament.

He says, "You're too young to have cancer."

"I agree – but I tend to think that it is always too young to have cancer!"

Opposite us is an elderly man who I guess to be in his late sixties. I then find out that he has just celebrated his 101st birthday. Dick and I talk a bit more. He tells me a friend of his son's was diagnosed thirty years ago with cancer simultaneously with his three-year-old son. I think it was with the same form of cancer for both of them. Fortunately both are still doing fine.

I head off to the Day Centre for those patients who just take the chemotherapy as a day procedure and I am put on a drip. Here Mary puts the drip into the veins in the bottom part of my arm. I warn her that although the ones on the top of my arm look relatively good, they consistently give problems. It appears that my veins are not up to much and resemble those of an old woman's.

Another nurse comes over and says out of the blue, "Your veins look like an old woman's."

I am asleep for the rest of the procedure and feel much better for it[279]. When I wake up I talk to a male nurse, Jack, about life which leads on to spirituality. He has started exploring Buddhism and tells me his brother-in-law went to a Vipassana course which he found helpful as well. I am the only one left for the last hour in the Centre so we end up going quite far down the track of a spiritual discussion.

At home Peter phones to see how I am going and refrains from gloating too much at the loss of England to South Africa in the World Cup. His family have been going through a difficult period as a close relative was found with a lump which caused concern. I am very pleased to hear now that it is nothing serious. However, Peter's managing director has been confirmed with incurable prostate cancer. His manager seems to have a very positive philosophy on life. He suspends judgement and appears to accept the situation. It sounds like the Buddhist idea of equanimity, "holy" acceptance of the situation. Coincidentally, I see a report on television that says 50 men die from prostate cancer in Australia each week. I send Peter some information on Epilobium, a herb which has a large amount of supporting, albeit anecdotal, evidence that it helps all types of prostate problems. Several men have reported it as curing them from prostate cancer. Epilobium is the only herb in herbology recognised as a "prostatelium", that is one specific to treating the prostate. I advise him to suggest to his boss he contact Hilde Hemmes[280], a well-known Australian Herbalist[281].

Peter and I conclude that when we judge, we move from being equanimous. It is very difficult to judge while remaining completely, and identically, happy with the various outcomes. Since we almost always perceive one option as better as or worse than the other(s), therefore we cannot remain in a state of total acceptance and are not being equanimous.

Olly is handling the situation very well but it is still having an effect on him. He is spending quite a lot of time up in his room on his own. Both my Mother and Ruth's Mother do not feel comfortable about this when I tell them over the phone. Conversely, I think it is a good way for him to deal with things. Also Olly's great sense of humour helps him to cope better with things and I hear him chuckling over an episode of the *Simpsons* as Homer says, "I am a good leader as I notice, when I am around, people have to work a lot harder."

I seem to be handling the high dose therapy very well in physical terms. People still express surprise that I am going through it. I believe it is because of the alternative things that I am doing, but my Mother is unconvinced. She tells me a middle aged lady who went through the same chemotherapy as her kept all her hair and seemed to handle it well too. However, I believe the blood type diet is helping me notably. Experts are arguing for and against it, yet parts could be checked relatively simply. I interpret the diet to predict that celiacs' disease would be significantly less common amongst type A's and type AB's than type O's and B's, although I have not seen Doctor D'Adamo mention this. Ruth has a mild form of the disease – she has been medically diagnosed with a gluten allergy, and she is a blood type O. (However, as predicted by the blood type diet, she can eat as much bread made from spelt flour as she wants without ill-effect.)

I also see a pattern indicating that dairy intolerance would tend to be rarer amongst blood type B's and AB's, and more common amongst type A's and O's. The three people I know with this intolerance, are these types. The blood type diet seems to suggest that true allergies to shellfish[282] are most likely amongst blood type A's and least likely amongst O's. Sure enough I and the other person I know with a major allergy to shellfish are blood type A's. My samples are small and you have to take into account the proportion of those eating wheat, dairy or shellfish, which may differ from the numbers in the population, but I think it is worth investigating.

Lisa phones to wish me well for my last chemotherapy. She has shown a great sense of optimism and consideration but her planning is not so good. I have a week to go! We talk about a number of things and I tell her the next stage is a check up to see if there is any cancer that can still be detected. In some ways, this process is going to be a lot harder mentally than the chemotherapy treatment was physically. I have got used to the discomfort of chemotherapy and the fortnightly visits to the hospital. Now I am to have tests which may indicate the duration of my life. I comfort myself by dwelling on the truth that whatever is, is. The test will not change the reality.

I see a Fox News report about the problems Gulf War veterans have had with illness since the conflict. It is thought that that as many as 160 000 of the 700 000 soldiers who served in Operation Desert Storm may have suffered some form of prolonged ill health[283]. In many cases the symptoms are extremely severe. There seem to be six main reasons being postulated. Soldiers being exposed to;

1 Chemical/biological agents used by Saddam Hussein or dispersed when Iraqi chemical munitions were demolished.
2 Significant doses of radiation from the depleted uranium in armour and anti-tank warheads colliding.
3 Toxins in thick oil clouds in Kuwait after the fighting.
4 The "cocktail" of vaccines given to protect them from potential biological warfare agents, including anthrax.

5   Pesticides and chemicals which combine to cause severe adverse effects.

6   Aspartame poisoning caused by drinking Aspartame which has been heated above 86 degrees Fahrenheit. Also known as Nutrasweet, Equal and Spoonful; apparently several thousand pallets of diet drinks were shipped to the Desert Storm troops and left in the heat for weeks. Jeanne Elizabeth Blum, in her revealing book *woman heal thyself* about Chinese acupressure and medicine, recommends never taking Aspartame (or Saccharine). It can break down into methanol, which then converts to formaldehyde of the class *"deadly poison"* (the same class of drugs as cyanide). It is also a carcinogen.

Jeanne Blum gave a lecture at a World Environmental Conference where she warned that if you were taking food or drink with Aspartame added, and you suffered any number of symptoms ranging from cramps, headaches or intense muscular pain, to dizziness, fatigue, depression, anxiety or memory loss, then "you probably have Aspartame Disease"!

While western medicine is looking for the one "culprit" it seems to me that all of these combined are potential factors although I think that vaccines are the most significant one[284]. The Germ Theory is not fact it is just an inaccurate model in the field of biology, just as Newton's Laws of Motion are inexact models in the field of physics. We need a new illness model to treat in our more complex medical environment just as we needed Einstein's Law of Relativity to better describe the complexities of momentum. Germs do not cause disease! Of course, the particular virus or bacteria is an important factor in any illness. However, the reason you suffer the dis-ease – any ill effects – depends on a whole range of factors and not all key ones are physical. Doctor Deepak Chopra, a Fellow of the American College of Physicians who has written several best selling books, described how cold viruses have been put directly into the mucous lining of volunteers' noses yet only

12% of these people suffered colds. This proportion was not increased by chilling the volunteers' bodies or doing any other purely physical intervention.

We recently watched the film *Apollo 13* and saw that the pilot Ken Mattingly was taken off the Apollo Mission because he got measles in his blood and medical specialists predicted that he would suffer the disease during the Mission. Then things went wrong for his buddies in space and he spent long hours in the simulator back on Earth to help work out what to do. Despite his exhausting work he never got the measles! The Germ Theory is an incomplete model.

Homoeopathy believes that experienced practitioners using the Mora machine in conjunction with equipment that can detoxify certain agents specifically – e.g. *Listen, EQ4*, or *Orion* – can help to alleviate the "Gulf War Syndrome".   Conventional medicine does not seem to have much to offer in this area yet, but it has not seriously looked at this approach as far as I know.

It is a time of visits and visitors. Sue comes around, and I ask her how I look.

She is hesitant but honest, "Not too great."

It helps as it gives me an accurate mental picture of where I am at.

Shortly afterwards Lisa comes around and says in reply to my question, "Pretty good," which aids me emotionally.

Later Don, a General Manager and friend I met at an aluminium smelting company, comes around with his two sons. Ruth bumped into his wife and told her of my situation. Don is now a barrister after initially studying as a solicitor and working in a range of roles. Don is always bursting with ideas and brings a new perspective with quick witted humour wherever he goes. At the moment he is trying to produce a film about the life of his grandfather who served as a stretcher bearer in the First World War. He studied art and played in a brass band before joining the Australian Army, where he served for 23 months before being blinded by mustard gas. I state,

> "That's a bit of a coincidence as the first attempt to treat my type of cancer, lymphoma, was by the great British surgeon, Bilroth, who used arsenic to try to cure his patients. But after World War I the first successful treatment of lymphoma with chemotherapy was achieved by using nitrogen mustard, another name for 'mustard gas'. Fortunately things seem to have improved markedly since then, as many thousands of chemotherapy drugs have now been developed and tested."

Don's grandfather returned to Australia married and later set up a family stain-glass window business. Although blind he continued to design and help produce stained glass windows. After his wife died, and more than forty years after being blinded, he had one of the first corneal transplants. He was then able to see from photos what his wife and the windows looked like for the first time. I am left wondering whether they matched what was in his mind. When I was trekking in Nepal in 1990 there were still about 400 men alive who had been blinded by mustard gas in the First World War[285]. I do not know how many are alive now.

I ask Don if there is a role for me in his film.

He replies, "Yes, you could be one of the old German soldiers who advances over the trench parapet and gets shot."

Somehow I don't think it is a role to die for.

Lying in bed on Sunday morning I again feel unwell. I have been thinking too much about my situation and have slept little. Rob comes in to see why I am not getting up. Then he notices that I do not have his large teddy bear next to me which he had given to me.

He asks, "Why don't you have it in your bed?"

And he retrieves it from the chair and places it firmly next to me. As he does so he pushes the little hand-sized teddy out of the way, saying, "That's no good – if it falls out of your bed you won't notice it. But you can't miss noticing this one falling out."

Trek – Day 15

Trekking Truism: All routes go up more than they go down.

1991: 8 December, Maimajhuwa Village, the Himalaya

I did some of my preparatory work, checking I had all my survey equipment and then noticed a beautiful five year old girl watching me with her doleful eyes … I quickly realized that she was a boy. The Nepalese dress young children up as the opposite gender to confuse the evil spirits and keep the children safe.

Every man and his yeti was there waiting for me to start the survey – thirty in all. I led the way to the source. It flowed at 0.225 litres per second so would provide nine taps at a gush. They of course want to go for ten. I had initially planned an open water system, rather than a closed one, as it would be easier to design, build and maintain. But the original information from the village said that the system was to supply 106 villagers. I was now told that it had to supply 300 school students as well. I thought it a toss up between a redesign and ordering a whole load of contraceptives.

A closed water supply system would be more expensive and the villagers agreed to provide the portering fees for materials from the nearest road head, Deurali; two and a half hours away by foot when carrying a load. The usual load is about 40 kilograms per man per journey. The Pradhan Panch agreed, firstly, that village tradesmen, such as carpenters and bricklayers, would provide their services free. Secondly, that all construction material, including sand, stone, aggregate and wood, would be provided by the village at no cost.

It sounded good and I weaved my way along a steep survey route, so steep in parts that we had to go uphill to go downhill. The cutters had done a superb job, far better than I had imagined given the time available. It looked like a bulldozer had ploughed its way through the trees, which grew on these slopes out of the ground for a short bit horizontally before twisting violently up towards the sky.

Chandra was with me as he knew the score well. I had not thought to bring pickaxes and crampons despite the fact that they could have helped, but then my travel insurance did not cover rock climbing … Instead I was happy to rely on his proven catching skills. I found it difficult to use the Abney Level on the steep slopes and got into some serious tree hugging. At one point my left hand was holding a tree behind my back, twisting straight up behind me. The Abney level was in my right hand and as I raised it to my eye my body shook. I was confident that these measurements were going to be accurate to at least 45 degrees.

Having seen the cutters' impressive work on these slopes I was confident that that the villagers would be able to dig in the pipes along this route. However, there were going to be difficulties as the ground might be too unstable to bury the water pipes. I tended to agree that there must be four rules for designing a water supply system. The trouble was that no one seemed to know what they might be.

As the spectators got bored, or I got past their house, they disappeared. I carried on as I was into the swing of things and did not want to break. We continued with an ever depleting band of disciples. I ended up finishing the last part of the survey down to the village school over ten hours later. Today is a lesson in the *3T's* – "*Things Take Time*". The usual problem I find when I do not suffer from the 7P's. I felt good to have completed the survey and it also meant that we were back on schedule.

I could not have failed to notice how critical leadership was here. The Pradhan Panch's style reminded me of Ratna's. It seemed a more "spiritual" approach to leadership – lighting the way. He seemed to appreciate the importance of diversity; it existed and so

**A young boy confuses me,
as he watches**

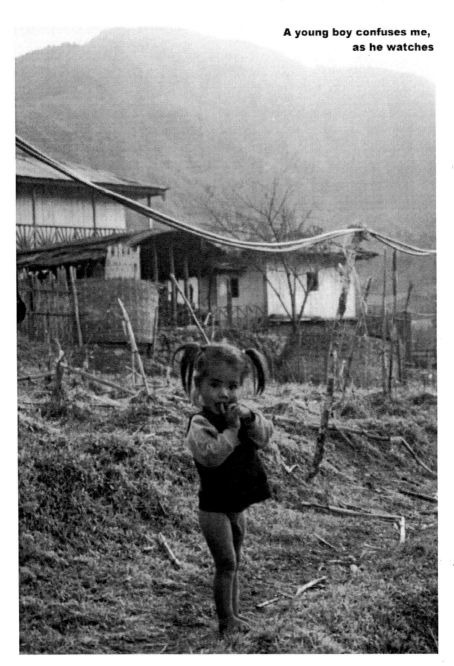

A House in Higher Hills

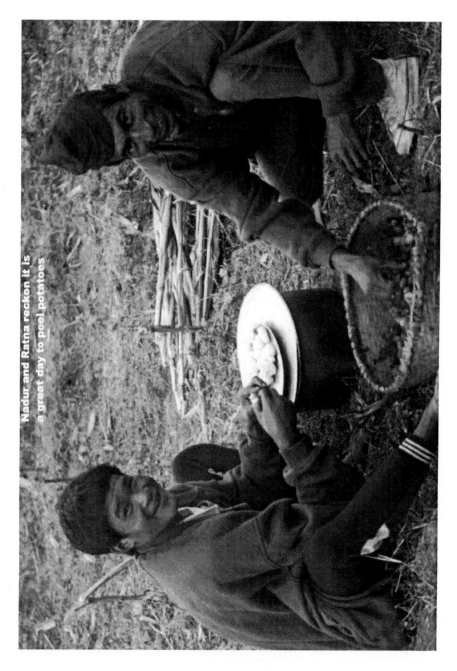

Nadur and Ratna reckon it is a great day to peel potatoes

A House in Higher Hills

had to be catered for. Subash and the other porters seemed to have differing expectations of what I should do as a leader. Chandra expected me to physically enable the way. In contrast Subash saw my role as more emotive and about encouraging the way, while for Nadur it seemed to be about me discovering the way.

It was chips and just three eggs for tea. I was on about six eggs a day and starting to cluck.

It reminded me of that famous poem I wrote: "Six eggs, six eggs, six eggs a day and yet I am thoroughly wasting away … "

My sum total of meat in the last fifteen days was twenty cans of tuna plus a few wads of some form of meat fat. I was rather looking forward to Christmas and turkeys.

I sat there listening to Subash and porters chattering in Nepalese. Later as I settled down to sleep, I ran through my calculations and I wondered whether I had made a mistake, perhaps I could still have supplied the village with an open system?

The Journey Inside – Step 14 – Not Who but How Am I?

"If you grab them by the balls, their hearts and minds will follow"
*General Westmoreland; his rationale for
the use of force in Vietnam*

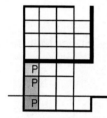

Selfish Levels – Influence

At the Level of Meaning the question "who am I?" Has little meaning – it is more "how am I?" How we act when relating to others ends up influencing or leading. If we are operating out of a sense of selfishness then it must be about influence, whereas leadership is a selfless motivation.

The British Army teach that there are three types of leadership; *Compulsion, Persuasion* and *Example*, in increasing order of effectiveness. However, the Chakra framework allows us to be more complete in understanding these forms.

Leadership is putting others first, *it is "selfless" rather than "selfish" behaviour.* Therefore true leadership can only be manifested at the 4th Chakra and above. However, there are three influencing motivations (focussed on oneself) below the 4th Chakra.

Leadership by Compulsion (*Survival*):
This form of "leadership" is simply influence by threat; it is about survival and a characteristic of the 1st Chakra; the Level of Survival. In its most extreme negative form it manifests as "death threats".

Leadership by Persuasion (*Power*):
This "leadership" is really a form of influence by argument, usually at an intellectual level, and is characteristic of the 3rd Chakra; the Level of Power. In its most extreme negative form it manifests as "blackmail".

Influencing by Reward (*Pleasure*):
There is also a characteristic form of influence manifesting from the 2nd Chakra; the Level of Pleasure, and that is influencing by "reward". It is appropriate at times too, but again is not leadership because of its "selfish" focus – getting someone to do something for our own sake. In its most negative form it is seen in the form of "bribery".

The types of influence are shown in the floor plan below:

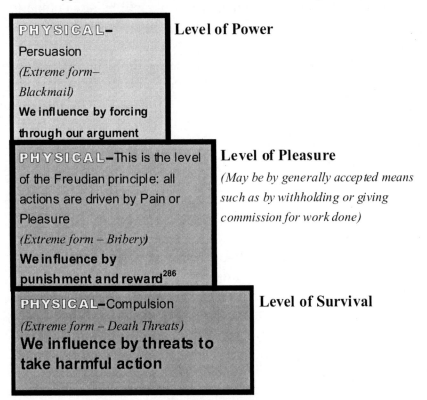

PHYSICAL– **Level of Power**
Persuasion
(Extreme form–
Blackmail)
We influence by forcing
through our argument

PHYSICAL–This is the level   **Level of Pleasure**
of the Freudian principle: all   *(May be by generally accepted means*
actions are driven by Pain or   *such as by withholding or giving*
Pleasure   *commission for work done)*
(Extreme form – Bribery)
We influence by
punishment and reward[286]

PHYSICAL–Compulsion   **Level of Survival**
(Extreme form – Death Threats)
We influence by threats to
take harmful action

A House in Higher Hills

Using the diagram on the previous page, identify which Rooms you spend a significant time in and put a circle in the Room or Rooms – noting the correct Level too.

1   Look at the Styles in the plan above.
2   Decide which one, or ones, you adopt significantly in your life.
3   Identify which of the Rooms it is in.
4   Go to Annex A, and look at the bottom three Levels.
5   Mark a circle in the Physical Room at the appropriate Level.

To decide which Rooms to circle ask yourself, "Which of these terms best describe my behaviour? Which of these descriptors would other close friends or relatives use about me, if any?"

If we are susceptible to bribery, then we will be susceptible to blackmail given the right circumstances, but not necessarily the other way around. This model suggests that when we are at the Level of Compassion, or higher, we remain uninfluenced by either. It is more difficult to explain how "death threats" are a lower form of energy than bribery and blackmail. The 1st and 7th Chakras are two ends of the same Chakra and so the Level of Survival has elements of the highest energy. In the short term, death threats can seem very powerful but this form of influence rapidly loses its power over time – it can have a very short "half-life". Death threats produce either a major response to negate them or an acceptance of them. Either way, at that moment, they lose their influence. Andy McNab, a British Special Air Service Sergeant, was tortured and continually threatened by the Iraqis with execution after his capture on a mission during the Gulf War.

After a few days of this he became resigned to death, "I thought: I've seen and done as much as I can. If it's going to happen, let's do it now [be executed] … I was not too worried about the actual dying bit … it would have been lovely to have the chance to say my farewells. What a way to go[287]."

A fundamental difference between influence and leadership is that influence only requires confidence, whereas leadership requires both character and confidence. In other words character is a prerequisite to leadership; as the Zulu proverb says, "I cannot hear what you say for the thunder of what you are."

CHAPTER 20

Good Leadership Involves Creating Leaders

1999: 25 October – 2 November

The workload is still very heavy in the office at the moment and I talk with Kevin about the possibility of my doing some assessment at home. Kevin has continued to work very long hours, but despite this, he has never put the slightest pressure on me to work more. Just the opposite in fact, wanting me to work only as much as I felt was "helpful" for me in my situation. It is a moment when I see things a bit more clearly.

We all lie somewhere on the continuum,

Selflessness

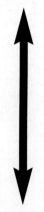

Selfishness

For most of us, we are somewhere in the middle, oscillating one way or another, depending on the situation we are in, or how we feel. Kevin is an accountant by background and shows that he invests in people too through his thoughtfulness. He is towards the top end, conversely, in my present predicament I am tending down towards the bottom of the continuum. Yet you can only "Lead" to the degree that you become "Selfless". It is a "necessary" but not "sufficient" condition for leadership. The first step is no guarantee of the second, but without it there is no second step.

To the extent that you are down to the end of "Selfishness", you can only influence, you may be a very good "politician", but you *cannot* lead. Trevor is a good example of someone who is intelligent and who influences well, but has yet to learn to lead. In fact many "world leaders" seem more like "world influencers". Only those Chakras with a selfless focus have a leadership style. The 1st, 2nd and 3rd Chakras are about influence. When I was in Nepal I met, physically or mentally (through the ideas I came across), the four leadership styles in the East – the monk, fakir, yogi, and the avatar. Each is associated with one of the top four Chakras. They also correspond nicely to the four leadership types in the West and this comparison is at Annex B[288]. Whatever the style, the East sees another requirement, "The principles used to lead a large group are the same as those used to lead a small group. It is a matter of organisation[289]."

"Selfless" type behaviour is not easy, irrespective of the situation. Another friend at work is weighed down with work, and clearly expects me to take on some of theirs.

Instead, I replied "Unfortunately not", remembering Oscar Wilde's words, "On an occasion of this kind it becomes more than a moral duty to speak one's mind. It becomes a pleasure."

I am feeling a definite sense of anticipation as I await my eighth and probably final chemotherapy. In many ways it is a lonely time for a lonely diagnosis. The support I get from family, friends, doctors – both conventional, and alternative, and from work, helps greatly. But in the final analysis I am the only one who can face this.

Joanna telephones me to see how I am going. She also asks about one of the projects and I promise to get back to her in a couple of days. I ask how things are going at her end and she mentions that a mutual friend and work colleague, Scott, has had a bad back injury and been off work recovering.

After her call, I send Scott a "get well card" saying, "I look forward to when we are both back on board at work."

I also attach the contact details for the excellent osteopath[290] (address) I have been using. I have been going to an osteopath, on and off, for a few years since a back injury ten years ago in Hong Kong. The exact location is where my primary tumour was located. I do not believe that this is a coincidence. Physically, the injury could have created a structural weakness and made me more predisposed to cancer at this point, or perhaps, much more esoterically, emotionally I have some issues at some level of compassion which meant I was "energetically" weak there and more susceptible to cancer? The idea linking cancer to the healing process going out of control is supported by a body of doctors who use nutritional therapy which includes vitamin B_{17}[291]. There is evidence that some cancers may result from the body's healing process not "switching off". B_{17} is the substance that helps the body's mechanism to do that, but once the tumour has become large it needs more than B_{17}. You may be told: not to be crazy and not to eat B_{17} (cyanoginic glycoside) as it has cyanide in it. However, the same people will tell you to eat Vitamin B_{12} (cyanocobalamine) which has the same cyanide radical. If you believe this warning, then beware of marzipan – it is commonly made by mixing apricot kernels (which have an extremely high B_{17} content[292]) and almonds!

It seems plausible to me that a significant number of cancers occur because of an injury. Smokers injure cells in their lungs repeatedly through inhaling toxic substances and hence are prone to lung cancer; research shows that mobile phones emit electromagnetic radiation which damages delicate ear and brain cells – hence the possible link to brain cancers. Colon cancers could arise from damage by substances we ingest which are toxic or turn toxic in the stomach. Constipation is a known increased risk factor for this type of cancer and means that the toxic chemicals are causing more damage as they remain in contact with the colon tissue for longer periods. Solar radiation damages the skin – hence the link to skin cancer – and high alcohol consumption causes liver damage and can lead to liver cancer. It may explain why racing cyclists, such as Lance Armstrong, have a heightened risk of testicular cancer because of repeated damage to their testicles while riding. Two acquaintances I know of were concussed a few years back and now have brain cancer. The patterns seem to be around us for all of us to see†.

Sunday is the Green Line Open Day. The Green Line is a co-operative venture which aims to supply organic and biodynamic food and produce, for families and individuals. I am sure that it is healthier to eat organic food but it is difficult and expensive to do so. So I just resolve to do it when I can. It is a good event and the food also tastes better than our usual non-organic food. It is a simply organised day with a comedian who gets Olly to come up and help him with his act. He tries to hold a rope while the comedian unicycles on it. Something which he finds hilarious, and my son's natural performing skills come to the fore.

There is also a composting demonstration, at the Open Day. It is very timely as ours is not working so I have "re-set" it after some advice from Peter on how it's done. He assures me that I must use a good starter. He says his urine works really well on his but unfortunately it seems a bit extravagant to fly him over from New Zealand to "wee" on our compost. Instead I plan to source it from here. Since chemotherapy may still be in my system and urine, I refrain from the temptation to have a go. Instead I get both my sons

---

† Note: I have been eating 5-10 apricot seeds daily for over two years and they have a very high concentration of B_{17}. I know of others who have been eating them for much longer than that and they say they feel better for it.

weeing on the compost at 20 cents a wee – much to their delight and Ruth's chagrin. I am now finding out how many times boys can wee when there is money in it … it is a fair few.

Chemotherapy does have the advantage of offering a good excuse not to drink your own urine. A disadvantage for Retired Indian Admiral L Ramdas who drinks his neat! The former Indian Prime Minister, Morarji Desai drank a glass of his own urine every day and remained healthy until he died aged 99 years. It may sound repulsive but each of us floated in amniotic fluid for nine months which is largely urine. Ramdas, his wife and daughter drink their urine, and he credits the therapy with helping him to maintain his health.

He explains, "There is nothing to be ashamed about. One only has to lower one's mental barrier, which is the result of brainwashing as a child. It demands tremendous courage and will."

I potter around the garden a bit and try to saw a small stump. I get about a third of the way through and I am absolutely knackered.

Rob comes over to see how I am doing and says, "I'll do it."

He tries, with my coaching, but he is finding it very hard to get the hang of using such a large saw which is almost as long as he is tall. My coaching probably needs improving too. Anyway, I decide to leave the sawing for a later date and go to pick up my other son.

When I get back it's done. Rob has done magnificently. The psychologist, William James, said that the deepest need in human nature is to be appreciated; and you can meet this need in others by recognising and understanding them. These can be addressed by raising self-esteem (operating from Compassion), and listening empathetically (where we are at the Level of Courage or Wisdom), respectively.

While it could be thought that using these processes is manipulative; it all depends on the intent. If I was given a wood saw and cut people's legs off instead, then the issue is with me not the tool, which may be very good. Anyway I try to raise Josh's self-esteem by telling him how well he did at such a young age in cutting a large log which I could not cut. I also give him A$20.00. (The President and CEO of DDI, William Byham Ph.D., in his book *Zapp! The Lightning of Empowerment*[293] outlines very clearly how to practically accomplish these important relationship requirements.)

Julie, the pastoral nurse, gave me the advisory booklet, *My Dad Has Cancer* and I now amend it. I rip out the pages which just seem to be too threatening for the boys. This leaves me with fourteen pages and I sit down with them in their bedroom, one at a time, and go through the story with them. It starts,

> "When Dad told me he had cancer, first I felt sad …
> Then I got really mad …
> Then I was very sad and confused."

It has a range of simple pictures to go with it. At each stage I ask Rob what he thinks the son is thinking.

He just says, "I don't know."

It understandably seems to be a bit of an uncomfortable story for him even without the more gory bits.

It goes on to talk about cells dying off, cancer being non-contagious and the three standard ways western medicine deals with it;

- Surgery,
- Chemotherapy,
- Radiotherapy.

I notice that they do not mention the fourth standard methodology which is included in countries like Germany. That is nutrition and I believe it is a critical omission.

I cut it down to ten minutes and add at the end, "You can also go to Chinese doctors and others."

Rob is pleased when it is over. My presentation skills for this sort of thing leave a bit to be desired. Now it is Olly's turn. He listens and shows great maturity while he sits with me.

Emotions seem to be contagious and one of our two cats, Sarah, also seems to be upset! She is "spraying" all over the house. We have tried a range of remedies to stop her over the last couple of months and now decide to take her to the *Animal Emergency Centre*, a privately run animal sanctuary. I do not want her put down as death is not my favoured option for anyone at present. We meet a man waiting in the queue, called Brian, who is trying to track down a lost dog. He looks at her in my homemade box and says he will take her if no one else will. Sure enough Sarah is not suitable for re-adoption, as she is too aggressive and rather than have her put down I ask Brian to take her. He cares for thirty stray cats at his own home, and many more at his factory.

Brian explains, "I don't care what sickness you have, whether animal or human, if you give the right care and attention then they have a good show of pulling it through.[294]"

Brian tells me about Flor•Essence (also mentioned by Doctor Soosay in the four herb/non-organic form of Essiac, when I was first diagnosed). In 1922 a white woman met a nurse, Renee Caisse, and told the story of how she was cured in 1892 of confirmed breast cancer, by a herbal remedy from a Red Indian medicine man. Renee noted down the formula as the mixture of eight herbs which was available locally. However, Renee forgot about this until her aunt was diagnosed with serious stomach cancer which had spread into her liver. She was operated on by specialists but they said they could do nothing more and gave her a maximum of six months to live. Renee started giving this tea to her aunt daily. It was just a year before the growth had gone and she was cured.

Renee went on to successfully treat many terminally ill patients One Doctor Leonardo, the Mayor of Rochester and widely acclaimed surgeon and specialist, visited her clinic and concluded (in Renee Caisse's words),

> "You've got it but the medical profession isn't going to let you
> do this to me … I could go home and burn them [the books he

had written]. It would revolutionise the whole treatment. They will never let you do it."

Renee's work convinced thousands of people and many doctors, and she ended up in partnership with Doctor Charles Brusche, JF Kennedy's personal physician, a highly respected specialist and co-founder of the largest medical facility in Cambridge Massachusetts. But her herbal remedy was not accepted by the medical authorities. This is despite the fact that independent doctors scientifically studying Renee's herbal treatment concluded that it prolongs life, relieves pain, breaks down the mass of growths, and is completely non-toxic. Renee continued her work although she had wanted the medical authorities to,

> "Make it available ... to the thousands of people that I couldn't reach at all, you see. I was so anxious for that, that nothing else mattered to me ... After seeing all those patients they still wouldn't accept that it was a cure[295]."

The Mora Machine can evaluate how beneficial or adverse foods or chemicals are for any particular individual, and it indicated that a mixture of organic flaxseed, sunflower and pumpkin seed, and a Chinese medicine given to me by Professor Wang, which I only know as ZZ-0089, were both extremely beneficial for me. Better than a whole range of other types of foods, vitamins and supplements tested on me. However, when my homoeopath checked some Flor•Essence which I had brought along, it registered as even more beneficial *for me* than these[296].

I resist phoning Peter up about the result of the 1999 Rugby World Cup semi-finals for about five and a half minutes. The New Zealand All-Blacks were convincingly and very surprisingly beaten by the French. Peter acknowledges it was a great match, with superb French play.

He even admits to letting out a potentially life threatening "Vive La France" in a room full of fellow Kiwis, albeit very quietly.

Nola is having farewell drinks as she is leaving her job as Aerobics Co-ordinator for a local YMCA Pool and Recreation Centre. I throw caution to the wind and decide to go for her farewell drinks. It is only the third time I have been out at night since June 10th. A number of people comment how well I look, although it is probably a matter of kindness or relativity as a few minutes later one friend says she has only just recognized me.

I stay only 50 minutes as I do not feel like kicking up my heels. Tony, another friend, comes over to talk for a bit. He tells me his father was diagnosed with cancer and given only three months to live a few years back. In the end he lived for three and a half years. That prediction was 1400% out and I wonder why make it, why tell someone they only have three months to live if not sure? Fear helps cancer, and that sort of prediction helps the fear. I presume it is out of a sense of honesty but predictions around cancer can be so way out is it not better to be optimistic?

I am convinced that a better and truer message for anyone with cancer is something like,

> "You have got a life-threatening illness but, as far as we can tell, you could live as long as ten or twenty years, but may only live for a few months. There is a lot you can now start doing to help with the outcome."

Twenty years ago, Peter, a family friend, (after retiring from the Royal Air Force) was diagnosed with cancer of the colon. It was found to have already breached the adjacent intestinal walls. On his subsequent discharge from hospital, and on asking the relevant junior medical staff as to his anticipated life expectancy, he was advised that five years would be the most likely maximum statistically-based forecast taking into account the medical category of his malignancy and, presumably, known records of similar cases available to the medical profession at that time. Peter remains fully active and he tells me how he remembers with gratitude the debt he owes to his surgeon for his outstanding skills, and also for the support of his family and friends. Peter is a gentle and considerate man and he tells me that, at the time, he made determined efforts before the start of each day, to maintain a positive mental outlook on the future.

Later, I lie in the bath that night in a state of flux, oscillating between some confidence that I will come through all this, and thoughts of dying. It's an uncomfortably interesting mix. But I am clear I want to still be around for longer. It is my opportunity to help my sons through their lives and to perhaps help others in some small way.

Sally phones up from England to see how things are going. Sally and I met at a university disco when we were both somewhat younger and she has remained a close friend since. She played Junior Wimbledon as a youngster but put tennis away when she went into further studies and a large manufacturing company. She is the sort of person who is pretty "out there" in life and who combines this with a very refreshing sense of humour. I tell her that things seem to be going in the right direction but I am not out of the woods yet. I add that my situation is not all bad, as I have now said to many others. Although I am not sure if I am saying this for them or for me?

She updates me on what has been happening with friends from Cambridge, which ones have gone to jail and which ones have not been found out yet… There are surprises both ways around. She wishes me all the best when I say my last Chemotherapy is due in a few days' time.

She adds, "You can now see the light at the end of the tunnel." I agree with the old line, "I hope it is not the headlamp of the oncoming train!"

Trek – Day 16

Trekking Truism: There is always one hour to go.

1991: 9 December, Maimajhuwa Village, The Himalaya

The air was clear and the strong smell of ploughed fields wafted into my tent. There was a low but constant generator-like hum from something, somewhere.

I had completed the recce but now I heard that the villagers wanted to discuss with me how to supply more people. They wanted the water supply system to supply 509 inhabitants plus the school students. We talked about it for an hour. The supply was good enough to provide adequate water for 106 adults and 300 school children, and the resulting estimated population growth over the next fifteen years, but would not support much more than that. I left them with this to think about and feeling more comfortable to have designed a closed water system. It would be more robust and should cope better with the potentially increased demands on it.

The track to Deuralis started narrowly but soon widened into a veritable highway for this part of the world. As usual the bridges varied in design. Most were warped bamboo or tree trunks. Good bridges for this part of the world. They had a natural grip from the dry bark. Many would have been built since the last wet monsoon which would have washed their ancestors away. There were areas with thick outcrops of trees but a lot of the land was denuded and the results of landslips were plain to see. It looked like God has given the hills some mighty karate chops.

We took a short cut off the track and rose to the hilltops surrounding us. Then the clouds started to thicken and the view became obscured. Ratna was struggling a bit but, in typical Gurkha style, would not hear of my taking any of his load.

We got to Deuralis at 3.30 pm which I had mistakenly thought was some major metropolis in the hills. It turned out to be a town the derelict side of barren. It has about twenty houses and did not sell most things.

A young ex-Gurkha soldier came up to us. He was one of the company disbanded in Hawaii a few years ago. Templer was a Colonel of the 7th Gurkhas and I was sure he would have been very sad at the incident. Typical of the Gurkhas he did not seem to hold any grudge towards the British or the Gurkha Brigade at losing his economic lifeline.

The Army is clear that to lead by example is better than persuasion, and far better than compulsion. Compulsion is just fear leadership and, "Correction does much, but encouragement does more[297]."

I sat with Subash and the porters, and we talked about the different cultures. Culture is linked to both values and norms, where values are about what people consider good or bad, and norms about what is considered right or wrong.

I bore in mind that Templer had found that there were certain things it was necessary to do irrespective of the culture you are leading in:

1 "Get the priorities right.
2 Get the instructions right.
3 Get the organization right.
4 Get the right people into the organization.
5 Get the right spirit into the people.
6 Leave them to get on with it.[298]"

Without further ado we took a scenic road out of Deuralis; heading towards Ilam, but then any road out was a good road. We stopped in the late afternoon and camped on the hillside. The grass was a touch boggy and the wind was getting up, bringing with it a low hum and chill. Very quickly the clouds went black above us, and coincidentally I heard on the World Service for the first time of Margaret Thatcher's resignation as Prime Minister twelve days earlier.

It was chip butties for dinner, Nepalese style, and Ratna cooked up another hillside special. Chandra and Nadur wanted to know about the ex-soldier we had met. Both were keen to join the British Gurkhas and I found it difficult to give them a sense of what had happened without giving them a misleading picture overall. Too often words fail to describe the reality. Instead I asked them what they hoped to get out of the military service they aimed for. I had found leading Gurkhas simple in some ways because they would accept your rank unless you worked particularly hard to get them not to. Despite this there was still more to leadership than that and they each had their individual needs.

The Journey Inside – Step 14 Continued – Not Who but How Am I?

"When a good leader leads the people respect and praise him;
The next best leader is one whom the people fear;
The worst leader is one whom they despise…
But when the very best leader leads,
The people say 'we did it ourselves[299]'."

Lao-Tzu: Tao Te Ching

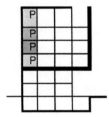 **Selfless Levels – Leadership**

B ritish soldiers have in the past divided officers into two types: "Go on" and "Come on[300]."

It is a succinct way to define the difference between influencers and leaders.

Roger Pearman, from the Centre of Creative Leadership in the United States, commented, "More skills are not enough… we fool ourselves that more skills will make us better leaders."

Leadership is about how we interact with people when focusing on others, not ourselves. It is what we do (or say), and the other side to "How I Am" leaves us with "Example" – the only "true" form of leadership. Leadership is not the same as management. The word "lead" comes from an Anglo Saxon word meaning "path" or "way". "Manage" comes from a completely different idea – the Latin word meaning "hand", as in "handling an object". Hence we may manage resources but we must lead people.

Leadership by Example can be demonstrated in four ways – each representative of one of the selfless Levels.

Leadership by Example through Service (*Compassion*):
Mother Teresa demonstrated this leadership by her Service to others.

"There should be less talk; a preaching point is not a meeting point. What do you do then? Take a broom and clean someone's house." She believed "To us what matters is the individual."

When asked what made her pick up the first child she replied, "If I'd never have picked up the first person, I'd never have picked up 42000 in Calcutta."

The British Army seems to agree as the motto of their Officer Training School – the Royal Military Academy Sandhurst – is *"Serve to lead"*.

Leadership by Example through Proficiency (*Courage*):
Sir Ernest Shackleton was a leader who showed his proficiency many times.

One of his men once said of him, "[He is] the greatest leader that ever came on God's earth, bar none."

In 1914 he set off to cross the Antarctic overland but his ship was trapped then crushed in ice. Shackleton and his men survived the next five months on a diet of dogs, penguins, seals and uncertainty. Shackleton initially led his crew to the safety of Elephant Island by rowing for seven days through pack ice. He then took five of his men in a twenty-two foot leaking lifeboat and sailed across 850 miles of the Weddell Sea, in winter, to get help for the rest of his men[301]. It is the stormiest ocean in the world, and after sailing through several gales and one full-blown hurricane they found that they could only land on the "wrong side" of the Island of South Georgia.

Shackleton then led two of his men across the intervening, never previously traversed, 10 000 foot mountain range taking one and a half days to reach help. In 2000, Reinhold Messner[302], one of the most famous mountaineers today, and two other highly acclaimed climbers repeated Shackleton's journey across the South Georgia Mountains. It took them three days using the latest hi-tech equipment.

Shackleton personally made sure that every single one of his men got home safely in the end.

Apsley Cherry-Garrard said of him[303];

> "For scientific discovery give me Scott;
> for speed and efficiency of travel give me Amundsen;
> but when disaster strikes and all hope is gone,
> get down on your knees and pray for Shackleton[304]."

Leadership by Example through Teaching (*Wisdom*):
Socrates understood that wisdom is not gained by someone teaching us but by our learning something. Hence Socrates emphasised questions to help others to find their answers.

He said, "You may have habits that weaken you. The secret of change is to focus all your energy, not on fighting the old, but on building the new."

When it comes to leading others at the Level of Wisdom we do this most effectively by asking effective questions.

Leadership by Example from Facing Ourselves (*Meaning*):
Leading by pure example is easily confused with leading by example through Proficiency. However, a story clearly illustrates the difference:

Gandhi was approached by a mother of a young boy who begged him to stop her son eating sugar. Gandhi hesitated then said, "Bring your son back in two weeks." The woman was confused but thanked him. Two weeks later she brought her son back. Gandhi looked the youngster in the eye and said, "Stop eating sugar."

Grateful but surprised, the woman asked, "Why did you tell me to bring him back in two weeks? You could have told him the same thing then."

Gandhi replied, "Two weeks ago I was eating sugar."

It is an example of *"meaning making"* – perhaps the ultimate form of leadership?

The types of leadership are summed up in the floor plan below:

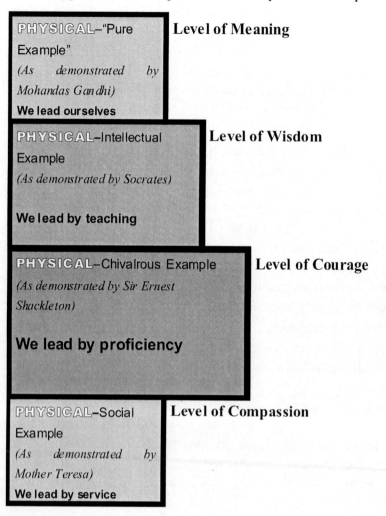

PHYSICAL–"Pure Example"
(As demonstrated by Mohandas Gandhi)
We lead ourselves

Level of Meaning

PHYSICAL–Intellectual Example
(As demonstrated by Socrates)
We lead by teaching

Level of Wisdom

PHYSICAL–Chivalrous Example
(As demonstrated by Sir Ernest Shackleton)
We lead by proficiency

Level of Courage

PHYSICAL–Social Example
(As demonstrated by Mother Teresa)
We lead by service

Level of Compassion

Using the diagram on the previous page, identify which Rooms you spend a significant time in and put a circle in the Room or Rooms – noting the correct Level too.

1   Look at the Styles in the plan above.
2   Decide which one, or ones, you adopt significantly in your life.
3   Identify which of the Rooms it is in.
4   Go to Annex A and look at the top four Levels.
5   Mark a circle in the corresponding Physical Room at the appropriate Level.

To decide which Rooms to circle ask yourself, "Which of these terms best describe me? Which of these descriptors would other close friends or relatives use about me, if any?"

Our world desperately needs more leaders while we seem to have more than enough managers and influencers.

Mark's Mansion explains why courage is probably the most easily recognisable form of leadership out of all four forms. It is because the Level of Courage's Main Room is the one through which leadership manifests – the Physical Room. Donald McGannon said, "leadership is action, not position", and *Mark's Mansion* gives greater definition to the first part of his statement, it indicates, "leadership is simply action for the sake of others."

The Director of Leadership Studies at the United Kingdom's Cranfield Institute of Management, Chris Keeble, succinctly clarified leadership when he said, "leaders love … managers manipulate".

CHAPTER 21

Chemotherapy Eight and A Journey Finishes

1999: 3–7 November

Chemotherapy number eight is here. I am feeling tired and a bit nervous about this chemotherapy, despite all the support. I have read that Gandhi said seven things may destroy us and it seems to me to be advice to keep to a higher Chakra:

"Wealth without work $[2^{nd} \rightarrow 3^{rd}$ Chakra?]
pleasure without conscience $[2^{nd} \rightarrow 6^{th}$ Chakra?]
knowledge without character $[3^{rd} \rightarrow 5^{th}$ Chakra?]
commerce without morality $[3^{rd} \rightarrow 4^{th}$ Chakra?]
politics without principle $[3^{rd} \rightarrow 5^{th}$ Chakra?]
science without humanity $[3^{rd} \rightarrow 4^{th}$ Chakra?]
religion without sacrifice" $[1^{st} \longleftrightarrow 7^{th}$ Chakra?]

In other words we need to add a "selfless" focus to the "selfish" one. I take some comfort from how Gandhi's link between religion and sacrifice supports my model. Sacrifice is to do with someone or something's survival, or lack thereof. Sacrifice is at the Level of Survival, and religion may be at this Level or at the Level of Meaning. The meaning of sacrifice is "to make complete", to integrate the spiritual part with the physical part and in my framework these Levels are linked by a ladder.

As I lie waiting for my next chemotherapy I understand more clearly that material things, even great wealth, cannot give meaning to life. In fact, nothing tangible can give meaning; not expensive cars, splendid houses, fine clothes or even children. (Many people have children whom they never see nor want to see.) Only the intangible can give meaning. For instance, the relationships you have with your children can give a very powerful sense of meaning; as can your feelings and your beliefs. This is where fundamentalist religions appear to me to miss the point. It seems that they take the symbol that is meant to represent the intangible truth and interpret it as a concrete reality.

For instance it is like someone telling you "They're on top of the world" and for you to think they are high on some physical object, and missing completely where they are emotionally, mentally or spiritually.

These thoughts are interrupted as my chemotherapy nurse for the day comes in. All the nurses at Cabrini have been highly professional and supportive; and I am happy to see it is Margaret who is my chemotherapy nurse again as I am particularly comfortable with her approach.

She asks how I am doing and I say: "I have not had so much fun in months. I plan to come back every Tuesday for years just to relive these happy memories."

Margaret goes through the list of initial questions on how I have been.

She asks: "Anything else?"

I say, "Yes, where is my certificate for completing eight chemotherapy sessions?"

She tells me she will get me a gold star, which she gets and I check if it is real gold.

It isn't and she says with feigned shock: "Get real; you're talking about the health budget here."

She hands me something to sign and reassures me by saying: "Don't worry, this just gives us Power of Attorney on your bank account should anything happen to you ..."

Margaret has not been watching the Rugby World Cup and I tell her of the surprise win of the French over the All Blacks, who seem to be playing more like the "All-Greys". I add that it is going to be an interesting change for the Australian team. They had the New

Zealand game plan and tactics all worked out but will now have to ditch that for the French game plan, which no one knows, including the French.

Marissa comes in to help. She asks if there is anything she can do.

"Yup," I reply, "you can take my chemotherapy."

Marissa is learning about chemotherapy treatment, so watches Margaret put my drip in and put some sticky tape over it as usual. Margaret then signs her name on it. I say I look forward to selling her work in the future. Margaret is transferring to work in the Day Chemotherapy Ward after 24 years in the overnight ward. A pretty good stint. I say in feigned surprise that she must then have started at 12 years of age. Marissa spots my desperate attempt to suck up to the nurse who is about to inject my drugs.

Marissa jokes, "You don't have to try so hard now, the drip is in!"

Margaret tests Marissa on the chemotherapy process. She asks Marissa whether DTIC (one of the chemicals I am injected with) is a vesicant.

She pauses and I jump in; knowing my stuff I say, "No, it is an irritant."

I ask Margaret whether she will accept my application for a nursing job. Margaret rejects it and then asks Marissa some technical questions about the drugs, about which Marissa shows a very good knowledge and about which I am happy to have none.

"So what happens if the patient goes into shock, Marissa?"

Marissa replies, "Immediately stop giving the drug, unless it is Mark whereupon you go down to the pharmacy for a quick resupply."

Marissa is tested on "Cannulation". I ask Margaret what Latin verb the word is derived from and express disbelief that she does not know.

I tell her "That's it; I have lost all faith in your treatment!"

I explain further, "It comes from the Latin root *'cannu'* meaning *'you are able to have'*, and *'lation'* a derivative of the word *'elation'*, meaning *'loads of fun.'*"

Marissa fields the questions about the side effects of Dicarbozin. These include things like hair loss, but I point out she has forgotten some of the other ones such as intense feelings of joy... I get the slight suspicion that I am interrupting the test session too much when they are discussing the side effects of Bleomycin.

Margaret says, "Yes, it can affect the patient's taste and smell. Sometimes the patient gets the sensation that the nurse has put a pillow over his face and is pushing down hard."

I decide to stop there for now, remembering "A closed mouth gathers no foot!"

Later, the lady who takes the food order comes up. I only have strawberries on my breakfast order and she asks whether I want anything else.

She is very helpful and keeps going through the whole list one item at a time, while I reply "No, nope, no thanks."

Finally we get to the end and I ask "Any champagne?"

She surprises me by saying, "Yes."

I reply, "No thanks."

I am in a double room and my roommate comes in. He is Travis, a 21-year-old man with a very rare form of liver and lung cancer. He looks very fit despite being almost bald. Apparently his cancer is so rare that there have only been 135 cases reported in the world. Despite this he seems very relaxed about his situation and I am sure he will be helped by his very positive mental focus. We talk about what we can do to help recovery. He shows me the vitamin pills he is on. Being the "Master", I go through them and confirm that they cover what I think is important.

Travis's father comes in a bit later. He is understandably very shaken by the whole turn of events. He says that Travis is supporting the whole family. I comfort him saying that I am sure Travis is doing the right things.

I leave the next morning, saying to the nursing staff, "Thank you all very much for all your kindness and help and I hope I never see you again … in an official capacity that is."

I feel relieved rather than happy to have finished this chemotherapy. I am learning the lesson I had when trekking the Himalaya, "The happiest people are those who have no particular cause for being happy except that they are so![305]"

It is the last treatment and I seem to have escaped the hiccups with the anti-nausea drugs but the increased dose is leaving more of its mark. I am feeling more nauseous and I am now losing my eyelashes and eyebrows. Fortunately this saves me from plucking them…

Both my sons have taken up writing books. Olly is writing a book about three boys, Max, Tim, and Tom, who find a Pirate Treasure Map. He is going to title it once he has completed it. I am helping Rob write his book called *The Magic School Bus Book* about a trip his class takes deep into the ocean.

He says: "It does not have to be true, all books are made up."
I reply, "No, some are true" and he remarks, "yes, of course like *let's eat right to keep fit*[306]."

I get the message that I have been pushing this point a bit too much.

One night I dream. "We all dream, we all must dream[307]."

It is thought to be the way the subconscious and conscious balance each other out. The subconscious makes sure your conscious life is in sync with it. At times it communicates (through symbols which is the only way it can) things that you are aware of at some level other than consciously. This may be the basis of premonitions. It is an old recommendation that to remember dreams at night you bang the back of your head lightly on your pillow three times and say to yourself each time, "I will remember my dreams tonight."

While I don't do that I still have two very vivid dreams two days after chemotherapy and get up at 05.15 am to write them down. The first is about accidentally swimming with white sharks and the second about being charged by a large female elephant, after her baby keeps following me.

The message could be, "Big animals don't like me, but small ones might" but I think that there a deeper meaning for me to find. The sub-conscious mind can only communicate in symbols. That is why effective advertising is often symbolic. It is accessing the sub-conscious, which is a very powerful influencer of one's actions. Subliminal advertising gives us an idea of how impactful this might be. Conversely, some experiments have found it to have no effect.[308]

So now I have come to a major point in my treatment; the last chemotherapy and I feel like I can stop trying to do the healthy thing so much. I am mentally less inclined at this stage to fight the side effects of chemotherapy with its nausea and other discomforts.

Lisa kindly lent me three books about "recovering" from cancer when I was first diagnosed. I do not feel the need to read two of them but *Quantum Healing*[309] is interesting. Doctor Chopra's experience with patients seems to show that the mind is a very important factor in any disease. He writes how in the spring of 1990, sociologists from the University of San Diego reported that Chinese mortality dropped by 35% the week before the Harvest Moon Festival. It is one of the major Chinese celebrations and one where special importance is placed on elders. Death rates climbed again when the festival ended. A week later they were 34% higher than normal.

A lady called Rodica phones me up. Edna had asked me if it was all right to pass my name to her.

Of course I replied, "Of course."

Rodica is in her early forties but has very advanced cancer and she says her doctor told her that there is little that can be done for her now. I find it difficult to know how to help her, as she is pretty well house bound. Talking with her, I face my own fears about cancer all over again. She tells me her background and I notice that she has had some of the experiences that Doctor Lawrence Le Shan had noticed were often reported by cancer patients. She tells me she has spent about A$80 000 on various alternative therapies, mortgaging herself to the hilt, but to no avail. I suggest that she try Flor•Essence and offer to leave the pack I have for her. She says she will consider it but is also set to try a new and, as yet, untested conventional therapy. In the end I never met Rodica or found out her full name, although I spoke to her several times on the phone. She picked up the Flor•Essence while I was out but found the powdered form too tiring to make. She died some six months later.

I have heard about a study in the UK in the 1990's, where patients were measured with all the medical prognostic factors known to be relevant. Then a correlation was made with psychological factors to see which were most predictive about who would live and who would die. Patients in comparable health and family circumstances, of the same age, and with the same severity of symptoms, were contrasted. Somewhat surprisingly, they found that there was no significant correlation between recovery and extent of family support, but some correlation with a positive attitude of the patient. However, there was a significantly greater correlation with "meaning". Those patients who believed that there was purpose for their being ill had a significantly better prognosis.

Ruth is instructing aerobics in the evening so I hire the science fiction film *Matrix,* which she does not want to watch. I am immediately struck by how it so cleverly parodies the archetypal meanings behind all the world's seven major religions. I also see a link with Buddhism, and its idea of life being an illusion seems apt. Buddhism does not say that there is "no reality" and presumably there must be. It is just that you cannot ever know what the underlying reality is actually like. When you listen to something, or use any of your senses, you do not actually hear, see, touch, taste or smell it. You use the electrical impulses triggering in your brain to create what you sense. When you look at something you cannot see it, only the image you create of it in your brain! This is one reason that, "We see things not as they are, but as we are[310]."

You may say "But you can compare your reality and check it is the same as others."

Nice idea but even if they coincide they may just be the illusion we are conditioned to see. I happen to be colour blind to a degree, as some men are, (women pass the gene on but are not affected by it). When I was first told as a ten-year-old that I see colours differently to other people, I thought, "What a load of rubbish."

I agree with others about the colours we see. Yet no matter how I see a colour if I am told it is "orange" and someone else is told it is "orange", we will always appear to agree that we are seeing the same thing when we are not. The same world is a different place depending on whom or what we are. If you had a shark's ability to sense electromagnetic radiation and smell then the world would intrude on you in ways you can only guess at. You would probably be confused if you could suddenly see like a chameleon – two eyes that can look in different directions! Some of our paradigms are "hard-wired" into us, making us see the world subjectively.

"To her lover, a beautiful woman is a delight; to an ascetic, a distraction; to a wolf, a good meal[311]."

That is not to say science is unimportant.

As a friend said to me, "Science shows us that there is an objective reality, and to strive to grasp even a bit of it can broaden our perspective and help us reach for a less-self centred world."

In *Matrix* the characters who are aware of the illusion can jump huge distances and run around vertical walls in the same way that "physical constraints" can be illusory in the real world. No one could break the "four-minute mile" for many years, possibly because it was universally believed to be beyond a human's physical capability. But once Roger Bannister broke it on 6 May 1954 (*in 3 minutes 59.04 seconds*), then John Landy broke it a few weeks later in 3 minutes 58 seconds, and several more runners quickly did likewise. Although you are constrained by some actual realities you may never reach them as your "beliefs" will limit you before any physical reality sets in! Playing a sport *"at home"* appears to give a huge advantage. Soccer teams in the English Premier League win almost twice as often at home as they do away – yet it is the same pitch, same game? There seems to be a non-physical effect, affecting the physical result[312].

In the film, Keanu Reeves lives in this grand Internet and is living a life of images fed to him. He is contacted by someone who has taken off the internet cables which feeds the illusion. This person has managed to get out of his pod and stepped into the real world *(become "liberated")*.

Keanu's character is dumped out of his pod by the controlling machines and now can see the world for what it really is; he has experienced the "real" reality *("nirvana")*. He gets beaten up by the machines' allies while his colleagues *(guardian angels, or "ariyas" – those ahead of him on the journey)*, who are standing around his physical body, mop his brow. He asks the head of this group of rebels *(his "guru")* how come people die when "killed" on the grand Internet, when it is just an illusion. His "guru" explains that the body cannot survive without the mind. At the end of the film Keanu is killed; however, he rises again having gained the experiential wisdom to go beyond the grand illusion in which life is experienced *(the "Matrix)* and remains beyond its grasp *("Buddhahood")*.

It all started with "release" because no matter how hard or cleverly you peer at the walls of the pod from the inside, you cannot see the world outside.

I do some reading practice with Rob later that evening. I give him a word and he spells it. I say "Hat", he goes H_A_T. I say "Mum," he goes M_U_M. I then say "Dad," he goes D_U_D! I quickly check the leather key ring which Olly gave to me.

It is almost exactly nine years since I came back from the land of the Himalaya to start a new journey. I am soon to find out whether I am officially in remission or not, but only time will tell whether I am "cured".

However, out of all of this I now understand a little better Lacordaire's words, "All I know of tomorrow is that Providence will rise before the sun."

Trek – Day 17

Trekking Truism: Always double, or halve, the time that you are told it will take to get to the next location.

1991: 10 December, Ilam, The Himalaya

Tradition plays quite a role in Nepal. Breakfast was looking very much like dinner, which usually looked like lunch. It was chip butties again.

The house next door appeared to keep some blind cocks. They started crowing at 3.00 am and finished at about 04.30 am. It then got light. Perhaps these cocks forecast instead?

We were surrounded by more greenery and I felt agreeably clothed by nature and Sergeant Joyce Kilmer's poem *Trees* seemed very apt. He was an American poet who died in action in France in World War I at the too young age of thirty-two.

There was only one road to Ilam from Deurali, so I guessed we had to be on it. However, we experienced some more classic Nepali directions from the locals. I asked for directions after one and a half hour's walking. I was told we had one hour to go. After a further hour's walking I was told there was one hour to go. Half an hour later we were told one and a half hours to go. I checked my compass. Fifteen minutes later I was told that Ilam was fifteen minutes away, only to eventually find out that it was thirty minutes away. We arrived at 11.00 am following a man into town who must have lost his donkey. He carried three tea bags on his back but they looked like they each weighed a good 10 kilograms.

I was surprised that Ilam was as small as it was. I was expecting some "metropolis" but it was very much a "one kukri town". We had a leisurely lunch for about £1.75. I doubted the restaurant cost that much more.

We walked up to the large tea factory and I was introduced to the "Three Tea Leaf" Theory. We went into a large, bare room where female workers performed the formidably boring task of separating the three different types of leaves into different sacks by hand, and the chaff into a fourth. They all remained pretty quiet in our presence. For this work they were paid a lot less than my porters, probably because they were women. There was a range of old, dilapidated looking tea-making machinery. Sieves and trays used for sifting and sorting tea, with large galley type wheels for operating it, lay rusting.

Out in the tea fields a handful of female workers walked amongst the tea crops picking tea. In this sea of green, their bright red clothes marked their paths. It looked a slow, methodical business.

I visited another English School. I had enjoyed my last school visit and had decided to see another school in the hills. Again it was a delight to see the kids smiling merrily away, just enjoying life as only children can.

Afterwards, Ratna suggested that we visit a Hindu mausoleum in the hills. It was beautifully set within the forest, like some lost jungle temple. The sombre grey walls were in stark contrast to the brightly painted yellow and red gates. Ratna and Subash told me more about Hinduism. The name is derived from the Sanskrit[313] word *sindhu* or "river", – specifically, the Indus. The mausoleum had inscriptions to major deities as well as some minor ones particular to the village. There was a large purposively grotesque Hindu statue with its bright colours rapidly fading. It was of the Hindu God, Ganesha, easily recognisable with his elephant head and six arms; he is the God of wisdom and prosperity. He is also the son of Shiva and Parvati, which was how he got his elephant's head. Shiva has a notorious temper, and after returning home from a very long trip away, he found Parvati in bed with a young man. Quick as a flash he cut the young man's head off. His wife was not too impressed to see her husband decapitate their young son and she forced Shiva to bring him back to life, which he could do but only by giving him the head of the first living thing he saw. This happened to be an elephant. I guess Ganesha has probably had enough of violence as his brother happens to be Kumar, the God of War.

Subash had told me that the Asian elephant, the largest mammal in Nepal at 2.75 metres high, is domesticated in this part of the world by first tying them to rubber trees with chains. After a time the elephants give up pulling. They can then be kept anywhere by putting a wooden stake into the ground and tying the same rope to it. The elephants do not try to pull away.

"So that is either proof that elephants are dumb animals or an insight into how easily we let ourselves become conditioned to behaving certain ways in life," he asserted.

There was lots of Nagri lettering, the Nepalese script, which I could not read[314]. It was covered with offerings, from the local villagers and the many birds.

This religious monument had nothing physically to compare with the great cathedrals of Europe and it would be easy to make the mistake that it reflected a less grand spirituality, forgetting the English proverb, "Some men go through a forest and see no firewood."

Subash had told me that Nadur was a Buddhist, but he now told me that he was a Hindu. I asked him about the change and he replied, "Sahib, it is the same."

He then gave me a Nepalese Divinity lesson. Some Hindus believe that Buddha was the ninth incarnation of Vishnu, the Preserver, taking human form. Vishnu has ten incarnations, incarnations being the different forms in which he appears. Buddha seems to be recognized as a godly person by the Hindu religion in

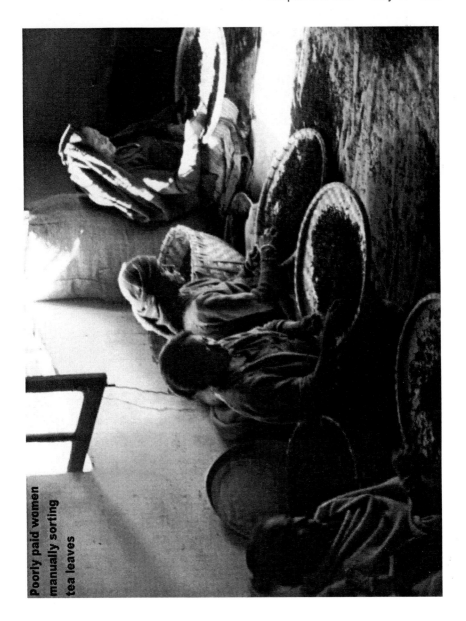

Poorly paid women manually sorting tea leaves

A House in Higher Hills

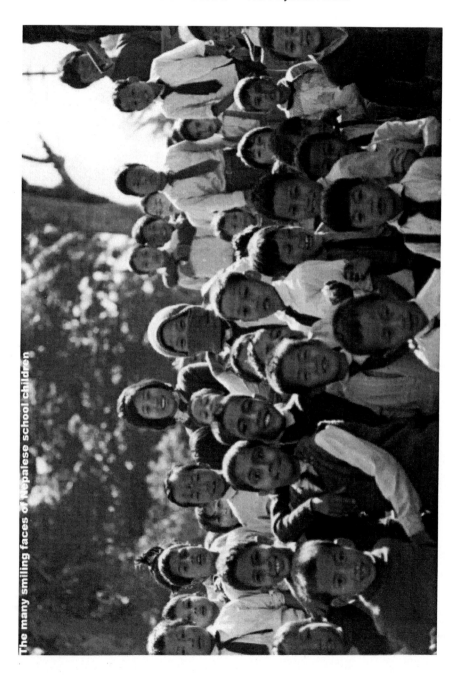

The many smiling faces of Nepalese school children

A House in Higher Hills

much the same way that Judaism recognizes Jesus. Yet Hinduism and Buddhism are very different on the surface (a bit like Christianity and Judaism). Hindus sacrificed humans in the past in the name of their religion as did Christians, whereas Buddhism emphasises the sanctity of all animal life, and seems more accepting of other religions. Perhaps Hinduism appreciates diversity in the way it attempts to help people to see the truth. Some of the Hindu gods may seem silly or even horrendous, but Hinduism uses an array of different symbols (its gods) so at least one will convey meaning in a way that any individual might need.

I asked them, "What is God like to you?"

For Nadur the most important question concerning God, religion or philosophy turned out to be Truth or objective knowledge. Ratna saw Love as the highest good, something that impacted humanity the most. Chandra believed that God was about "right action" – where Truth and Love meet? The question I posed did not seem to interest Subash that much. Perhaps he would have been more interested if she had been very well endowed!

These religious perspectives could have been generalized into four types: either focussed on the intellectual role of "Reformer", the visionary one of "Prophet", or conventional one of "Minister". While for Subash the more healing role of "Samaritan" seemed applicable as he always appeared ready to comfort his fellow man.

Back in the town we went through small markets where women were selling freshly cooked food. With a fire to roast the food on, two women wearing simple shawls squatted down to talk and to sell to passers by. I asked their permission before taking a photo of them – something that is the polite thing to do in Nepal – while young children came up to me smiling and chattering.

Later we had a celebratory drink. Carlsberg was on offer but I stuck to Tongba to which I was now rather partial. The attraction at our bar was an impromptu floor demo of Taekwondo kicks by two ten-year-old Gurkhas. As they whirled around they laughed infectiously and showed us their repertoire. It was a fairly heavy session although everything closed even earlier than in Kathmandu. We had run out of open bars by 8.30 pm.

The porters bought a chicken from a local house, then dispatched it and made dinner. I saw some of the action and became a vegetarian again. The monotony of the food seemed unlimited. I was hoping to be able to suffer from something like "arachibutyrophobia[315]" in the near future.

Reading *The Mountain Kingdom*[316] that night, I wondered several things: how my photos would compare, at this remarkable place, and whether I might ever return.

The Journey Inside – Step 15 – What Is My Purpose?

"It's not what happens to you,
It's what you do about it that makes the difference"
W Mitchell; ex Mayor, Managing Director, pilot, US Congress nominee. (He was extremely badly burned and recovered only to be permanently crippled in a later accident)

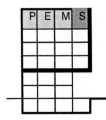

Level of Meaning – Logotherapy

The 7th Chakra is linked to the spiritual, which is above thought. So attempts to rationally describe or define the spirit scientifically are bound to failure. Apparently, surgery has been carried out specifically to try to locate the spirit in the brain. Not surprisingly it was unsuccessful, as it is a bit like trying to find the music by taking apart a radio. Author, and lecturer in Strategic Leadership Management at Oxford, Danah Zohar talks of the "God-spot" – which is a small node of brain tissue just behind the temples, and which she believes is connected with spirituality. She sees this as the part which gives us *SQ* – Spiritual Intelligence. This goes beyond *IQ* and *EQ* and is the part of us that produces a "quest for meaning". It also fits into the location, identified millennia ago, of the 7th Chakra.

After World War II and his experience of being imprisoned in the Nazi death camps of Auschwitz and Dachau, Viktor Frankl came to see the link between meaning and survival, (in Chakra terms – the connection between the 1st and 7th Chakras).

He devised Logotherapy, a psychotherapeutic treatment based on "Finding meaning in life", and it is the psychology which typifies this Level.

He believed everyone had to detect rather than invent their meaning and this psychological treatment confronted the patient with, and reoriented them towards, the meaning of their particular life. He found that the more we try for it as a goal the more we will miss it. It will only happen by our not being concerned about it. It can actually occur because we have forgotten to think about it. He believed that the striving to find a meaning in one's life is the primary motivational force in all of us.

Viktor describes in his book some of his painful experiences, including the murder of his wife, parents and brother in the Nazi concentration camps. From all these experiences he came up with the different ways to find meaning in life in his book, *Man's Search for Meaning*317. They are shown on the next page.

Floor plan for meaning

Look at the "Floor Plan" overleaf and turn to Annex A at the back of this Book again to look at how Purpose is defined at this Level.

 1   Look at the Purposes in the floor plan on the next page.
 2   Decide which one means the most to you.
 3   Identify which of the four Rooms it is in.
 4   Go to Annex A and look at the seventh Level.
 5   Mark an "→" in the corresponding Room at that Level.
 6   *Mark only one room with an arrow at this Level.*

To decide which Room to arrow at this Level, look at the floor plan on the next page and the verbs associated with each Room.

Ask yourself: "Which of these do you most want to achieve in your life, if any? Which of these is most important to you?"

EMOTIONAL–Love	SPIRITUAL–Truth
(Aim)	*(Aim)*
To experience something or encounter someone – *such as experiencing truth or beauty, or the love for a human being or animal*	**By the attitude we take towards unavoidable suffering –** *Meaning may be found by turning human predicament or personal tragedy into triumph. However, where suffering is avoidable the meaningful thing is to avoid it*
PHYSICAL–Right Action (One Way)	MENTAL–Right Action (Another Way)
(Aim)	*(Aim)*
To do a deed–*such as supporting a charity at home or in some far off land*	**To create a work–***such as writing a book through which others may better understand life*

The four aspects of this floor plan are not too different from the four areas the ancient Greeks pursued in their philosophy — Goodness, Beauty, Truth and Unity.

As a guide, if you see your highest aspect as "Action" then if it is a mainly physical deed put an arrow in the Physical Room. If it is mainly a mental work, then arrow the Mental Room. Some "works" are harder to place as they lie in both these Rooms, such as forms of art like "sculpting". Choose the Room that is most applicable to you. "Right action" features in two of the Rooms and both combined, make the third way by which Viktor believed we could discover meaning in our lives.

Viktor stressed that we should not search for suffering, where suffering is avoidable the meaningful thing to do is to avoid it! However, when it is unavoidable it can help us to go into the Spiritual Room.

Logotherapy focuses on the external meanings to be fulfilled by the person in the future; it is at the Level of Meaning. In contrast, therapies like psychoanalysis look more at the past and concentrate on the person introspectively and at the lower, "selfish", Levels. Psychoanalysis can identify past conditioning and therefore may enhance self-awareness. This might be very helpful. However, it is only a necessary, not sufficient condition to doing something about it; as the Japanese proverb cautions, "To know and not to act is yet to know."

At first sight Logotherapy and Viktor's ways of finding meaning in life may seem contradictory to Eastern approaches. However, it fits well with Buddhist philosophy which says that our mind is conditioned to create our experiences, and by being aware and equanimous to these experiences we can come out of conditioning. This takes us out of suffering. Therefore the more extreme the experience, the greater the opportunity we will have to find meaning in it.

The Last Rites symbolise this Level in the Christian Sacraments. It may not sound like that attractive an option but it can also represent the changes at points in our life: a metaphorical "last rites". Either way it symbolizes the end of one journey and the start of another, and this can take place many times in a single human life.

We can sum up Logotherapy as, "A man or woman needs, in life, a mission that matters", a sentiment echoed in *The Alchemist*[318] about the journey of a shepherd and the transforming power of our dreams.

CONCLUSION

"When we come to the edge
Of all the light we have
And we must take a step into
The darkness of the unknown,
We must believe in one of two things:
Either we will find something
Firm to stand on
Or we will be taught to fly."

Anonymous quote from a support organisation for
people living with cancer[319]

This concludes these particular three journeys in my life and Part II – the next book – describes each of the Home-Comings.

BOOK 1

"There are two types of fool;
The one says it is old therefore it is good,
The other says it is new therefore it is better"

The Talmud

Final Decade of the Millennium

This discussion about allopathic versus alternative medicines may appear to be more about the Mental Room than the Emotional one. However, we view the world through our paradigms and beliefs, and moving these around may be more an emotional than intellectual exercise.

In a number of ways, I differed from the conventional medical view on how to treat serious illness, but I was grateful for the very professional treatment and advice that was provided to me by my doctor, oncologist and Cabrini Hospital. Western medicine has some excellent tools for the diagnosis and treatment of acute illnesses, but there are other great tools in the "toolbox" called medicine and these may be more appropriate at times. Life is a series of journeys and it seems to me that medical progress is cyclic too. Wendy sends me an email titled *A Short History of Medicine*[320] which describes this well.

"Doctor, I have an ear ache ... "
1000 BC – "Here, eat this root."
500 BC – "That root is heathen, say this prayer."
1850 AD – "That prayer is superstition, drink this potion."
1960 AD – "That potion is toxic, take this antibiotic."
1990 AD – "That antibiotic is ineffective, swallow this pill."
1999 AD – "That pill has side-effects. Here, eat this root[321]!"

I think that my oncologist prescribed to me the appropriate chemotherapy treatment given my state of health and my type of cancer. I also greatly appreciate his support for my decision to take high doses of vitamin C[322] and for recognising that I might not need radiotherapy. The use of chemotherapy has pros and cons, and I am convinced that certain strategies – particularly around nutrition – can help a person's body cope with an infusion of toxic chemicals.

I believe chemotherapy is appropriate at times but that western medicine generally uses it too much and too often (although I prefer the idea of it to radiotherapy[323]). It has been described as a massive "free radical" attack on the body which aims to kill cancer cells; but what do free radicals cause? The immune system is the mechanism which protects the body from disease and cancer cells; yet what does chemotherapy do to the immune system? It looks like a double whammy. I believe that conventional medicine's general approach to treating cancer would be more effective if it involved a much wider range of methodologies.

The risk is that experts in any field will focus solely on their particular expertise in a situation. "He that is good with a hammer tends to think everything is a nail[324]."

In 1990, a cancer biostatistician Doctor Ulrich Abel, concluded after polling hundreds of cancer doctors,

> "The personal view of many oncologists seems to be in striking contrast to communications intended for the public… many oncologists would not take chemotherapy themselves if they had cancer[325]."

It appears surprisingly easy to see why we have the current *"cancer epidemic"* and the increase in numerous other serious diseases too. Firstly we tend not to spend enough time giving our bodies what they need. TCM[326] provides a model that succinctly, if not obviously, explains what that is. This philosophy believes that the body needs to have its five major systems in balance for good health.

Each system is linked primarily to certain organs and each must be equally "energised". The "immune system" (*liver/gall bladder*) by balancing rest with exercise; the "circulatory system" *(kidney/bladder)* by drinking at least one litre of pure water daily; the "respiratory system" *(lungs/large intestine)* by breathing in fresh air properly; the "endocrine system" *(heart/small intestine)* from smiling and getting sunlight on the retina[327]; and the "digestive system" *(stomach/spleen-pancreas)* by getting the 60 minerals, 16 vitamins, 12 essential amino acids and 3 EFA's (*essential fatty acids*) we need daily.

When it comes to food, it seems useful to remember there is no one diet that suits everyone and nutritional impacts should not be underestimated. After writing this Trilogy I read a summary of the "world's most comprehensive" review of diet and cancer that was published jointly in 1997 by the American Institute for Cancer Research and the World Cancer Research Fund.

Chaired by John D Potter MBBS Ph.D. the panel producing the report[328] estimated that 30-40% of cancer cases throughout the world are preventable "By feasible dietary means", which supported previous findings that "Inappropriate diets cause around one-third of all cancer deaths."

The TCM model predicts getting too much or too little of one "system" will tend to lead to dis-ease through imbalance.

Secondly, we are toxifying our bodies and minds. Mankind has always suffered this to a varying degree but it is getting more pervasive. Physically this is through substances we put into our body, such as mercury amalgams, food additives, fluoridation of water, excessive fats and vaccinations (not just that "diphtheria, tetanus, pertussis" vaccine contains small amounts of mercury – and there is no safe level of mercury). This is in addition to continuously increasing the amount of toxins in the environment. We can compound this by doing rather silly things like mainlining carcinogenic substances into our bodies, as I did – following a medical recommendation to inject tinc benzene into blisters[329]. It was pretty painful and rather spoilt all the care I had taken to avoid ingesting toxins by other means.

Our skin is our largest organ, and is not impervious to substances put onto it; otherwise diet and nicotine patches would not work. (A four gram droplet of VX nerve agent on the skin can kill an adult.) Researchers are even trying to make clothes which are impregnated with medicines or medicinal herbs so that the body is constantly medicated via the skin! Yet we happily apply toxins to it every day; "884 of the chemicals available for use in cosmetics have been reported to the government as 'toxic substances'[330]." A number of them are very common and are found in many shampoos, toothpastes, anti-perspirants, bubble baths, soaps, shaving creams, hair sprays, makeups, perfumes, sunscreens, dishwashing liquids, etc.

This concurs with part of John Potter's summary in the worldwide cancer review where it concluded that the key factors around whether people get cancer or not, are environmental rather than genetic[331]. Chemotherapy is a regular dose of toxic chemicals which, if my analysis is correct, would make a *triple whammy!* I have tried to get a minute drop of a chemotherapy agent in a sealed glass vial from various medical authorities to carry out a homoeopathic detoxification. This has been without any prospect of success at the time of publishing this book, and the way at least one medical establishment described these cytotoxic[332] drugs to me when asked for a drop made them sound extremely dangerous.

It makes sense to be clear of the cure rate before deciding to go ahead with any treatment, and no expert or anyone else should make the decision for us. Difficult as it is to be in that situation.

A beautiful and wise speech which is attributed to Chief Seattle is almost certainly only vaguely similar to Seattle's 1854 speech and was penned by Ted Perry in 1971 for a film about ecology.

However, the words are prophetic and remain relevant. A very small part of it goes:

> "Whatever befalls the Earth – befalls the sons of the Earth. Man did not weave the web of life; he is merely a strand in it. Whatever he does to the web, he does to himself… One thing we know, which the white man may one day discover – our God is the same God … He is the God of man, and His compassion is equal for the red man and the white. The Earth is precious to Him, and to harm the Earth is to heap contempt on its Creator … Contaminate your bed, and you will … suffocate in your own waste."

We cannot pollute the world without poisoning ourselves. Many people seem to think that because pollution does not poison us quickly, therefore it is not killing us.

Others see the problem more clearly. "It is in the nature and essence of industrial civilization to be toxic in every sense… We are faced with the grim prospect that the advance of cancer and of civilization parallel each other[333]."

It may seem to be an over-emphasis of the affects of pollution but about 60000 people die each year in the United States alone from just "particulate air pollution" – the result of smoke in the air[334].

Modern society has become increasingly focussed on progress in the material world and, in this way, distracted from the other aspects of life. Experience tells us that life is best when in balance – "everything in moderation". The secret is to know what degree is "balance". Progress for progress sake leads to disaster to people and planet. Real progress is progress for the sake of all people and living things.

"Progress" is otherwise illusory, and leads to forms of "emotional" toxification, such as the stress which arises from "Not seeing things as they are."

The mind is important and one double blind statistical study apparently found that a placebo was as effective as a common drug used for treating Parkinson's[335]. What was more surprising was that the researchers found that the people taking the placebo had the same *physical* changes in the brain as those "caused" by the drug. Perhaps the belief was the cure? At the Chelsea and Westminster Hospital in London, studies around the affect of music and art are showing measurable improvements on the health of patients.

"For the first time we have established physical and biological evidence for the influence of art on healthcare[336]."

It is not surprising that double blind statistical studies contradict each other on the efficacy of vitamins and other more gentle interventions. They assume that only one variable is changed, an unrealistic assumption when dealing with a group of humans, unless they all have the same blood type, body type, genetics, number of mercury amalgams and vaccinations, diet, food quality, exercise, lack of sleep, fresh air, parasites, mental/emotional states (stress, optimism etc), not to mention potentially major one off factors, such as exposure to a high doses of radiation/chemicals. Modern medicine has to use better statistical methods such as MVT (multivariable testing). This can not only analyse a range of factors at the same time, but can also identify the effects of combined causes. Some medical establishments have used it already. Saint Luke's Hospital in Kansas City reduced the mortality rate associated with Warfarin, a drug that prevents blood clotting, and which is a widely used rat poison! Using MVT they were able to test seven possible factors which did not register as significant when tested individually. However, some in combination proved critical and this led to a 68% improvement in the use of the drug. Yet MVT is not a new methodology and it was first described in *The Design of Experiments* by the great British statistician and biologist, Sir Ronald Fisher, in the Nineteenth Century.

The effects of "toxification" in our modern society are pretty stark and getting worse. In the US in 1998, one million people died from heart disease, and more than 16 million North Americans suffered from diabetes, killing 300 000 of them. There were over one million people in the US diagnosed with cancer and, of those diagnosed, 50% are expected to die within 5 years. About 730 000 people had a stroke and it was predicted that 150 000 would die from it – leaving many of the "survivors" in a vegetative state. So over 1.5 million people are dying annually in the US from the "Four Diseases" of modern society and the rate is similar in the rest of the western world[337]. Recent studies have even suggested that pollution may be seriously damaging the descendents (offspring not born or even yet conceived) of those exposed to pollutants[338].

One way to treat or stop certain diseases might therefore be to detoxify our bodies and minds.

The best methods I know for the former are: homoeopathy, colonic irrigation and fasting[†] – "Fasting is the greatest remedy, the physician within[339]."

I found homoeopathy to be a phenomonal medical therapy in a whole range of ways and one that can detoxify the body of potentially anything. I also believe colonic irrigation is well worth doing and that TCM is an excellent medical therapy with the right doctor. Some good quality foods and supplements[††], such as vitamin C[340], also help the detoxing process. One of the ways Flor•Essence appears to be of great benefit to people is by helping their bodies to detoxify.

Doctor Max Gerson[341] has had remarkable success for many years working on the basis of detoxifying the body to help cure

---

[†] Fasting techniques can be extremely effective but the better they are, the harder they are to do. Professional medical advice should always be sought if fasting more than 24 hours, or if you have a health problem.

[††] Always seek professional medical advice before consuming high doses of any vitamin, or mineral, as some are very toxic in large doses.

cancer, but his results seem to have been largely dismissed by conventional medicine. When his therapy has worked for terminally ill people, ranging from Ian Gawler to the Oxford University don, Gearin-Tosh, and many more besides, some have dismissed it as "luck" or "coincidence". The reality is no one knows for sure, and the remark may just be a sign of the arrogance – which as we have already determined is a manifestation of fear. It lacks the courage to face the fact that there may be a very different but more effective approach.

If you are seriously ill then you may want a wise and skilled, but humble medical practitioner; one who is open to the field of possibilities and who remembers the Talmud's advice, "Train your lips to say as often as possible – 'I don't know.[342]'"

We can detoxify our minds by meditating in any way we find helpful. So we can see things as they really are; the meaning of Vipassana in Pali[343]. It may be by traditional eastern methods, including Qigong, Tai-chi, Transcendental Meditation, and some forms of yoga; or more common Western ways such as by walking, jogging, sailing, painting, golf, knitting and reciting poetry which can all be forms of meditation. Unfortunately watching television and playing computer games are not.

If we still suffer an illness then we have the full range of complementary and conventional medicines to help us.
In the words of Professor Avni Sali[344], "Why use one hand when you can use both", and the other hand includes specific nutrition.

I believe that a very strong immune system will greatly help although not guarantee immunity from cancer, not least because we can always toxify our body or mind too much for it to cope. For instance, no matter whom we are, if we are exposed to high enough radiation, for long enough, then we will get cancer if we do not die first. Also detoxification will not necessarily lead to a spontaneous remission, because by the time we have cancer we have toxified ourselves very heavily, one way or another. I believe this approach is an important step to take in maintaining health or getting over cancer – although there are no guarantees in either case. It would be quite reasonable to ask why I and others should know what some experts appear not to. Sometimes non-specialists – those outside the field – are better placed, often because of the experiences they have had. In 1992 I watched the British Minister for Agriculture, Fisheries and Food[345] go on television to pronounce that experts were confident that British beef was safe, even though BSE (Bovine Spongiform Encephalitis) had been detected in it. Then one of the Minister's children was filmed eating a hamburger.

I doubt I felt much different to many people when I turned to Ruth and said, "In a few years time we will know that there is a definite risk with that."

The information was staring us in the face – the virus had already jumped two species (from sheep to cows to cats) – and it had been shown scientifically that beef infected with BSE which was well cooked, still had the active virus[346]. The same seems to be happening with the link between synthetic toxins and cancer. There is the counter argument that if these commonly used toxins were a factor then everyone would get cancer or serious disease. However, we know from the studies around smoking that this counter argument is flawed.

Surely too many of us are unnecessarily living too short and dying too long? Yet I believe that there is always hope in who we are and what we do. The human body has evolved over hundreds of thousands of years to survive and given the right environment it has an incredible ability to recover. Millions of people alive today are testament to this. To resist cancer and other serious diseases we want to make our immune system as strong as possible and it may help us if we understand a New Illness Model, one focussed on health and which is presented in Part II – the sequel to this book.

BOOK 2

"If you want one year of prosperity, grow grain.
If you want ten years of prosperity, grow trees.
If you want one hundred years of prosperity, grow people."

Chinese Proverb

Nepal is a constitutional monarchy of southern Asia, bounded on the north by the Tibetan Autonomous Region in China and on the east, south, and west by India. Its positioning between these two regional Goliaths has given this Davidian nation a fine line to walk, and it has significantly influenced its history.

Nepal is also one of the poorest ten countries in the world and its population is growing at 2.7% annually. Military service remains a very important source of its income and Gurkhas serve in the Singaporean Police, and British, Nepalese, Bruneian and Indian armies. Approximately 100 000 Nepalese serve in the Indian Army alone.

Unfortunately, poverty remains a major problem, "Access to primary education is low, children under five suffer from malnutrition, mortality rates are high, literacy rates among women are depressing and the prevalence of HIV/AIDS is increasing alarmingly[347]."

BOOK 3

"What is to give light must endure burning"

Viktor Frankl MD, Ph.D.

Each of us tends to value one Room most highly at each Level, and the floor plan for each Level can be generalised as:

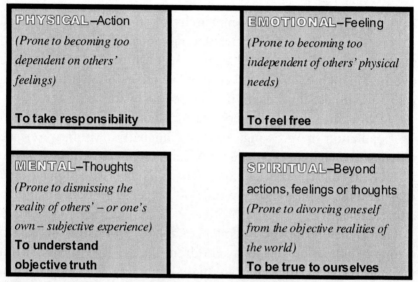

PHYSICAL –Action	EMOTIONAL–Feeling
(Prone to becoming too dependent on others' feelings)	*(Prone to becoming too independent of others' physical needs)*
To take responsibility	**To feel free**
MENTAL–Thoughts	SPIRITUAL–Beyond actions, feelings or thoughts
(Prone to dismissing the reality of others' – or one's own – subjective experience)	*(Prone to divorcing oneself from the objective realities of the world)*
To understand objective truth	**To be true to ourselves**

There is a dichotomy in these values or purposes which may not be obvious. I highly value "taking responsibility", which in some ways stops me gaining significant responsibility. For instance it makes me reluctant to delegate and therefore limits the magnitude of the enterprises in which I get involved. The contradiction is that in order to gain more (significant) responsibilities, we need to hand over (lesser) responsibilities. A friend of mine highly values "feeling free"; however, this tends to stop her from entering fully into relationships as she feels that that ties her down. The result is that she may never have the freedom to choose to have children.

Some people need to live life to understand it, others have to understand life to live it. However, if we value "understanding objective truth" too highly then we may forever remain a spectator and thereby miss the experiential wisdom to truly know it.

Oliver Wendell Holmes[348] once said, "I wouldn't give a fig for simplicity on this side of complexity, but I would give my right arm for simplicity on the far side of complexity."
I believe that one example of the simplicity he sought is that *love* is essentially selflessness *(which* "Is the dissolution of the separateness of mankind[349]" and is a healthy adult state) and its opposite, *fear,* manifests as selfishness (and is about maintaining this separateness from other beings).

From each of these two fundamental emotions arise three Basic Human Motivations, and *Mark's Mansion* sums up the range of our drives as intents to either:

- Act for ourselves *(Survival)* or to act for others *(Courage)*
- Feel for ourselves *(Pleasure)* or to feel for others *(Compassion)*
- Think for ourselves *(Power/Intelligence)* or to think for the sake of others *(Wisdom)*
- "Be" – not consciously act, feel or think *(Meaning)*

This model brings to life the wider implications of "Teaching a man how to fish" rather than "Giving him a fish". This is shown more fully at Annex C.

This model suggests that we all have different Purposes at various Levels, in life, unless we move out of our House – which is what may happen if we lose our minds. It also indicates that if we are not in a state of love then we must be operating out of fear. We can only be in one state, just as we can only be either "pregnant" or "not pregnant". However, unlike pregnancy we can oscillate between these two states very quickly and may only be in one of these states for a few seconds! Conversely we may stay at one Level and/or one Room for days, months, years... This is how neuroticism might be defined in this model. It is where someone remains in one Room despite their environment suggesting they should move around a bit more, but this only happens at Rooms in the lower three Levels. Our behaviour may be important but, at the end of the day, our intent is the most important. Two people may each cut a man in a way that causes both men to die – but one is a mugger trying to rob him, the other a surgeon trying to save him.

Our inner life is more important than our outer one.

There may be critical changes in the former without any change in the latter, and hence the Zen Buddhist saying, "Before enlightenment, chopping wood, carrying water; after enlightenment, chopping wood, carrying water".

This book has been a journey through the Mental Room – about self-awareness. That is a "necessary but not sufficient" step towards going to where you want to go in life. Knowing where you are in relation to Kathmandu can help you to get there, but you still need to take action. *Mark's Mansion* is one of many "self-awareness" models, and like any of the others, it will not carry you to Kathmandu – or anywhere else. You need to do the work and it provides a well signposted way. *Mark's Mansion* is more about character than competence, more about motivation than intelligence.

But then I tend to agree with Nehru[350] when he said, "The older I get, the more I judge people by their character, not by their ideas."

Friends have kindly said to me that I am being courageous in the way I have taken this. Kind as these words are, I do not think it has been really a matter of courage on my part. Courage is best defined as putting oneself at avoidable risk *for others' sake,* whether this is physical, emotional or mental. Bravery focussed on ourselves is not at the Level of Courage at all. Putting ourselves at avoidable risk for the sake of ourselves may just be a risk to gain control for ourselves, which is operating at the Level of Power.

In my case it was more to do with the 1st Chakra and operating at the Level of Survival.

Although it has also given me a sense of meaning (and the 1st and 7th Chakras are connected), and Viktor Frankl recognised that one way to find meaning was "By the attitude we take towards unavoidable suffering".

It has been about turning personal misfortune into some form of personal accomplishment as I endeavour to remember the 4L's – to *Learn* from the past, to *Live* in the present and to *Layout* (as in plan) the future – applying positive emotions *(Love)* to as many of the phases of time as I can.

In the Emotional Room we tend to live in the past and the present, but may neglect the future. If we stay too much in the Spiritual Room then we might ignore lessons from the past. The Physical Room is a good place to live, but be there too much and we can forget about the past and future. In the Mental Room we are pretty good at noticing all phases of time but can lose sight of the other Rooms! My learning for now is that everyone we meet on our journey is a fellow-traveller, a friend, although occasionally they may hide it well, and that coincidence is an overused explanation. We all are students and instructors in life but the trick is to know whether the moment is for learning or teaching. The greatest learning for me has not been in gaining new information but in breaking old paradigms. It has not been in seeing new things but in seeing the new in things.

There are about *6 billion*[351] different profiles to *Mark's Mansion* if you have followed my process, and in Part II the implications of your "House" are discussed in more detail.

Jung suggested that the goal of "individuation[352]" meant that we have to transcend *"type"*, and this aligns with the Indian idea, "Everyone is a house with four rooms, etc." In *Mark's Mansion* model this means going into all four Rooms at all seven Levels. If you want ideas on how to explore Levels further then at Annex D is a list of books which may help you.

To move purposefully towards the Truth, we must know what it is. Life may still stop us going directly to it, but if we do not see it, then we will only get there by accident and all too easily "Hurry off as if nothing has happened."

As we come home we are at first faced by the words "Sapere aude – dare to be wise" – for the sake of ourselves.
But as we ponder on it for longer we see that it means have the courage to know for the sake of the rest of the World. There's a minefield of information around but we each have to walk, or tiptoe, through it ourselves.
We all have to spend some time at the Selfish Levels otherwise we would not survive; for a start we would starve. However, we will only be fulfilled in life to the extent that we pay attention to the *Lush* side of life. What matters most is the degree to which we: *L*ead by example, *u*nderstand, *s*ave and *h*elp other living things, and in this way achieve the 3M's on our Journey – *Make More Meaning*.

Afternote

"The first step is to measure whatever can be easily measured... The second step is to disregard that which can't be easily measured or give it an arbitrary quantitative value. This is artificial and misleading. The third step is to presume that what can't be measured easily isn't really important. This is blindness. The fourth step is to say what can't be easily measured really doesn't exist. This is suicide!"

McNamara's Fallacy; Robert McNamara was US Secretary for Defence 1961-1968

My Mother went on to have three chemotherapy treatments and radiotherapy but these did not cure her cancer. John was very disappointed saying that they had tried the best that medicine had to offer. I agreed in part, as she went to a hospital recognised as one of the best oncology establishments in Europe; but I also begged to disagree.

I replied, "She has had the best that ONE medicine has to offer."

If one full course of chemotherapy fails then following it up with stronger chemotherapy treatments may be appropriate as a stronger dose may be required.

On the other hand it may show a lack of imagination and fit one definition of insanity, "Doing what you have always done and expecting vastly different results."

Some of the things I did, such as taking 1000 times the RDA for vitamin C, might seem a bit mad too, but then perhaps real lunacy is, "Knowing what to do but just not doing it ..."

We all have large gaps in our knowledge and someone once said that, "We all differ in the extent of our knowledge, but in our infinite ignorance we are all the same."

Specialists have an important part to play in this world, but do not forget that the Ark was built by novices and the Titanic by experts!

John has recounted to me how he quickly identified several problems in my Mother's treatment which were not brought up by the specialist medical staff. For instance shortly after another of her chemotherapy courses, which in turn was three and a half weeks after completing five radiotherapy sessions to the chest, John noticed that her pulse rate was very high all the time. He mentioned this several times to several clinicians at the hospital, but they did react to his concerns about it. So he searched the World Wide Web and came across an article which mentioned that a few incidents had been reported where patients who had chest radiotherapy, like my Mother's, had incurred heart muscle damage when given one of the chemotherapy drugs afterwards. John pointed this out to a senior registrar who immediately ordered another heart scan to compare the results with those obtained from a similar scan taken prior to treatment. This scan indicated that her heart muscle was impaired and the senior registrar had the treatment stopped straight away.

My mother bore with grace and humour the pain she suffered in the last four years of her life, and I would like to express my deep gratitude to John for the magnificent way that he looked after my Mother during this time, up until she finally succumbed to cancer.

ANNEXES

"It is what you learn after you know it all that counts"
John Wooden; writer

A – MARK'S MANSION

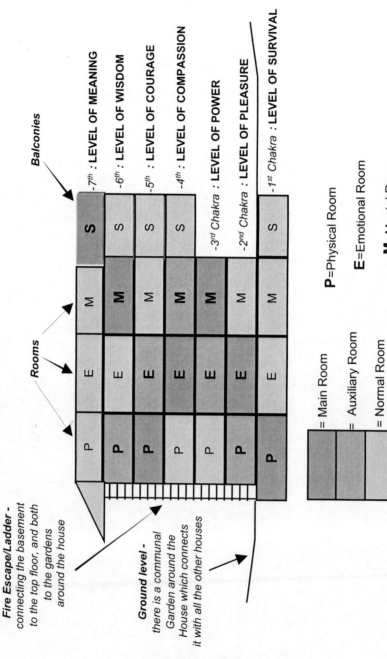

Balconies

Rooms

Fire Escape/Ladder -
*connecting the basement
to the top floor, and both
to the gardens
around the house*

Ground level -
*there is a communal
Garden around the
House which connects
it with all the other houses*

-7th : LEVEL OF MEANING
-6th : LEVEL OF WISDOM
-5th : LEVEL OF COURAGE
-4th : LEVEL OF COMPASSION
-3rd Chakra : LEVEL OF POWER
-2nd Chakra : LEVEL OF PLEASURE
-1st Chakra : LEVEL OF SURVIVAL

P=Physical Room
E=Emotional Room
M=Mental Room
S=Spiritual Room

= Main Room
= Auxiliary Room
= Normal Room

A House in Higher Hills

B – LEADERSHIP STYLES AT DIFFERENT LEVELS

Energy Source	Western Style (Eastern Style)	Example	Purpose In the West	Purpose In the East	Leadership Style
Meaning	Exceptional visionary (Avatar)	Mohandas Gandhi	To lead oneself	To remove all conditioning from the mind thereby attaining "enlightenment"	We lead by example (inspiring)
Wisdom	Prudent philosopher (Yogi)	Socrates	To understand	To control the mind in order to develop focussed attention	We lead by teaching (changing)
Courage	Expert explorer (Fakir)	Sir Ernest Shackleton	To save	To follow a tortuous physical discipline so as to develop an iron will	We lead by proficiency (facilitating)
Compassion	Mindful mentor (Monk)	Mother Teresa	To help	To develop a profound and intense love of God, and so love everyone	We lead by service (coaching)

C – THE IMPLICATIONS OF HOW WE "FISH"

Basic Human Motivations	Fishing Analogy	State of Mind	Who the Focus is On	Stage of Life
Meaning				
Wisdom	Educate and equip a person to make rods and you make a difference to a community	Interdependence *(As defined by Stephen Covey)*	"We" *(Responsibility)*	Adult *(Maturity)*
Courage				
Compassion				
Power	Teach a person how to fish and you feed them for a lifetime	Independence	"I"	Adolescent
Pleasure				
Survival	Give a person a fish and you feed them for a day	Dependence†	"You" *(Blame)*	Child *(Immaturity)*

† Counter-dependency is a rebellious form of dependence - however it is still a "controlled" state, it is just in this case the dependent person tries to do the opposite to the focus of their dependency.

A House in Higher Hills

D – BOOKS EXPLAINING TYPOLOGIES

Level	Typology	Associated Psychology/ Biology (*Mark's View*)	Intellectual Wisdom – *Books*
Meaning (*linked to Survival*)	Different philosophies	Logotherapy	*The Monk and the Philosopher*[353] by - Jean-Francois Reveland Matthieu Ricard
Wisdom	Myers-Briggs Type Indicator	Jungian	*I'm Not Crazy I'm Just Not You*[354] by Roger Pearman and Sarah Albritton
Courage	The Enneagram	(Ram Dass†)	*PERSONALITY TYPES: Using the Enneagram for Self-Discovery* by Don Richard Riso
Compassion	Temperament Theory	Abraham Maslow	*Please Understand Me II*[355] by David Keirsey
Power	Movement Types	Adlerian	*Our Inner Conflicts*[356] by Karen Horney
Pleasure	Physiognomy	Freudian	*WHO AM I? Personality Types for Self Discovery*[357] edited by Robert Frager – Professor of Psychology at the University of California
Survival (*linked to Meaning*)	Twelve Archetypes	Darwinian	*Man's Search for Meaning*[358] by Viktor Frankl

†Ram Dass was originally a Professor at Harvard University called Dr Richard Alpert. *Ecstatic States* is a very insightful video discussing his beliefs – Contact *Wiseone Edutainment*, Tel: +61 2 9371 3933.

ENDNOTES

1   Mark Twain; American Author.

2   Doctor I Soosay
    Camberwell Medical Centre
    984 Toorak Road
    Camberwell
    Victoria 3124
    Australia
    Tel: +61 3 9889 5885

3   *You Can Heal Your Life* by Louise L. Hay - ISBN: 1561706280 (Gift Edition; September 1999): copyright © 1984 & 1987. Published by Hay House. (*Over 3 million copies sold worldwide*). All Rights Reserved.

4   Hay, Louise, Ibid.

5   Ectomorphs characteristically have a long limbed and slim build, and often find it difficult to put on weight. I, my Mother and my uncle are all blood type A's and I read a few years later of a "[Blood group] association... validated in multiple studies and... generally accepted in medical science... Blood group A's greater susceptibility to most cancers" – pg xviii in *Eat Right for Your Type Complete Blood Type Encyclopedia* by Dr Peter J. D'Adamo with Catherine Whitney.

6   Deepak Chopra, M.D.

7   British Army saying.

8   In 1997.

9   French-born Jesuit priest, scientist and philosopher.

10 A good friend, Elwin, tells me a few years later of John J Scherer's "*four major feelings*" – *mad, sad, glad and scared*. Scherer was the associate director of the Whitworth/LIOS Graduate Centre for Applied Studies at Whitworth College, Washington, and a core faculty member for the MA program in Applied Behavioural Science.

11 Short for pommy which is Australian and New Zealand slang for a British person. Its origins are uncertain, unlike the American term for a British person – limey – which originates from the British Navy forcing its sailors to take lime-juice to stop scurvy.

12 "*Hi*" in Japanese.

13 *Home web page*: www.noni.com.

14   See *Island Noni*, by Neil Solomon, MD, Ph.D. published by The
      Woodland Health Series – Telephone USA (800) 748 2996. In *Anti-
      cancer Activity of Noni in Mice with Lung Cancer*, A Hirazumi, 1994.
      Mice implanted with cancer cells and fed Noni lived more than twice as
      long as those which were not. This effect was even more pronounced
      when conventional anti-cancer medication was administered as well.

15   Pronounced "chee".

16   Nepalese for "land at the foot of mountains"; It is pronounced "tear'-
      rye". (Tear as in "*to rip*"). This southernmost region is an area of plains,
      swamps, and forests. The alluvial soils of the Terai are fertile, unlike
      those of the mostly barren uplands. Other than the Terai, the only sizeable
      area of flat land is the Valley of Kathmandu, a basin in the centre of the
      country. The wildlife of the Terai inhabits humid areas and includes
      leopards, deer, elephants and tigers.

17   Statistic from World Vision.

18   Definition of Spiritual in the **Concise Oxford Dictionary.**

19   From the book **No Ordinary Moments**. Copyright © 1992 by Dan
      Millman. Reprinted with permission of HJ Kramer/ New World Library,
      Novato, CA. www.newworldlibrary.com

20   Professor Yong-Qiang Wang
      235 Camberwell Road
      Hawthorn East
      Victoria 3123
      Australia
      Tel: +61 3 9882 2782
      Fax: +61 3 9882 4816

21   Pronounced "Chi-gung" and often spelt this way.

22   Nutricorp Industries Pty Ltd, PO Box 3 Flinders Lane, Melbourne,
      Victoria 3000, Australia – Tel: +61 3 9629 7488 and Fax: +61 3 9629
      7482, email: lcameron@nutricorp.com.au

23   Lane WI & Comac L, 1992. Published by the Avery Publishing Group
      Inc, New York.

24   *Alternatives in Cancer Therapy*, Pelton R & Overholser L 1994.
      Published by Simon & Schuster, New York.

25   *Shark Liver Oil: Nature's Amazing Healer*, Neil Solomon MD, Ph.D.,
      Richard Passwater Ph.D., Ingemar Joelsson MD Ph.D. – Kensington
      Health 1997.

26   These results were reported at the First International Symposium on Ether Lipids in Oncology, held in West Germany in 1986.

27   American Society of Clinical Oncology report in 1999 titled, *The Effects of Alkylglycerols on Cellular Growth and Sensitivity to Chemotherapeutic Agents in Tumour Cultures.* Firshein R, Brohult J, Rothstein-Rubin R – The Firshein Centre for Comprehensive Medicine, NY.

28   No longer operating.

29   For anyone who finds my description of Vipassana meditation too compelling to miss there are sites all over the world and contact details are on the *Home web page:* www.dhamma.org.

30   Printed by: Dharma Press, 1241 21st Street, Oakland, California 94607.

31   Nepalese for stone; pronounced "*dhun'-go*".

32   Written by Thomas O Jordan Jr, 2nd Edition.

33   Richard Holloway, the former Anglican bishop of Edinburgh, commented on the similarity of Christianity, Islam and Judaism, saying, "***[they are all] carriers of important human values, such as justice and mercy and forgiveness***". These are in essence the same as the spiritual qualities Buddhism advises us to cultivate; compassion, mercy, forgiveness, patience, and so on.

34   The purpose of this book is not to explain NLP however a major part of NLP is training in sensory awareness. It is being aware of internal images, sounds and feelings. See *Introducing NLP News – Linguistic Programming* by Joseph O'Connor and John Seymour.

35   More information can be found on the Vipassana website at www.dhamma.org.

36   A number of people have claimed that they have been cured of cancer or other serious illnesses by eating Sunrider foods. An example is *Florence Chavez's Story*. According to the testimonial she was diagnosed with breast cancer in November 1987 and told that she would have to have her breast removed, followed by the other a few years later. She heard about Sunrider and decided to take large amounts of Sunrider foods and not undergo any surgery, chemotherapy or radiotherapy, despite repeated advice from doctors that she must have the surgery to stay alive. She was X-rayed months later and doctors found that "***no tumour or malformation was noted***". She was still cancer free when last checked in August 1989.

37   *The Defenzol Story: A Gift From The Sea – Natural Immunity From The Ocean*; ISBN: 0-473-05375-6.

38   From the Latin, *"I shall please"*.

39   Conducted by Charamlambox A. Gogos, M. D.

40   The United Kingdom's Independent Expert Group on Mobile Phones, headed by Sir William Stewart, released a report in May 2000 on the possible effects of mobile phone technology. Articles in the **New Scientist** 26 October 2002; pg 9, and 11 January 2003; pg 7, identify more research which deepen fears over mobile phone safety and raise the prospect that even the tiniest doses of radiation can be dangerous and may trigger cancer.

41   There is a study suggesting that you get more radiation by using a "hands free" attachment rather than listening into the phone directly. It seems to me to be an example of the "dopeler" effect – the tendency for stupid ideas to seem smarter when they come at you rapidly! However, whether or not this is true, there is an innovative device – called the **Safe-T-Fone**, which uses a cleverly designed sound tube to connect the phone remotely to the user's ear, thereby removing the problem of an electromagnetic radiation producing device next to, or in, the ear. **Australian Distributor**: Red Telecommunications +61 3 9428 9848/1800 676 888 & **UK Distributor**: Acoustic Phone Technologies Ltd +44 870 162 3007.

42   A game where there is one person "on" who stands between the start line and end line. Everyone else starts behind the start line and has to make it past the end line without being tackled to the ground or held in the air for 10 seconds.

43   *Adam Lindsay Gordon – The man and the myth* by Geoffrey Hutton; ISBN 0-571-10921-7. Reprinted by permission of Faber and Faber Limited, London.

44   This is a small surveying device – a "pocket sized" theodolite.

45   Sultan Assawal Bolkiah of Brunei's net worth as of 1997.

46   Nepalese for "certain" or "real"; pronounced "puk'-ka".

47   Pg 87, *Nepal*, ed. 4 © **Lonely Planet Publications** ISBN: 0-86442-704-2.

48   *The Myth of Nine to Five: Work, Workplaces & Workplace Relationships* by Scott, T. & Harker, P. (2002) Sydney: Richmond. Reprinted by permission of Phil Harker and Ted Scott.

49   Since then the rare condition of compulsive punning has been called Forster's Syndrome.

50   Hay, Louise, Ibid.

51   Page 21 of *Psychology as an exercise in paradox*.

52   Colon Irrigation Australia Pty Ltd
      38 Glenferrie Road
      Malvern
      Victoria 3144
      Australia
      Tel: +61 3 9509 2133
      Fax: +61 3 9509 2122

53   *The Tissue Cleansing Through Bowel Management*, Excondado, CA, USA. More information can be found on websites such as The Wolfe Clinic at www.thewolfeclinic.com/newsletter0207.html.

54   Most advice seems to suggest that the vitamin C should be in the form of calcium ascorbate.

55   **The Ecologist**, Vol 28, No. 2, March/April 1998, p 95.

56   This amount is much more than recommended by most conventional and alternative medical practitioners. Always seek professional advice before consuming large doses of any vitamin. Such large doses can be problematic as if the vitamin C is even slightly contaminated then you will be ingesting quite high amounts of the contaminant.

57   *Vitamin Safety – 4th Revised Edition 1989*; F. Hoffmann – La Roche & Co Ltd, by John Marks MA, MD, FRCP, FRCPath, FRCPsych, Fellow, Tutor and Director of Medical Studies, Girton College, Cambridge University.

58   *Vitamin C – The Master Nutrient* by Sandra Goodman Ph.D.; ISBN: 0-87983-571-0.

59   **New Scientist**: 10 August 2002 No 2355; pg 23. In an excellent analysis on the implications of research indicating that an underactive gene might explain why some abused children turn into abusive adults, David Concar explains that such a scientific explanation is incomplete and may not be useful because the environment is always such an important consideration.

60   Gigantopithecus.

61   A leading British psychologist.

62   Saville Holdsworth's definition used for its Occupational Personality Questionnaire.

63   Bouchard, T. *Genetics and Evolution: Implications for Personality Theories, by Thomas J Bouchard* (Chapter 2) and *Measures of the Five Factor Model and Psychological Type: A Major Convergence of Research and Theory*, James Newman (Ed.), CAPT: 1993, 20-41.

64   *Motivation and Personality* by Maslow, © 1970. Reprinted by permission of Prentice-Hall, Inc., Upper Saddle River, NJ.

65   Cabrini Hospital
183 Wattletree Road
Malvern
Victoria 3144
Australia
Tel: +61 3 9508 1444
Fax: +61 3 9500 9453

66   See www.drlam.com/WhatIsAging.cfm. Some research suggests that less than 0.5% of the human population have bad genes causing degenerative diseases, yet 68% of the population eventually die from a degenerative disease.

67   *Beating Cancer with Nutrition*, Doctor Patrick Quillin; p 6.

68   *Understanding the Chakras* – ISBN: 1-85538-009-9. Published by Thorsons – An Imprint of HarperCollins Publishers.

69   Adapted from *On the Psychology of Military Incompetence*, by Norman Dixon – pg 169: ISBN 9 780712 658898.

70   We can see this link from the two tables – love covers the same four Chakras as selflessness, and fear covers the same three as selfishness.

71   Extroversion, emotional stability, openness to experience, conscientiousness and agreeableness.

72   The elephant, lion, rhinoceros, Cape buffalo and leopard, are known as the "Big 5" for hunters who shoot in Africa.

73   I personally believe that all animals have a consciousness and the more evolved they are, then the bigger it is. This is one way to differentiate between animals and plants – animals are living organisms with a consciousness, and plants are ones without. Eastern philosophies, especially Buddhism, have recognised for thousands of years that animals have some form of consciousness. Now western science is finding evidence too. For instance scientists at the University of Cambridge, Doctors Nicky Clayton and Nathan Emery, have observed the ability of birds, when hiding caches of food, to use memories of past experiences and plan for the future. This has traditionally been considered in the West to be unique to humans, and it is indicative of conscious thought.

74   *Anatomy of the Spirit* by Caroline Myss: ISBN: 0-7338-033-5. Reprinted by permission of Harmony Books, Random House, Inc, New York.

75   By all accounts an extraordinary person and psychiatrist.

76   Someone who bites their fingernails.

77   Nepalese for death or time; pronounced "kaal".

78   The Endocrine System is the name given to the structure which controls the use of chemical messengers (hormones) to regulate the continuous function of the whole human body.

79   *The disease burden associated with overweight and obesity.* Must, A. et al; JAMA 1999. 282:1523-29. Also **The Economist**, 31 Aug-6 Sep 02, commented, *"Independent of the implications of being overweight, diet also plays a role in other illnesses, such as cancers of the bowel, colon and prostate".* (pg 25).

80   My Mother suffered a relapse and went down with cancer after my bout so if John is right that I should recover well because my Mother did, then it might indicate that I should also go down a second time with cancer?!

81   *Home web page*: www.sunrider.com.

82   *Home web page*: www.usana.com. A Nobel Prize winner, Doctor Myron Wentz, is the President and Founder of USANA Health Services. I personally believe that Usana's vitamins are good quality and studies show that vitamins can have an anti cancer effect, for example: *Antioxidants reduce the risk of cancers of the lung, uterus, cervix, mouth and gastrointestinal tract*, **Am. Journal of Clin. Nutr. Suppl.** to 53(1):346S 1991.

83   Examples include; *Antioxidants slow ageing and reduce degenerative disease* in the **American Journal of Clinical Nutrition, Supplements** 53(1):373S, and *Professor Ames of Berkeley endorses Antioxidants in cancer prevention*, the **Journal of the American Medical Association** (JAMA) 273, 1995.

84   For instance Doctor Hahn's report in **Advanced Experimental Medical Biology** 1994; 336:241-251.

85   Also called Allopurinol.

86   The Australian College of Herbal Medicine's education program for doctors is now recognised by the Royal Australian College of General Practitioners. Studies estimate in Australia that 70% of people have used complementary medicine.

87   **New Scientist**: 8 June 2002 No 2346; *Newswire – "Duped by Drugs"*: pg 7. Research by Jim Nuovo and Joy Melnikow.

88   Written by W.H. Sheldon Ph.D. Copyright © 1942 by Harper and Brothers. Contact W. H. Sheldon Trust.

89   *Vitamin Safety – 4th Revised Edition 1989*; Marks, John, Ibid.

90   Produced by MicroOrganics. This Spirulina in certified as organic.

91   Nowadays I add liquid chlorophyll to this mixture which I find even better. I use QMEDICINALS High Strength Chlorophyll.

92   The two polysaccharides are rhamnose and glycogen. *One gram a day caused total regression of mouth cancer lesions in 44% of male tobacco chewers.* Harvard Study. In a clinical study of under-nourished, radiation poisoned children from Chernobyl, Spirulina decreased urine radioactivity in **83%** of cases.

93   Not his actual name.

94   There are only three channels we can use to communicate. Research shows that the words used are the smallest mode making up about 10% of the communication. The effect of the body language – the gestures, eye contact and facial expressions – communicates about 60% of the message, with tone – the pitch, volume, pauses and pace of speech – communicating the remaining 30%. With the advent of modern communications and mobile phones we only have about 40% of the total package (the listener cannot see the body language), and emails leave us with only the words – about 10%. There are several studies in this area and an example is *Inference of Attitudes from Non Verbal Communication in Two Channels* by Mehrabian and Ferris, reported in the **Journal of Counselling Psychology** Vol 31, 1967, pages 248-52, 55/38/7. It quotes the figures 55%, 38% and 7% for body language, tone and words respectively.

95   Mind you I got that wrong as he is part of the first American team to win.

96   **New Scientist**: 18 May 2002 No 2343; *Beyond Organics*, pp 33-47.

97   **New Scientist**: 4 January 2003 No 2376; *New year, new debate*, pg 3.

98   **New Scientist**: 18 May 2002 No 2343; Researchers in Canada have found canola plants that are resistant to three different herbicides, although commercial seeds carry no more than a single resistant gene.

99   **New Scientist**: 20 July 2002 No 2352; pp 38-41. Reduced fertility rates mean that the Earth's population may start declining. One UN projection peaks at 7.5 billion in 2050 then has the population imploding.

100   Xue Dayuan, a scientist and adviser to Greenpeace at the Nanjing Institute of Environmental Sciences, commented in 2002 that researchers found it took bollworms, a cotton eating caterpillar, only about five years to develop resistance to toxins produced by GM cotton plants which were meant to protect them from this pest.

101   **New Scientist**: 25 May 2002 No 2344; pp 42-45. The report indicates that safely disposing of used radioactive material presents major problems.

102   The Gaia Theory – describes how Earth appears to act as a living organism with self-regulating mechanisms. EF Schumacher's book *Small is Beautiful* (ISBN: 0-349-13132-5) looks further at some of the implications.

103   **New Scientist**: 23 November 2002 No 2370; *Stray genes spark anger*: pg 7.

104   **New Scientist**: 28 September 2002 No 2362; *Genetically engineered fungus bites back at the crops it's meant to save*: pg 7.

105   Tel: (Australia) 1300 133 868 Email: info@geneethics.org – *home web page*: www.geneethics.org

106   www.holisticmed.com/ge/trypt.html

107   The Norwegian adventurer.

108   Produced by Tim Flowers of Sussex University.

109   **New Scientist:** 18 May 2002 No 2343; pg 47.

110   Joseph Mallord William Turner; the great English artist.

111   More information on the Holmes-Rahe scale of stress ratings can be found in Chapter 9 of Doctor Walter Doyle Staples' well reasoned book, *Think Like A Winner!* ISBN: 0-87980-433-5: copyright © 1991, published by Pelican Publishing Company. The original reference is **The Journal of Psychosomatic Research**, Vol II: TH Holmes and RH Rahe, Social Readjustment Rating Scale. Copyright © 1967.

112   Ralph Waldo Emerson; US Poet.

113   Zurma
16 Barbour Street
Waltham
Christchurch,
New Zealand
Tel: +64 3 379 3555/ Fax: +64 3 379 3553
It sells a range of good quality essential oils – 100ml bottle of organic lavender in a cold pressed carrier oil is NZ$7.50. (2002 price)

114   Americans are on average getting under 7 hours of sleep a night, whereas just over a century ago the average amount of time spent sleeping was over 9 hours a day.

115   Contact the US National Sleep Foundation for more information on sleep studies.

116   Adaptation of the title of Susan Jeffers' motivational book; *Feel The Fear And Do It Anyway*.

117   I think there are three sources of humour, each with a specific intent: either to gain a sense of superiority/power, to experience physical pleasure from the laughter, or to relieve stress in life threatening/ black situations. The first is characterised by "put down" or aggressive humour and is commonly the motivation behind racist, ethnic or sexist jokes. The next type are jokes commenting on the absurdities or ironies in life and their pleasure results from the endorphins released. However, the British sense of humour excels when it comes to facing hardship and life-threatening situations. So humour originates from one of the three selfish drives - Power, Pleasure or Survival. I tend to believe humour around Survival connects to Meaning and is the most powerful. Conversely, Rod Martin, a leading humour researcher and the director of the clinical psychology program at the University of Western Ontario in Canada believes that there are four basic styles of humour: Aggressive, Affiliative, Self-enhancing and Self-defeating. He thinks that each style of humour may be beneficial for one aspect of mental health while being detrimental to another.

118   Cornejo, 1995 and Davis, 1984.

119   Post traumatic stress disorder.

120   Creator of Peanuts.

121   *TEMPLER – Tiger of Malaya* by John Cloake; ISBN: 0-245-54204-3. Originally published by Harrap Limited, London.

122   Nepalese for "*old man*"; pronounced "burr'-row man'-chay".

123   The Gurkha Welfare Trust is a registered charity (No: 1034080) and does a huge amount to provide individual aid through welfare pensions, medical assistance and hardship grants to Gurkha ex-servicemen of the British Crown and their dependants. Tel: +44 20 7251 5234/ Fax: +44 20 7251 5248/ Email: secretary@gwt.org.uk.

124   This story, and other Eastern parables, is described more fully in *The Art of Living – Vipassana Meditation* by William Hart; ISBN: 0-06-063724-2. It also describes the philosophy behind Vipassana with great clarity.

125   One Table from AWAKENING THE HEROES WITHIN by Carol S. Pearson. Copyright © 1991 by Carol S. Pearson. Reprinted by permission of HarperCollins Publishers Inc.

126 *The invention of primitive society*, by Adam Kuper – published by Routledge.

127 Sometimes called a "nocebo".

128 US Food and Drug Administration.

129 **JAMA** (15 Apr 98). Also **JAMA** (Vol 284, 26 Jul 00) reported that western health care is responsible for 225 000 deaths annually (the third leading cause of death in the USA).

130 Doctor V Coleman, The Betrayal of Trust, EMJ, 1994.

131 **JAMA** 1998; 279: 1200.

132 William James.

133 Shin-Huang-Ti.

134 Written by John Gray, Ph.D.

135 *Gifts differing: Understanding personality type*; Myers IB (with Myers, PB) (1995). Palo Alto, CA, USA: Consulting Psychologists Press, Inc.

136 Lord Acton – the great 19th Century historian.

137 World Health Organisation.

138 World Health Organisation. Environmental Mercury. Criteria 118. Geneva 1991.

139 Dichlorodiphenyltrichloroethane – developed by Swiss chemist, Doctor Paul Müller.

140 *Cancer: Cause & Cure* by Percy Weston; ISBN 0-646-40313-3.

141 Documentary *The Cutting Edge: The Miraculous Poison – A History of DDT* (Denmark): In summary, it describes how when DDT was first developed it was seen as a blessing, with the scientist who discovered it receiving the Nobel Prize in medicine in 1948. Yet sixty years on we are discovering the extremely harmful effects of this chemical on all life.

142 In 1992.

143 **New Scientist**: 23 November 2002 No 2370; *The Last Word – "Plant Poser"*: pg 65. Cyanobacteria, also called blue-algae (although not really algae), were responsible for initial oxygen production and still are the main source of ongoing oxygen production.

144 Reproduced with permission from *Nepal*, ed. 5 © **Lonely Planet Publications** 2001.

145 Cloake, John, Ibid.

146 At the Battle of Waterloo a RHG (Royal Horse Guards) officer was sent post-haste by his colonel to report the regiment's success in driving off the French cavalry of Napoleon's Guard. Despite losing his helmet on the way, he saluted the Duke of Wellington who was gratified enough to tell

the young officer that in future the RHG (now incorporated into the Blues & Royals) could salute their seniors when bareheaded — but not return salutes.

147   Deepak Chopra M.D. In **Talk Language** (ISBN: 0-9593658-1-8) by Alan Pease it notes that, *"of the 40000 impulses… [you] receive each second, you can only pick out a few on which to focus your attention."*

148   *The Rising Curve – The rise in average IQ scores*; Ulric Neisser (ed.) (Washington, DC: American Psychological Press, 1997). Daniel Goleman, the author of *Working with Emotional Intelligence*, has been highlighting this issue for several years now.

149   *Are America's Children's Problems Getting Worse? A 13-Year Comparison – The decline in children's emotional intelligence*: Thomas Achenbach and Catherine Howell (**Journal of the American Academy of Child and Adolescent Psychiatry**, November 1989).

150   Strictly speaking a theory is different to a model: a model gives a representation describing **what** is happening, while a theory predicts **why** it happens. However, the usage and definitions of these terms seem to be changing.

151   Written by Roger R. Pearman & Sarah C. Albritton: ISBN 0-89106-096-0. You can purchase this book from Davies-Black Publishing, an imprint of CPP, Inc. Palo Alto, CA 94303 www.daviesblack.com.

152   J. Churton Collins.

153   ISBN: 1-86350-029-4.

154   *The Conquest of Cancer*, Doctor Virginia Livingston Wheeler, pp 101-2.

155   The British National Health Service gives the same advice.

156   Written by James C Collins and Jerry I Porras.

157   Environmental Health Consultant.

158   From the 74th Congress, 2nd Session.

159   For instance, *August Celebration* a study by Linda Grover, reported that in 1948 an average bowl of spinach had about 150 milligrams of iron, while in 1998 the same bowl contained only 2 milligrams.

160   From the Dumfries and Galloway Royal Infirmary and University of Strathclyde.

161   **European Journal of Nutrition**, Vol 40, p 289. Also Jens-Otto Andersen, a professor at the Royal Veterinary and Agricultural University in Copenhagen, Denmark, has been studying plant physiology for the last 20 years. He has said that, *"**I think there has been a very slow depletion**"

of vitality in plants since World War II. What we do with conventional agriculture is that we over-emphasise the growth of the plant, because that is where the money is, and we always focus on the bottom-line profit".

162   Also may be spelt "homeopath".

163   Written by Doctor Peter D'Adamo with Catherine Whitney – ISBN: 0-7126-7784-4.

164   ISBN: 1-876462-09-4.

165   **New Scientist** 28 September 2002; pg 20. Recent research suggests that this percentage, which has long been regarded as accurate, may in fact be less than 95%.

166   Both the blood type and high protein, low carbohydrate diets have their critics. For instance, Professor John Dwyer, head of the School of Medicine at Sydney's Prince of Wales Hospital says of D'Adamo's theory to support the blood diet, *"the whole premise is nonsense"*. Doctor Rosemary Stanton, a nutritionist, says of the high protein, low carbohydrate diet, *"this diet is unproven, potentially harmful and nutritionally lacking"*. (See the **Australian Reader's Digest** September 2002, pp 66-69). Contradicting this, is the experience of many people who have found these diets to significantly help their health and fitness, and to lose weight.

167   Note: In *Please Understand Me II* this is described as the source of self-confidence not self-esteem. However, in my model it appears more appropriate to swap the source of self-confidence and self-esteem.

168   Note: In *Please Understand Me II* this is described as the source of self-confidence not self-respect. However, in my model it appears more appropriate to swap the source of self-confidence and self-respect for Artisans.

169   *Please Understand Me II* ISBN: 1-885705-02-6. Reprinted by permission of Prometheus Nemesis Books, California.

170   Called the Sun Chlorella Corporation.

171   *Chlorella – Gem of the Orient* by Doctor Jensen, has more information.

172   Doctor Joe Reich
27 Denmark Hill Road
Camberwell
Victoria 3123
Australia
Tel: +61 3 9882 1347

173   Also called Aciclovir.

174   Hay, Louise, Ibid.

175   ISBN: 0 85572 3203. Reprinted by permission of Michelle Anderson Publishing Pty Ltd, Melbourne, Australia.

176   Written by Doctor Carl Simonton and Stephanie Matthews.

177   *The Holistic Approach to Cancer* by Ian CB Pearce; ISBN: 0-85207 211 2. Reprinted by permission of The CW Daniel Company Ltd, United Kingdom.

178   *Childhood energy intake and cancer mortality in adulthood.* Must A, Lipman RD: Nutr Rev 1999; 57:21-4.

179   Centers for Disease Control, 1999. (www.cdc.gov/nccdphp/).

180   *Learned Optimism* by Martin EP Seligman Ph.D., ISBN: 0-09-182568-7. Reprinted by permission of Knopf Publishing Group, Random House, Inc, New York.

181   Study by researchers from Columbia University and New York's Psychiatric Institute – written up in the **Journal of the American Medical Association's Archives of General Psychiatry**.

182   This fictional book written in 1954 describes in detail the very nasty exploits of a band of young children who are isolated on an island. It follows their striking transition from being civilized to becoming barbaric. This book suggests that man has an inherent capacity for evil and is not naturally moral.

183   Keirsey, David, Ibid.

184   Keirsey, David, Ibid: *Chapter 7 – Mating* (in particular – page 209, second paragraph).

185   Research has indicated that attraction is associated with certain physical/ relatively objective characteristics which can be understood in terms of "evolutionary advantage". First of all, not only are body features which form after puberty associated with increased attractiveness, but also increasing facial symmetry is linked to it, as this in turn is linked to a more symmetrical body as a whole which has been found to indicate increased fertility. Secondly, it has been found that our smell indicates key things about our biological makeup, and we tend to be attracted to others whose smell indicates that they have opposite genes to us. The more opposite, the better the offspring's immune system is likely to be, and the more attractive the potential partner turns out to be. Smell can also indicate when women are at their most fertile, and provides some hormonal information about men. Finally partners with more resources

or better "status" tend to be considered more attractive because they can better look after the offspring. Therefore older men with more resources and buying power seem to be more attractive to women probably because they will be able to better provide for any offspring. Conversely young women tend to be more attractive to men as they are more fertile and more likely to be able to have children (whether the men consciously want more children or not).

186   I am in good company, as I read three years later in *The Art of Happiness* by Howard C Cutler, MD about his discussions with His Holiness the Dalai Lama; ISBN: 0-7336-0858-2. In this practising psychiatrist's discussions with the Dalai Lama, the Dalai Lama outlines a similar belief.

187   Skivvies are a British/Army term for underpants.

188   Doctor Clif Sanderson
www.broadviews.com
www.fengshuimanual.com
email: clif@compuserve.com.

189   *Web page*: www.broadviews.com.

190   *Web page*: www.fengshuimanual.com.

191   William Shakespeare; **Hamlet – Chapter 1 Scene v**.

192   *Healthy Life Expectancy* – The World Health Report 2001 produced by the World Health Organisation listed healthy life expectancy at birth for Nepalese men as 48.7 years and Nepalese women as 49.1 years. The corresponding figures for Australians were 70.1 and 73.2 years.

193   Nepal Microsoft (R) Encarta. Copyright (c) 1994 Microsoft Corporation. Copyright (c) 1994 Funk & Wagnall's Corporation.

194   My own experience tells me that we can all predict things. Apparently 90% of people report having had the experience of predicting the telephone ring. Scientifically this is sometimes explained by déjà-vu – the impulse of the ear nerves carrying the sound reach the brain from one ear faster than the other. So the brain believes it "knew it was going to ring". But plausible explanations are not always the right ones. Several years ago, Ruth and I agreed we would tell each another before the telephone rang. Two weeks later, I did and sure enough it rang about three minutes later. It was the only call we had all day and we were not expecting any calls. Could I do it again? Probably not "on demand", it would then have to be an objective truth, whereas this is a subjective truth. But it is a truth all the same.

195   Seligman, Martin Ph.D., Ibid.

196   Pronounced "khukuri".

197   Eric Fromm escaped the Nazis and came to the United States towards the end of the 1930s. His two books on personality, *Man for Himself* and *Escape from Freedom*, influenced many psychologists. After the Second World War, he headed a movement along with Abraham Maslow and Carl Rogers, called The Third Force in psychology which tried to soften the harsh view of Man as portrayed by Behaviourism and Psychoanalysis.

198   Ball, IL (2002) **MBTI Australian Data Archive Project**. Psychological Type Research Unit, Deakin University, Melbourne, Australia. This data is drawn from a population of over 17000 people in a range of employments; however it has a significantly higher proportion of managerial and professional employees in it, compared with the Australian population.

199   Keirsey, David, Ibid.

200   **New Scientist** 13 July 2002 No. 2351; pp 34-7. Marc Bekoff, a biologist at the University of Colorado in Boulder, USA, has evidence suggesting that animals can distinguish right from wrong. He describes how they can sometimes act unselfishly and with a sense of fairness.

201   Summary of *1986 Seville Statement on Violence* signed by twenty top scientists.

202   Research conducted by C. Daniel Batson and Nancy Eisenberg.

203   **New Scientist** 21/28 2003 No. 2374/5; p 8. About 50 million Americans will not be able to take the vaccine because of suppressed immune systems or other risk factors, and these people, as well as healthy people, may catch the disease from those vaccinated. (An immunosuppressed Israeli who lived with someone who was vaccinated is recently reported to have become seriously ill). **The Australian Financial Review**, 27 September 2002, on pg 17 commented, *"[the smallpox vaccine has dangers itself with] some experts warning that one out of every two people may be at risk of serious side effects"*.

204   Australian Vaccination Network - Fax: +61 2 6687 2032 *Email*: info@avn.org.au – *home web page*: www.avn.org.au.

205   **JAMA**; May 94 Vol. 271 No. 20.20

206   Bovine Spongiform Encephalitis.

207   Information through the AVN website.

208   Clay pigeon shooting.

209   Adler was a leading psychoanalyst and contemporary of Sigmund Freud.

210   From OUR INNER CONFLICTS: A Constructive Theory of Neurosis by Karen Horney. Copyright © 1945 by W.W. Norton, Inc., renewed © 1972 by Renate Mintz, Marianne von Eckardt and Brigitte Horney Swarzenski. Used by permission of W.W Norton & Company, Inc.

211   Eastern Proverb.

212   Euphobia = "*Fear of hearing good news*", a euphemism used in the Army to describe shooting someone.

213   Horney, Karen, Ibid.

214   The Theosophical Society is a non-sectarian body of "seekers after the truth", which promotes brotherhood and strives to serve humanity. Its Melbourne address is (the bookshop is on the second floor):
lst Floor
126-128 Russell Street
Victoria 3000
Tel: +61 3 9650 3955
Fax: +61 3 9650 4894

215   I won decisively although the Australian champion was a more skilful exponent at taekwondo than I.

216   The science of the action of drugs on the body.

217   **New Scientist** 21 September 2002 No. 2361; pg 10. *Is there a safe limit for weedkillers?*

218   I have gone to a practitioner who uses a Vega machine for therapy thrice before, and found it very helpful once, quite helpful once, and no help the other time. My Homoeopath's Mora machine I have found consistently extremely helpful. It is worth noting that my Father has been going for many years now to a practitioner who uses a Vega machine, and has found it very helpful for him.

219   Experiments show that large placebo pills work better than small ones and coloured ones work better than white ones. Homoeopathy pills are usually very small and white, unlike many pharaceuticals! The BBC science program *Horizon* broadcast an investigation into homoeopathy in November 2002 called *Homeopathy – the Test* which cited some evidence that it worked while ending with an experiment showing a "supposed" theoretical basis was flawed, like the 1988 investigation by *Nature*. (The experiment's design meant it could not disprove homeopathy.) Professor Madeleine Ennis of Queen's University of Belfast, a sceptic of homoeopathy, said that statistically the *Horizon* experiment was incapable of making any kind of definitive conclusion.

220 Written by Tom J Chalko MSC, Doctor Eng. Sc – who cured himself of cancer following a program of detoxification and meditation: ISBN 0 0646 23407.

221 **NEXUS** Volume 2, Number 2 – February 1991.

222 d'Raye, Tonita, *The Facts About Fluoride*, PO Box 21075, Keizer, OR 97307, USA.

223 ISBN: 0-9535012-4-8. More information can be found out about chemicals and pharmaceuticals, by contacting **Credence Publications** on the World Wide Web or at PO Box 3, Tonbridge, Kent TN12 9ZY, United Kingdom.

224 d'Raye, Tonita, ibid.

225 *How to Save Your Teeth*, page 139. Facts from Citizens for Safe Drinking Water.

226 Red Seal Natural Health Ltd, 46 Honan Place, PO Box 19-046, Avondale, Auckland 1230, New Zealand. Telephone: +64 9 828 0036.

227 Red Seal also produce a toothpaste called *Baking Soda* and on this packaging it states, *"**New Zealand research shows that the reduction in dental decay is just as great in non-fluoridated areas as it is in fluoridated ones**"*.

228 Instead this toothpaste uses a milder coconut-based foaming agent called Decyl Polyglucose.

229 491 Burke Road, Camberwell, Victoria 3124, Australia. Telephone: +61 3 9822 9131.

230 *Home web page*: www.taekwondo.com.au

231 Francois-Marie Arouet.

232 Anonymous. Perhaps by the same person who noted that the difference between mechanical and civil engineers is that the former build weapons and the latter construct targets…

233 MM stands for the Military Medal, which was the most widely awarded gallantry medal in both World Wars. It has now been withdrawn and is no longer awarded, which is a shame as it was reserved for non-commissioned soldiers and ensured that their gallantry was recognized.

234 Ganju Lama died on 30 June 2000 aged 77 years.

235 *The Anatomy of Courage* by Lord Moran.

236 ISBN: 0-14-008574-2, published by Penguin Books.

237 From PERSONALITY TYPES: Using the Enneagram for Self-Discovery. Copyright © 1987 by Don Richard Riso. Reprinted by permission of Houghton Mifflin Company. All rights reserved.

238 Shamwari Game Reserve turned out to be a magnificent game park. There I found out that some lions are kept in an enclosure when they have become familiar with people. They know that humans are separate to the vehicle and they become too dangerous to let out. I expect this makes them "enlightened lions". They see the world a bit more for what it is! See *Website*: www.shamwari.com for more information.

239 From THE MONK AND THE PHILOSOPHER: Copyright © 1997 by Jean-François Revel and Matthieu Ricard. Reprinted by permission of HarperCollins Publishers Ltd, London.

240 It is an extract – the 1st and 3rd verses – from *Life's Clock* by Robert H Smith written about 1932. We have made all efforts to contact the owner of the copyright and please contact us if you are the owner and we will settle any reasonable claims in good faith.

241 St. Andrews Place, East Melbourne, Victoria 3002, Australia.

242 US Department of Health and Human Services Public Health Service National Toxicology Program – http://ehp.niehs.nih.gov/roc/toc9html.

243 Doctor Martin Luther King, the Baptist minister and ardent fighter for civil rights through non-violent means, commented that race was the least significant distinction among different people. (He was assassinated in 1968).

244 Joel Barker recounts this story in more detail in the video *Paradigm Pioneers*; produced by Charthouse. Coincidentally I sat next to a world expert in this field at a lunch in 2002 who corroborated this story.

245 Heart Specialist at the University of Maryland.

246 Doctor Timothy Lobstein's degree was in psychology and his doctoral thesis concerned the overlapping area between physiology and psychology. He is editor of **The Food Magazine** and co-director of The Food Commission.

247 The **British Committee of Medical Aspects of Food Policy (COMA)**.

248 Although it might conceivably be applied to the foetus of pregnant woman who eat "fast food". **New Scientist** 1 February 2003 No. 2380, pp 27-29; described how the evidence is "*piling up*" that people can get addicted to fast food.

249 Elizabeth Somer, nutrition expert and author of *Food and Mood*.

250 **New Scientist** 11 January 2003 No. 2377; pg 7. *DISPATCHES – Prozac for Kids*.

251 Edgar Watson Howe.

252 In fact almost all my film was eventually developed intact and 33 out of the 36 negatives were developed thanks to some adept developers in Hong Kong.

253 Descartes – *"I think, therefore I am"*.

254 Cloake, John, Ibid.

255 *The Alchemist* by Paulo Coelho; ISBN 0-06-250218-2.

256 *Facing Your Type*, Wernesville, PA: Typrofile Press, 1982 and MDA Consulting Group, Inc, Minneapolis, MN.

257 We have made all efforts to contact the owner of the copyright and please contact us if you are the owner and we will settle any reasonable claims in good faith.

258 Gawler, Ian, Ibid.

259 Female Sherpa.

260 1997 figures.

261 Clarified butter made from the milk of buffaloes or cows.

262 Anthony Robbins' philosophy is explained more in his bestseller and highly readable book, *Awaken the Giant Within*.

263 Sheldon, W.H., Ibid.

264 Diener's research indicates that it only takes an annual income per head of US$8000 for money to stop being a factor in happiness in the USA.

265 Tests and surveys on happiness and personal strengths can be completed on the Web site www.authentichappiness.org and then compared with thousands of American results. Diener's research suggests that Scandinavians have the highest "life satisfaction" in the world.

266 The age of menarche (the age when a girl has her first period) has dropped from 14/15 years in 1900 to 11/12 now. It is not known for sure what is causing this. Exposure to substances ranging from hormones in chicken or beef to oestrogen mimicking substances in shampoos and plastics may be a factor. Research from the Australian Royal Women's Hospital suggests mental factors, such as exposure to childhood violence/trauma, may also reduce the age of menarche.

267 *Dietary Calcium; adequacy of a vegetarian diet*. **American Journal of Clinical Nutrition**; Weaver CM, Plawecki KL, 1994; 59 (Suppl):1238S-41S.

268 There is some research in the USA by Connie Weaver and Dorothy Teegarden at Purdue University, and by Michael Zemel, the chairman of the Nutrition Department at the University of Tennessee which suggests that a diet rich in dairy foods significantly helps with weight loss, so

there may be other reasons to consume dairy apart from increasing ones calcium intake!

269   Peter Rendel, M. A. (Cantab).

270   Telephone: +61 3 9786 0266/0772 5844.

271   Also called asturia or asturia-spelt flour.

272   It was farmed at least 5000 years ago.

273   Hildegard von Bingen lived 800 years ago.

274   Aristotle (who lived around 350 BC).

275   French for *"Lion-Hearted"*. He was King of England from 1189-1199.

276   Don Richard Riso, Ibid.

277   Those who know typologies well might notice that the Rooms do not necessarily relate to the same Room at another Level. For example the Compliant Type of Karen Horney's Movement Types is in the Emotional Room at the Level of Power, but can be Enneagrams 1, 2 and 6, and so may be thought of as either in the Physical, Emotional and Mental Rooms at the Level of Courage.

278   This or similar descriptions are in several biographical descriptions of Hitler.

279   Strangely enough the after effects also seemed to be markedly less unpleasant in the days following this chemotherapy.

280   Telephone: +61 8 8264 2453 or fax: +61 8 8263 2033.

281   To the best of my knowledge Peter's managing director never tried Epilobium and unfortunately he has since died.

282   Some apparent allergies to shellfish may be due to iodine or because of toxins trapped in the shellfish.

283   *The Washington Post* reported that the US Government has funded 224 research projects costing some US$213m to try to find the cause and best treatment for the illness.

284   This seems to be supported as apparently soldiers who prepared for the Gulf, but did not go, have also suffered the symptoms. For more information on Aspartame search the World Wide Web. A Google search provides interesting reading. A sixth possible factor has been identified, the anti-chemical warfare tablets – called NAPs tablets in the British Army. All soldiers had to take these tablets to protect them from nerve agents and they have not undergone full trials to evaluate their safety.

285   This statement is from Denis Winter's comment before 1990, saying that there would be 400 men still blind in that year.

286   The leadership training program *Leading Successfully* from Blessing
      White differentiates between rewards, which promote more of a
      behaviour by introducing something desirable or taking away something
      undesirable, in response to someone committing the action; and
      punishments, which aim to reduce undesirable behaviour by introducing
      these the other way around – introducing something undesirable or taking
      away something desirable.

287   Extract from BRAVO TWO ZERO by Andy McNab published by
      Bantam Press/Corgi. Used by permission of Transworld Publishers, a
      division of The Random House Group Limited. Andy McNab ended up
      surviving captivity.

288   Almost a year after coming up with my model on leadership and
      presenting it, I read a short summary about Peter Kostenbaum and his
      new book, *Leadership: The Inner Side of Greatness*. He sees four
      strategies to "great leadership" which equate to my four Rooms, and his
      strategies seem to fit pretty well with the upper four Chakras and the
      conclusions I have arrived at independently.

289   *Art of War*, by Sun Tzu: ISBN: 0-19-501476-6.

290   David Parker
      Osteopath
      27 High Street
      Kew East
      Victoria 3102
      Australia
      Tel: +61 3 9857 0599

291   Vitamin B_{17} is also called Amygdalin or Laetrile. Three years later I was
      talking to an excellent physiotherapist, Ross Smith (*The Balaclava–St
      Kilda Physiotherapy Centre*; Telephone +61 3 9527 7532). He has been
      to the Olympic Games five times in an official capacity – three times as
      the Chief Physiotherapist for the Australian Olympic Team – and he
      commented that he had noticed a similar link himself with Australian
      Rules Football players getting tumours at the site of injuries, e.g. after
      suffering testicular injuries.

292   In Australia you often have to sign a waiver to say you will not eat the
      apricot seeds before buying them! Other foods which are generally high
      in vitamin B_{17} include elderberries, wild blackberries, mung beans, fava
      beans, cassava, bitter almonds, macadamia nuts and eucalyptus. "Wild
      foods" tend to have higher concentrations of B_{17}. *The Little Cyanide
      Cookbook (Delicious Recipes Rich in Vitamin B_{17})* by June de Spain has

more information. Robert Pollock in his very well researched book, *Good Luck Mr Gorsky*, explores many "urban myths"; however, he seems to fall for one when he says, "one American man died of cyanide poisoning after eating a cup of apple seeds". This example is often quoted but there does not appear to be any information suggesting it is true (for instance no name or medical report). For up to date details on "urban myths" see www.snopes.com

293   ISBN: 0-449-00282-9. It has sold about 5 million copies worldwide.

294   Sarah has settled down dramatically over the months under Brian's care.

295   Rene's life is recounted in the book by Doctor Gary L Glum called *The Calling of an Angel* (Silent Walker Publishing, PO Box 80098, Los Angeles, CA, 90080) which also tells of the documented recoveries of thousands of cancer patients who had been certified in writing by their doctors as incurable.

296   Flor•Essence is the organic, full eight herb formula. It is obtainable from **Flora Manufacturing & Distributing Limited, Burnaby, BC V5J 5B9, Canada**. It is imported into Australia by *NTP Health Products, 17 Blytheswood Avenue, Warrawee, NSW 2074*. (My homoeopath does not sell it – for those who may view the result with some cynicism).

297   Goethe.

298   Cloake, John, Ibid.

299   A more exact translation can be found in chapter 3 of *Tao Te Ching* **translation by Victor H. Mair**; ISBN 0-553-07005-3. Published by Bantam Books, New York.

300   These are descriptions British soldiers have used as far back as at least the Napoleonic times. In terms of the British Army's three ways to lead: "*go on*" is either compelling or persuading, and "*come on*" is about example.

301   IMAX has an epic film describing this feat of endurance, called *Shackleton*.

302   Information about Messner's expeditions and climbing feats can be found at www.jerberyd.com/climbing/climbers/messner/ .

303   Paraphrase of the judgment by Apsley Cherry-Garrard, as summed up by Sir Edmund Hillary and others.

304   Extract from SOUTH – THE STORY OF SHACKLETON'S LAST EXPEDITION – 1914 by Sir Ernest Shackleton published by Ebury. Used by permission of The Random House Group Limited.

305   WR Inge; author.

306   Written by Adelle Davis – published by Allen & Unwin.
      ISBN: 0 04 641017 1
307   Patrick Oliver.
308   Subliminal programming was first used publicly in the film the *Picnic* in
      1956. Adverts encouraging the consumption of Coca-Cola and popcorn
      were flashed onto the movie screen during the film every 5 seconds for
      1/3000th of a second. Although these subliminal messages were not
      perceptible to the human eye, it was claimed that they had had a dramatic
      effect, with increased sales of Coca-Cola and popcorn – 18% and 56%
      respectively. Other experiments by television stations did not show a
      significant effect but the general public were very concerned about
      potential brainwashing, and this type of advertising was banned.
309   Written by Deepak Chopra, M.D. Published by Bantam Books; ISBN: 0-
      553-34869-8.
310   Henry Major Tomlinson; English novelist and essayist.
311   Zen poem.
312   **New Scientist** 11 May 2002 No. 2342; p 18. Another factor identified in
      this report, which may be giving home teams an advantage, is the affect
      that a home crowd seems to have on biasing neutral referees towards
      decisions favouring their teams. Evidence supporting this idea is that in
      sports where the refereeing is more clear cut, such as non-team sports
      like golf, players show no advantage when competing at their home
      ground.
313   Sanskrit is the ancient language of the Hindu civilisation and religion, in
      much the same way that Latin is the basis of European language and
      culture.
314   Nagri is the original form of written Nepalese, although Roman Gurkhali
      (English letters) is increasingly used in the British Army.
315   Fear of peanut butter sticking to the roof of the mouth.
316   ISBN: 0-911977-07-4.
317   From *Man's Search for Meaning* by Viktor E. Frankl © 1959, 1962,
      1984, 1992 by Viktor E. Frankl. Reprinted by permission of Beacon
      Press, Boston.
318   Coelho, Paulo, Ibid.
319   Source: **Australian Fitness Magazine**, Vol 14 No 4 2001.
320   We have made all efforts to contact the owner of the copyright and please
      contact us if you are the owner and we will settle any reasonable claims
      in good faith.

321   I am indebted to the original author.

322   I did not specify to my oncologist exactly how many grams of vitamin C I would be taking each day.

323   Also, my understanding is that radiotherapy produces free radicals in the body and suppresses the immune system.

324   Abraham Maslow.

325   *The Cancer Chronicles*, December 1990. Doctor Abel is from Heidelberg, Germany.

326   Traditional Chinese Medicine.

327   Early morning or evening sunshine is best and it may help not to wear sunglasses at these times?

328   Entitled *Food, Nutrition and the prevention of Cancer: a global perspective*, it was produced by a panel of 16 leading international scientists and United Nations observers, who worked for three years to review some 4500 scientific and other expert studies which looked at the cancer risk from dietary patterns and related factors under varying conditions around the world.

329   As a chemical engineer I knew that benzene is a known carcinogen but I made the assumption that medical procedure would not allow this to happen and that tinc benzene must be some safe compound. Only later did I find out that tinc benzene is simply benzene in alcohol.

330   **American National Institute of Occupational Safety and Health.**

331   I have not read the review *Food, Nutrition and the prevention of Cancer: a global perspective*, but have only read an outline of it by Health Research Pty Ltd, 11 Carrington Street, Adelaide 5000, South Australia – called *The Global View.*

332   Poisonous to living cells.

333   *Cancer: Nature, Cause and Cure*, Berglas, Doctor Alexander; Paris 1957.

334   Estimate by the US Environmental Protection Agency – reported in *The Australian Financial Review Special Report on Occupational Health & Safety* – 22 August 2002.

335   This information was broadcast on an Australian radio news report.

336   **New Scientist** 22 June 2002 No. 2348; pp 39-41. Said by Rosalia Lelchuk Staricoff who heads the Chelsea and Westminster Hospital's research into the clinical effect of art.

337   *Your Health is in Danger by Robert G. Allen: Special Report – Your Health Today* produced by the Churchill Trust in 1998.

338   **New Scientist** 14 December 2002; pg8. *Pollution triggers genetic defects.*

339 Paracelsus – 15th Century physician who established the role of chemistry in medicine. *The Miracle of Fasting* written by Paul C Bragg and Patricia Bragg is a very good treatise on how to fast properly.

340 Remember the quality and type are critical when taking high doses. Most advice I have read in this area recommends taking calcium ascorbate. Calcium is a very important mineral for the body generally and this form is not as acidic as some other forms.

341 *A Cancer Therapy; Results of Fifty Cases*; Gerson M, 1958: Totality Books, California, USA.

342 Translated from the **Talmud** – the body of Jewish civil and ceremonial law – by Pavel Florensky.

343 Pali was the language spoken in India at the time of Buddha. Sanskrit was exclusively a literary language.

344 Professor Sali founded Swinburne University's Graduate School of Integrative Medicine, and spearheaded the recently opened Swinburne University Hospital in Melbourne, Australia.

345 John Selwyn Gummer.

346 **New Scientist** 28 September 2002; pg23. Ingenious ways are being used to predict how many people will die from vCJD, the human form of BSE, however the current prediction is that 100 000 people in Britain could have died of vCJD by 2080.

347 *Millennium Development Goals – Progress Report 2002*; published in Nepal by the Nepalese Government and the United Nations Development Programme.

348 Author and professor of anatomy and physiology.

349 Quoted by Ted Scott and Phil Harker.

350 Indian Statesman and Prime Minister (1947–64).

351 This is without differentiating the different Types within Rooms for Archetypes and Enneagrams.

352 Carl Jung used this term to describe the process of self-development in which an individual integrates the many facets of their psyche to become who he or she really is – to fulfil their potential.

353 ISBN: 0-7225-3650-X.

354 ISBN: 0-89106-096-0.

355 ISBN: 1-885705-02-6.

356 ISBN: 0-393-30940-1.

357 ISBN: 1-85538-425-6.

358 ISBN: 0-671-66736-X.